FROM THE LIBRARY OF BERKELEY COLLEGE

New York:
NYC (Midtown and Lower Manhattan)
Brooklyn • White Plains

New Jersey:
Newark • Paramus • Woodbridge
Woodland Park

Berkeley College Online:
BerkeleyCollege.edu/Online

Berkeley College®

MARKETPLACE
OF THE
MARVELOUS

Also by Erika Janik

Apple: A Global History

Madison: History of a Model City

A Short History of Wisconsin

*Odd Wisconsin: Amusing, Perplexing,
and Unlikely Stories from Wisconsin's Past*

MARKETPLACE
OF THE
MARVELOUS

The Strange Origins
of Modern Medicine

Erika Janik

BEACON PRESS, BOSTON

Beacon Press
25 Beacon Street
Boston, Massachusetts 02108-2892
www.beacon.org

Beacon Press books
are published under the auspices of
the Unitarian Universalist Association of Congregations.

17   16   15   14   8   7   6   5   4   3   2   1

This book is printed on acid-free paper that meets the uncoated paper
ANSI/NISO specifications for permanence as revised in 1992.

Text design and composition by Wilsted & Taylor Publishing Services

Library of Congress Cataloging-in-Publication Data
Janik, Erika.
  Marketplace of the marvelous : the strange origins of modern medicine / by Erika Janik.
     pages cm
  Includes bibliographical references and index.
  ISBN 978-0-8070-2208-5 (cloth) —ISBN 978-0-8070-2209-2 (ebook) 1. Alternative
medicine—History. 2. Medicine, Magic, mystic, and spagiric—History. 3. Medicine—
Specialties and specialists—History. 4. Medicine—History. I. Title.
  R733.J33 2014
  610—dc23   2013023296

For Matt

The doctor of the future will give no medicine but will interest his patients in the care of the human frame, in diet and in the cause and prevention of disease.

THOMAS EDISON

Prevention is preferable to cure.

HIPPOCRATES

CONTENTS

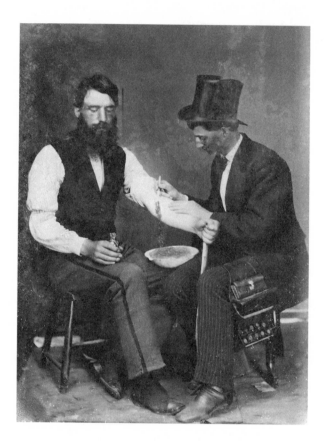

Medical knowledge was limited in the nineteenth century, so both regular and irregular doctors used methods often dangerous and of dubious scientific validity. Bloodletting was among the most common regular treatments, and venesection its most extreme form, in which doctors would slit open a patient's vein and catch blood in a bowl. (The Burns Archive, New York)

Medicine at the Crossroads

Riffling through a box of family photos and letters, I found a small cardboard tube enclosing a tightly rolled sheet of paper with lightly stained edges. I carefully pulled it from the tube and began to gently unroll the paper. Swirls began to appear along the border as well as an official-looking seal, a certificate of some sort. "The Kellberg Institute for Hygiene, Massage, and Medical Gymnastics" it read across the top. Medical gymnastics? An image of a woman in a blue hospital gown vaulting over a hospital bed, her gown flapping open immodestly in the back, popped into my head. Who did gymnastics for medical reasons?

Below the school name it read Corinne Newmann, the date, May 12, 1916, and her apparent specialty: water therapeutics. It seems my great-grandmother did.

I soon learned that medical gymnastics is still around—we just call it exercising today. Swedish immigrants in Chicago founded the Kellberg Institute and offered instruction in the Swedish gymnastics system developed in the early nineteenth century by Swede Per Henrik Ling to promote health and healing. Ling developed a method of medical calisthenics after noticing how his own daily exercises had healed the joint injuries sustained from his strenuous fencing hobby. His regimen also incorporated massage; Ling is the Swede behind Swedish massage.[1]

The mainstream medical community did not exactly welcome Ling's system with open arms—outright disdain for his presumption of medical knowledge might be more accurate—yet his system found widespread approval among the general public and a vast group of independent healers with their own divergent ideas of disease, health, and wellness. And yet we now take it for granted that exercise is fundamental to good health.

How did that happen? What other now widely accepted ideas began on the margins of medicine?

These questions led me deep into the history of what we would now call alternative medicine but what was often known in the nineteenth century as unorthodox or irregular medicine, and at less kind times, quackery. But the more I read, the more difficult it became to determine what was quackery and what was simply a bold innovation.

Take hydropathy, or the water cure, which advocated the importance of water to health. Patients did all kinds of odd things like taking cold baths outdoors and wrapping themselves in cold wet bandages as a means of washing away disease. But hydropaths also advised drinking eight or more glasses of water a day. I tried to remember the last time I didn't fill my own water bottle several times a day with the vague notion that I did it to keep healthy. This idea, too, came from a quack?

Wading still deeper, I found nineteenth-century irregulars advocating cleanliness and diets of fruits, vegetables, and whole grains, prescribing medications with few side effects and made of natural ingredients, and hypothesizing on the connection of both the mind and body to one's overall well-being—nothing that would seem out of place in modern discussions of health and wellness.

At the same time, the more I read about mainstream, or regular, medicine—as it was known at the time—the less regular it seemed. Many of the therapies practiced by these doctors seemed at best odd, and at worst more quackish than the quacks. Bleeding, induced vomiting, blistering, and sweating, often to painful and sometimes deadly degrees, were the primary tools in the doctor's bag. The reasons for prescribing bleeding over vomiting for any given patient seemed to depend more on the doctor's inclination, training, or mood than anything we would recognize as sound evidence today. At the same time, regular doctors lampooned hydropathy's concern for daily baths and regular water consumption, just as they had disdained Ling's exercise regimen.

And then there was Missouri physician John Sappington, who

manufactured and sold his own brand of pills for fever in the 1830s. "Doctor John Sappington's Anti-Fever & Ague Pills" bore all the marks of the classic patent medicine, and Sappington of the snake oil salesman: he kept the ingredients secret, he advertised in newspapers and magazines, and he made a fortune off of its sale. But Sappington's pills also proved quite effective, particularly against malaria, as one of its secret ingredients was quinine, the first effective treatment for the disease. His regular colleagues denounced him as a quack, but Sappington's pills made him one of the first people in the United States to use quinine to successfully treat malarial fever.[2] How could he be a quack? Or was he a regular doctor who also sold patent medicines, making him what—an irregular regular?

The more I read, the more confused about these distinctions I became. These weren't the stories I was used to hearing. Most accounts of early American medicine focus tightly on embattled doctors valiantly protecting the public from harmful—and even deadly—medical charlatans and quacks. The nineteenth century was not called the "golden age of the quack remedy" for nothing, right? But here were quacks advising patients to drink water and prescribing patent remedies with active ingredients that really worked. Calling one group regular and everyone else irregular seemed far too simplistic and even misleading.

The contest between regular and irregular medicine brought me into nineteenth-century America, where I found a medical landscape both contentious and wildly hopeful. It was a time when healers of all kinds—regular, irregular, quacks, and everything in between—vied for public favor as the criteria for practicing medicine seemed to be no criteria at all. Phrenologists read character on the topography of human skulls, mesmerists transferred animal magnetism through a hypnotic stare, and Thomsonians found all the drugs they needed growing just outside their doors. These healers fought to win the right to heal the bodies and minds of a people in a new country with their own ideas of who to trust. In an era when reformers banded together to try to remake religion, abolish slavery, outlaw liquor, open free schools, and grant women rights, it seemed only natural to me that some would focus on improving the quality of health care. So why hadn't I heard these stories before?

Many of the nineteenth century's healing claims seemed just as ridiculous and unbelievable as I'd always supposed. Why would people think that the shape of their heads revealed anything about their character? Or that sickness resulted from a lack of internal heat? But millions of Americans, educated and not, rich and poor, did believe, or at least hoped these cures would work. And as the contradictions stacked up before me, I wondered where some of these irregular medical systems had even come from in the first place. Which caught on and why? What made them believable? And how did modern medicine, which appears to be a conglomeration of regular and irregular therapies, emerge from this nineteenth-century maelstrom of competing claims?

My own feelings of incredulity fit the tenor of the times. Hard-eyed skepticism and zealous belief ran hand in hand throughout much of the nineteenth century. The era fairly throbbed with new ideas, technologies, and sciences, each seemingly more novel, unbelievable, and glimmering with possibility than the last. Few could resist giving at least some of these novelties a try.

On a fall afternoon in 1873, writer and humorist Mark Twain arrived at the London offices of a fellow American. In town for a series of lectures, Twain had seen an advertisement for Lorenzo Niles Fowler, "practical phrenologist" and decided to investigate.

Phrenology wasn't new to Twain. He remembered the itinerant phrenologists from his childhood in Hannibal, Missouri, giving demonstrations and offering advice. These travelers were "popular and always welcome," satisfying the townspeople with "translations of their characters," he recalled. Nearly everyone received positive readings. "I still remember that no phrenologist ever came across a skull in our town that fell much short of the [George] Washington standard," wrote Twain.[3]

Phrenology wasn't new either, but by the 1870s, its massive wave of popularity had long since crested in the United States. Devoted phrenologists could still be found, though, courting true believers and those who perhaps just ardently wished to believe that character could be scientifically "read" on the skull and possibly even improved.

Entering Fowler's Ludgate Circus office, Twain "found Fowler on duty, amidst the impressive symbols of his trade … all about the room stood marble-white busts, hairless, every inch of the skull occupied by a shallow bump, and every bump labeled with its imposing name, in black letters."

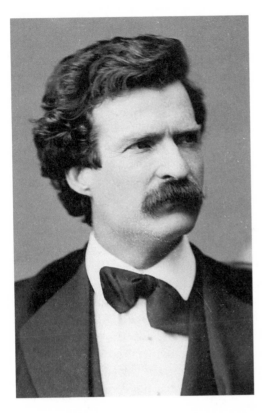

Mark Twain was both an enthusiastic experimenter and vocal critic of irregular medicine throughout his life. He tried many such medicines on himself and his family in an endless quest for better health, and many irregular therapies appear in his stories, often satirically. (Mathew Brady, 1871, Wikimedia Commons)

Twain paid Fowler for a reading. It's not clear whether he attempted to disguise his physical appearance. Well known by this time for his short stories, lectures, and best-selling travelogue *The Innocents Abroad, or The New Pilgrims' Progress*, Twain cut a fairly recognizable figure. Either way, Fowler gave no indication that he recognized Twain. In fact, Twain complained that Fowler "fingered my head in an uninterested way and named and estimated my qualities in a bored and monotonous voice."

The reading was fairly typical, a balanced mix of neutral and positive traits, save for one spot particularly galling to the famed humorist. "He found a cavity, in one place; a cavity where a bump would have been in anyone else's skull," recalled Twain. "He startled me by saying that that cavity represented the total absence of the sense of humor!"[4]

Twain's colorful report of his analysis in his *Autobiography* is the only remaining record of his visit; the original chart does not seem to have survived. Although he clearly twisted the results for a good joke, Twain, whose interests ranged "from protoplasm to infinity" according to one biographer, remained both dubious about and fascinated with phrenology, among other irregular healing methods, throughout his life, submitting to at least two other evaluations and writing phrenology into many of his stories and essays.[5]

Twain wasn't alone. In a world where an invisible electric substance could transmit messages over telegraph wires, and where mechanical looms operated by a single person could do the weaving of forty women in a single day, who could really say that phrenology wasn't at least plausible?

In this fast-changing world, Americans wrestled with hope and doubt in their daily lives, but perhaps nowhere more than in matters of health. Nineteenth-century lives billowed with peculiarly named aches, epidemics, and invalidism: Quinsy. Catarrh. Bilious fever. Ague. King's evil. Flux. Neurasthenia. Nearly everyone, it seemed, suffered. Abraham Lincoln shepherded the country through its great civil cataclysm while battling his own severe depression.[6] Louisa May Alcott wrote *Little Women* and *Little Men* while suffering from what she believed to be the terrible effects of the mercury prescribed to treat the typhoid fever she contracted during the Civil War. Harriet Beecher Stowe experienced attacks of hysteria so severe that she remained bedridden for weeks at a time in the years before she wrote *Uncle Tom's Cabin*.[7] Charles Darwin wrote *On the Origin of Species* while confined to his home, a vigorous young man done in, according to his doctor, by "intellectual labour and moral anxiety" that turned him into a reclusive invalid by age thirty-three.[8]

Sickness, both physical and mental, was a major part of being alive. Large segments of the population suffered poor health most of their lives. Filth pervaded daily life. Water was often polluted. Food preparation and storage were unhygienic. Garbage littered streets and yards along with animal droppings and the bodies of animals that had simply dropped dead. Privies and cesspools overflowed. All created breeding grounds for mosquitoes, flies, and other disease-carrying pests. Malnutrition and poor housing, particularly in rapidly growing urban areas, only magnified health problems and spawned epidemics. Infants died of diarrhea and dysentery from contaminated food. Deaths from tuberculosis, scarlet fever, diphtheria, smallpox, and cholera occurred so regularly that they were considered a matter of course. Not every disease killed, though. Others simply made life exceedingly unpleasant and painful.[9]

But even when a sick American visited a regular doctor, he rarely received an effective treatment. Scientifically valid medical knowledge was limited, and modern methods to sort out effective from ineffective and even dangerous treatments did not yet exist. Doctors did not understand the role of viruses and bacteria in causing disease, how most organs functioned, or the significance of personal contact and insects in the spread of infectious disease. Most people, including doctors, rarely washed their hands and did not think twice about sharing forks and cups. Medical advances of the period tended to occur in areas of theory, classification, and diagnosis, but not cures. For the average patient, these advances offered little immediate benefit beyond fancier and sometimes more specific names for their malady. Doctors made diagnoses by asking questions, observing the patient's appearance, taking the pulse, and examining, and sometimes even tasting, urine; few performed physical exams. Lacking both the understanding and the correct therapeutic measures, doctors could only respond to symptoms and speculate about the cause of disease.[10]

Regular doctors practiced a form of medicine known as "heroic," a name that came not from the efficacy of the treatment or the prowess of the administrator but from the magnitude of the intervention. Doctors bled, blistered, and purged to draw disease from the patient. The most extreme form of bloodletting was venesection, in which a doctor would slit open a vein and catch the pint or two of blood in a bowl. Doctors also applied blood-sucking leeches and employed a spring-loaded device called a scarificator that delivered a series of moderately deep cuts to the skin from rows of sharp steel blades at the flick of a release lever; it was developed in the eighteenth century as a more merciful bleeding tool. Blistering involved placing hot plasters or irritating chemicals onto the skin to raise sores that were then drained. Doctors purged patients with large doses of medicines containing mercury, antimony, and arsenic. The effect was always drastic and noticeable. And it was just what patients wanted. Sick people in every time and place want to feel better and will seek out the treatment or healer that makes that desire a reality. Everyone could agree that heroic treatments did something. Emetics purged, diaphoretics sweated, bleeding bled and changed the pulse. These treatments instilled confidence in the doctor's skills, and confidence could stimulate remarkable recoveries in patients. Anyone could see that bleeding "worked" because it nearly always produced some change in the condition of the sufferer that could be interpreted as progress, though it might also have been a strong placebo effect or simply a different symptom brought on by difficult-to-control treatments that were prone to infection.[11] Bleeding and purging could cause a patient's blood pressure to drop by decreasing blood volume and oxygen delivery to tissues. Too much, though, could cause organ failure and eventually death. Blistering opened wounds on the skin that could become infected, particularly in these unsanitary times, and spread to the bloodstream, which could also cause organ shutdown and death. Leeches, on the other hand, are still used in medicine to remove excess blood, helping doctors do everything from preventing clotting to reattaching severed fingers.[12]

Heroic approaches to healing reflected contemporary thinking on how disease worked but also an ancient cosmology. Medical theory of the time held that external symptoms revealed the disease, so anything that changed symptoms was viewed as potentially useful. These ideas went back thousands of years to the Greek physician Hippocrates and the Roman physician Galen, who proposed that the body consisted of four humors (black bile, yellow bile, blood, and phlegm) that needed to be kept in balance to be healthy. Every person had his or her own temperament or mixture of humors that could be thrown off balance by a variety of factors, including diet, lifestyle, or environment. The symptoms that people complained of and associated with sickness were not the actual disease but a sign of an internal imbalance that needed adjustment. Fever, for instance, was believed to result from too much blood, so anything that could reduce or eliminate it, usually bloodletting, was viewed favorably.[13]

Most of the medicines in active use were also known for their harsh effects. Some we would now think of primarily as poisons, such as the derivations of mercury used to purge and sweat patients. Leading emetics to produce vomiting included ipecac, tartar emetic, and sulfate of zinc. Powerful laxatives to clear the bowels included calomel and the root of the jalap plant. Of these, calomel, or mercurous chloride, was among the most dreaded of drugs. Doctors believed that this powerful cathartic flushed disease from the body and stimulated the cleansing power of the liver. But as a compound of mercury, calomel was also toxic. Patients given doses over a period of several weeks developed swollen mouths, ulcerated gums, and uncontrolled drooling. A 1720 prescription for a patient suffering from swollen joints called for two doses of calomel, followed by bleeding twelve to fourteen ounces of blood. After a day of rest, the patient received two more shots of calomel, more than enough to cause acute mercury poisoning. Doctors considered the visible oral damage and extreme salivation proof that the calomel had worked by producing a physical response that differed from that of the disease. Horrible side effects were considered necessary evils on the path to health.[14]

With these treatments, the real wonder is that most people survived. But many people did improve, enduring both their sickness and its treatment. Doctors viewed recovery as confirmation of the effectiveness of their therapies and as proof that their underlying theories were valid. In truth, many illnesses, particularly most infections, simply went away on their own. Thousands of years earlier, Hippocrates identified the body's innate ability to respond to illness and even restore itself to health in some cases. This capacity was given the Latin name *vis medicatrix naturae*, "the healing power of nature." Mainstream doctors from antiquity onward held nature in high regard but by the late eighteenth century, that esteem had become little more than lip service. Most doctors enthusiastically pursued heroic interventions when they could. They did not necessarily deny nature's power, but few believed that she alone could cure.[15] To claim otherwise, though, would have been career suicide for doctors, an admission that medicine was redundant or worse, helpless in the face of nature's supremacy. Well-known colonial American physician Benjamin Rush advised medical students at the University of Pennsylvania to "always treat nature in a sick room as you would a noisy dog or cat" by "driv[ing] her out at the door and lock[ing] it upon her."[16]

Nature often had no answer for chronic illnesses, however. Even after surviving a disease, many people lived with compromised health for the remainder of their lives, as did Louisa May Alcott after surviving typhoid fever and its brutal, if well-intended, medical treatment. Disease became a part of life, and many people treated themselves for the aches and pains of everyday living. Do-it-yourself medical books, medical almanacs, and family recipe books abounded with recipes for healing salves, prophylactics, and popular herbal remedies. Many American colonists had brought their favorite manuals along with them, like Nicholas Culpepper's *The Complete Herbal* or E. Smith's

The Compleat Housewife; Or, Accomplish'd Gentlewoman's Companion.
Treating yourself was more convenient and cost less than a visit with
a doctor, if one could even be found within a day's journey from home.
For some, home care was a powerful way to democratize medicine
and spread knowledge. John Wesley, better known as the founder of
Methodism, was among domestic medicine's biggest proponents. In
1747 he published *Primitive Physick: Or, An Easy and Natural Method
of Curing Most Diseases,* his own low-cost and nontechnical medical manual that instructed users on how to turn kitchen staples into
medicine. Onions, honey, and licorice could treat coughs; apple water, asthma; whey and raisins, nosebleeds. He also recommended the
unusual application of toasted cheese as a bandage to staunch bleeding.[17] For millions of Americans, these domestic guides functioned as
primary care doctors.

Armed with these guides, women served as "Dr. Mom" long before
marketers invented the term. Since the earliest colonial days, women
acted as their family's doctor, nurse, and pharmacist, providing most
home medical care and nearly all birthing assistance. Many women
had an impressive knowledge of herbal remedies, traditional rituals,
and preventative measures passed down through families, found in
books, and gained through firsthand experience. The technical simplicity of contemporary medicine made it possible for women, and
others who were at the time denied any formal education, to offer
many of the same services as a doctor.

Although these alternate healers, and alternate forms of health
care, had long existed alongside doctors, many more Americans began
to turn away from regular medicine in the nineteenth century. It was
not so much that medicine had changed as that American culture had
changed after independence from Britain.

Early Americans demonstrated a stubborn attachment to the idea
that every person possessed the common sense to take care of him- or
herself. The conditions of life on a new continent had forced colonists
to improvise and make their own way in a rough and challenging new
environment. As a result, Americans became proudly self-directed,
self-reliant, and confident in their own judgment. This did not mean
that no one ever sought the advice or counsel of others but it did
foster an environment that prized individual good sense. Breaking
away from British control only bolstered American confidence in the
power of personal freedom and a concomitant distrust of authority,
elitism, and control.

The rise of Andrew Jackson, a poorly educated man from the backwoods of the Carolinas, to the presidency in 1828, seemed, to many Americans, to herald the triumph of the common man, equality, and democracy in the new country. The Jacksonians denounced the moneyed aristocracy and espoused a democratic ideology predicated on equality, although this equality remained restricted to white males. Under Jackson, free white men finally earned the right to vote as rules requiring property ownership fell. Celebrations of democracy and the right of the people to have a say in all aspects of life shot through popular culture even as the Jacksonian policies simultaneously supported sexual, racial, and ethnic subordination and exclusion. Slogans such as "knowledge is power" and "knowledge, like money, depends on circulation" became the catchphrases of the day. New technology made print cheaper, so books and newspapers proliferated. Public libraries, political parties, and associations devoted to literature, science, and philosophy encouraged the spread of ideas. This democracy of knowledge covered a wide range of topics, including health and science. These events and institutions spurred an egalitarian ethos among many Americans that clashed with the exclusivity of medical knowledge and skill claimed by regular medicine.[18]

The growing feeling that people could decide for themselves was not limited to medicine. Democratization significantly reshaped religious attitudes as well, as nineteenth-century evangelicals like Charles Grandison Finney, Lyman Beecher, and Francis Asbury focused on sin as a human choice rather than an inherent part of human nature. With salvation no longer left in God's hands alone, an individual could save her soul by turning away from sin to embrace moral action and God's grace. This emphasis on personal choice opened the door to new religious groups like the Latter-day Saints, Millerites, and Seventh-day Adventists who questioned religious orthodoxy and offered more contemporary and personally empowering alternatives as they competed with older denominations for adherents.[19]

Other people and institutions seized on the democratic impulse to propose social innovations that they hoped would usher in a better world. All of the transformations remaking the nation promised so much hope but came laden with challenges. Poverty, lawlessness, and overcrowding gripped city and town alike. Inequality persisted. To solve these problems, reform organizations dedicated to sanitation, abolition, dress reform, vegetarianism, and countless other issues formed around the country. Utopian communities like the

Transcendentalist Brook Farm in West Roxbury, Massachusetts, and those of Robert Dale Owen at New Harmony, Indiana, and John Humphrey Noyes at Oneida, New York, attempted to remake society. Most of these communal experiments disintegrated quickly, but these reform efforts nonetheless raised expectations about the possibility of perfecting both human nature and its institutions.[20]

All of these disparate reform efforts shared one overriding goal: to match American reality with American ideals. Early Americans evinced a remarkable faith in the boundlessness and perfectability of the nation. The path to perfection naturally began with the individual. Ralph Waldo Emerson counseled, "Nothing can bring you peace but yourself. Nothing can bring you peace but the triumph of principles."[21] Reformers of all kinds encouraged Americans to work toward the perfection of their individual lives, believing that this would have a cascading effect that uplifted all of humanity.

In this dynamic environment, it's hardly surprising that irregular medicine flourished. When these systems first arose, the country's medical marketplace was already among the most varied in the world. Medical practice in the eighteenth century had been loosely organized and lightly regulated, an activity in which just about anyone could—and did—participate. All tastes and budgets could find a medical system to match. People relied on doctors as well as midwives, lay healers, herbalists, and Indian doctors skilled in the use of native plants. Ministers, often the best-educated people in a community, received frequent calls to heal the body as well as the spirit. Trained doctors were in short supply. The problem was particularly severe in the South and the West as people moved farther and farther into the frontier. Before the telephone, a doctor had to be summoned in person. A farmer traveling eight miles to town for help could lose a whole day of precious work. Even then, there was no guarantee that the doctor would be home. As a result, responsibility for medical care often fell on the sick themselves.[22]

While Americans had frequented a variety of healers since colonial days, in the nineteenth century, medicine became a war zone as health came face-to-face with a growing commercial society. The capitalist marketplace spawned a business sector of medicine that vended medical services and remedies on a large scale. The pace of change in other health fields only accentuated the lack of progress by regular doctors. For the first time, healers who had generally practiced alone began to band together. Thomsonians, mesmerists, homeopaths, and hydropaths led the first offensive, while osteopaths, chiropractors, and Christian Scientists launched a second advance later in the nineteenth century.[23] Each had different therapies, theories, and techniques, but they all wanted to overturn and supplant regular medical practice—or at least, that's what regular doctors tended to believe. "These systems, however widely they differ in character, all agree in one thing—they are all at war with what they term the 'regular' profession," reported Worthington Hooker to the Connecticut Medical Society in 1852. "And this war, which is one of extermination, they have prosecuted from the beginning."[24]

Irregulars identified regular medicine with overly aggressive therapies based on old and speculative ideas. They derisively nicknamed regulars "drug doctors" and "knights of calomel and the lancet." Bloodletting and heroic dosing—and in many cases, drugs altogether—were virtually banished from most irregular practices. Irregulars claimed that common sense and their experience with an alternate form of healing—often gained through some kind of conversion experience—had completely discredited regular medicine's damaging and depletive therapies. Most relied on natural remedies and proclaimed nature the source of both the strongest treatments and the most effective preventative medicines. They presented their case to Americans in simple and direct language that reinforced the era's widespread belief in intuition, practical sense, and accessible knowledge, while exploiting regular medicine's weaknesses. Irregular doctors were no more equipped to cure than regulars, but their treatments tended to be milder, cost less, and cause fewer side effects.

The proliferation of medical systems and alternative routes to wellness spoke to the lack of scientific advancement and to American hunger for new and potentially more effective treatments. Irregulars speculated on the cause of disease and devised coherent and unified theories that made sense of many confusing and often vague symptoms. They promised a clear path to health and wellness. In many ways, irregulars could make greater claims to scientific authority than regular medicine. Most based their theories on their own observations and experimentation, a method generally considered the most modern form of scientific induction of the time. Irregulars observed the effects of certain drugs or procedures and then made claims based on what they saw. They even got a few things right.[25]

Even before the irregular assault gained force, regular medicine as a profession had started to lose status. "Medicine has ever been and is now, the most despised of all the professions which liberally-educated men are expected to enter," lamented the *Medical Record* in 1869.[26] Most doctors commanded little respect. Some could barely scrape together a comfortable living and took on second jobs, usually farming, to get by. One dissatisfied doctor even took to robbing stagecoaches on the side, but he was eventually captured and imprisoned.[27] Jokes about doctors filled newspapers and magazines. When a nation abounds in doctors, one wit said, it grows thin of people.[28] English journalist William Cobbett remarked that American physician Benjamin Rush's penchant for extreme bleeding and purging regimens was "one of those great discoveries which are made from time to time for the depopulation of the earth." Even Thomas Jefferson got in on the critique, attesting that doctors tended to be ignorant, uneducated, and extreme in their therapies, especially considering how little they actually knew about health and disease. Looking to the future, Jefferson hoped "that it is from this side of the Atlantic, that Europe, which has taught us so many other things, will at length be led into sound principles in this branch of science, the most important of all, being that to which we commit the care of health & life."[29]

Stories of medical men grave robbing for anatomical material and dissection also did little to win public favor to the medical profession. One of the most notorious incidents occurred in New York City in April of 1788 when medical student John Hicks allegedly waved a cadaver's arm at some children peering through the window of a hospital dissecting room. Hicks then called out, "This is your mother's arm! I just dug it up!," likely unaware that one of the children had recently lost his mother. The boy ran home and told his father, who exhumed his wife's coffin and found it empty. As the story got out, an angry mob gathered around the hospital. Hicks and his fellow students and teachers ran as the crowd broke into the hospital. One doctor and five students remained inside, determined to protect a valuable specimen collection. James Thacher, a physician who witnessed the riot, reported that the mob found several human bodies "in various states of mutilation. Enraged at this discovery, they seized upon the fragments, as heads, legs and arms, and exposed them from the windows and doors to public view, with horrid imprecations." Bands of rioters moved across the city reporting what they had seen inside the hospital as they searched for Hicks. To protect the medical students from the crowd, Mayor James Duane had several escorted to jail. The unrest continued overnight and into the following day until eventually more than five thousand people gathered outside the jailhouse throwing rocks and demanding retribution. Finally, the governor sent the cavalry charging up Broadway to break up the jeering crowd. In the end, at least three and as many as twenty people died in the riot or from wounds sustained in the melee.[30] The New York Doctors' Riot, as it came to be known, was not the first or the last medical riot—others broke out in Philadelphia and Baltimore—and public anger at doctors lingered long after the disturbances ended.[31]

Standard medical practice was partly to blame. Medicine in 1820 was little better than it had been in 1700. Heroic interventions remained the doctor's primary tools, just as they had for centuries. Most of the methods to truly understand disease had yet to be discovered. Medical science was not completely stagnant, of course. Physicians and scientists continued to discover more about the body's structure and function, but they had little in the way of new treatments. Many regular doctors sought to draw a line between themselves and those they saw as quacks by proclaiming their devotion to science, but in truth, the boundary between regular and irregular medicine was hazy at best.[32] British physician Matthew Baillie remarked, "I know better perhaps than another man, from my knowledge of anatomy, how to discover disease; but when I have done so, I don't know better how to cure it."[33] Doctors watched helplessly, and not without a bit of jealousy, as scientific discovery and progress rapidly remade nearly every other aspect of nineteenth-century life. The complete ignorance of the cause of disease prevented effective methods of healing or even lessening symptoms, creating a dilemma for doctors trying to heal those who hungered to be well.

Public dissatisfaction with doctors was likely not helped by the poor training most received. Medical schools often had minimal entrance requirements, and degrees could be granted in as few as six months. Most doctors, though, had attended no medical school at all. Medical schools of any kind were slow to develop in the United States. The first medical school, at the College of Philadelphia, opened in 1765, more than a century after the founding of Harvard in 1636. Before 1840, only a third of practicing doctors in New England had attended medical school or completed an apprenticeship.

The number was far lower in the West and South.[34] Poor training persisted throughout the nineteenth century. It was so bad that one physician bemoaned in the *Medical Record* that "after a man has failed in scholarship, failed in writing, failed in speaking, failed in every purpose for which he entered college ... there is one unfailing city of refuge—the profession of medicine."[35]

Medical licensing systems, weak as they were, were mostly repealed in the 1820s and 1830s. This encouraged the rise of irregular movements by eliminating the legal boundaries between regular and irregular medicine. Many colonies had chartered medical societies in the eighteenth century with the power to administer licenses that placed a nominal penalty on practicing without a license. But even when in force, these licensing systems did not require doctors to demonstrate any of the principles or practices of medicine. Under pressure from proponents and practitioners of irregular medicine, nearly every state legislature removed restrictions on medical practice in the nineteenth century. These irregular healers seized on the democratic spirit of the time to protest restrictions that they said limited choice and fostered elitism. Unlike Europe, where medical practice received some state and institutional support, the United States adopted a laissez-faire approach to medicine. Irregular healers claimed that their common sense and personal experience with alternate forms of healing completely discredited heroic medicine and its terrible side effects. "The practice of physic requires a knowledge that cannot be got by reading books; it must be obtained by actual observation and experience," proclaimed botanic healer Samuel Thomson.[36] Irregulars reminded regular doctors that the first rule of Hippocrates had been to do no harm: only pain and suffering resulted from bleeding, blistering, and purging. Refusing to submit to the pretenses of regular medicine, irregular healers believed in their own right to practice and in the public's right to choose how and by whom they were treated.[37]

Regular doctors viewed these irregular systems with derision. They considered irregular medicine a random mix of inert and sometimes dangerous therapies passed off as legitimate on a gullible and unknowing public. "This subterfuge cannot avail," lamented physician Caleb Ticknor. "Call himself by what name he will, a quack is still a quack—and even if the prince of darkness should assume the garb of heavenly innocence, the cloven hoof would still betray the real personage."[38] But who qualified as a quack was a matter of perspective.

Irregulars were "quacks" in the eyes of regulars. In these prescientific times, a quack was always that other guy whose methods seemed improper, unscientific, or deceitful to someone else. That someone else often happened to be losing business to these so-called quacks.

Regular doctors were not ignorant of the shortcomings of their therapies. Harvard professor and regular physician Oliver Wendell Holmes, one of the century's most outspoken, shrewd, and witty critics of irregular medicine, demonstrated a surprising evenhandedness in his assessments of his own brand of medicine. He despaired of the lack of progress and innovation in medical science. In 1843, Holmes ignited fierce controversy among regulars for his contention, contrary to popular belief, that physicians often transmitted the contagion of puerperal fever, a deadly infection now known as postpartum endometritis and contracted by women during or shortly after childbirth, to their patients. He also decried the overuse and abuse of drugs by regulars. He placed some of the blame, though, on patients who pressured their doctors to do something with big effects as well as the particularly grandiose American character found in doctors and patients alike. "How could a people which has a revolution once in four years, which has contributed the Bowie-knife and the revolver, which has chewed the juice out of all the superlatives of language in Fourth of July orations, and so used up its epithets in the rhetoric of abuse that it takes two great quarto dictionaries to supply the demand; which insists in sending out yachts and horses and boys to out-sail, out-run, out-fight, and checkmate all the rest of creation," asked Holmes, "how could such a people be content with any but 'heroic' practice? What wonder that the Stars and Stripes wave over doses of ninety grains of sulphate of quinine, and that the American eagle screams with delight to see three drachms of calomel given at a single mouthful?"[39] The *American Journal of the Medical Sciences* acknowledged that "the majority of physicians over-medicate" despite "all that has been written on this subject," and more than a few regulars denounced their field's neglect of nature's healing power.[40] Nature, according to physician Worthington Hooker, was a "good, kind angel, hovering over the bed of sickness, without fee, and often without even any acknowledgement of her services" as she "saves the life of many a poor patient, who is near being drugged to death by some ignorant quack, or some over-dosing doctor."[41]

Until the second half of the nineteenth century, though, most regular doctors did not seriously question the efficacy of their remedies and even fewer experimented with anything other than increasing the dose or expanding the range of ills a remedy could treat. Regulars maintained their commitment to heroic therapies for many reasons. Primarily concerned with asserting and consolidating its power as a profession, regular medicine as a whole tended to be less open to new ideas, particularly those that might diminish confidence in its power in the eyes of patients. Heroic treatments caused big effects that emphasized a doctor's authority and control over the situation. Heroic therapies also made regular medicine distinct, a point that became more important as irregular healers grew more numerous and medicine more competitive. As irregular medicine grew in strength and size, it was only natural for regular doctors to rally around their depletive therapies as a mark of cohesiveness and group identity.[42]

From the perspective of the average American and despite protests to the contrary from regular doctors, regular and irregular medicine were often indistinguishable. The professional and educational qualifications for both were minimal and the scientific proof for any treatment virtually nonexistent, so people made choices based on their common sense, convenience, finances, and personal experience. They cared only who made them feel better. For most patients, the decision to seek care rested on a multitude of factors, such as cost, expediency, and their personal relationship with the healer. The sick paid close attention to their own illnesses and actively chose among the burgeoning marketplace of healers, regular and irregular. People often tried one and then another and another. An implicit trust in doctors and medicine was not common before the mid-twentieth century. Whether a doctor earned a degree or completed an apprenticeship mattered less to most people than his ability to instill hope and practice confidently. Americans wanted results, and when regular medicine failed to deliver cures as quickly, easily, or cheaply as they sought, they were not afraid to turn elsewhere.[43]

Regular and irregular doctors differed most dramatically on one issue: women. Since colonial days, women had performed nearly all of the tasks that professionally trained doctors, nurses, and pharmacists later assumed. But as regular medicine became more organized in the nineteenth century, many regular doctors dismissed traditional female healing practices as ineffective, irrational, and even dangerous. Prevailing ideas about women's health and anatomy also worked to exclude women from practicing medicine. The common theory of female anatomy and physiology placed responsibility for all female physical and mental symptoms on a woman's reproductive organs. Ruled by reproduction, women were deemed too irrational, emotional, and intellectually inferior to pursue professional careers. Some regulars may also have feared that female doctors would steal their business. Even more, the very image of a professional person seemed to challenge women's acceptance in medicine. In the early nineteenth century, a professional was by definition a man and medicine a profession of gentlemen; a professional female physician thus represented a contradiction in terms.[44] As a result, nearly all regular medical schools and medical societies barred women from entry until the late nineteenth century and many into the twentieth century.

Those women who did pursue a career in regular medicine faced discrimination and outright hostility. One of the most egregious incidents occurred in 1869 when students from the Woman's Medical College of Pennsylvania received permission to attend the Saturday morning surgical clinics at the all-male Pennsylvania Hospital in Philadelphia. When the women arrived, the male students greeted them with angry jeers, whistles, and groans. Some men even threw stones. "Ranging themselves in line, these gallant gentlemen assailed the young ladies, as they passed out, with insolent and offensive language, and then followed them into the street, where the whole gang, with the fluency of long practice, joined in insulting them," reported Philadelphia's *Evening Bulletin*. "During the last hour missiles of paper, tinfoil, tobacco-quid, etc., were thrown upon the ladies, while some of these men defiled the dresses of the ladies near them with tobacco juice."[45] Though opposition to female doctors rarely became violent, women, nevertheless, faced a discouraging path in their chosen field.

Irregular healers tended to take a different view. Many welcomed women practitioners and established coeducational medical schools. For some, welcoming women served the practical purpose of building market share. Others championed a woman-positive message that celebrated women's unique skills and intelligence. Healing highlighted the "feminine virtues" of nurture, altruism, and morality that made women good wives and mothers. Most women physicians shared that view, believing they were better positioned to protect and improve the health of women and children. They saw themselves as a link between the practice of medicine and women's everyday lives.[46] Like their male counterparts, female doctors treated patients, presented case reports, debated therapeutic methods and innovations, and read medical journals.

Allowing women to participate in medicine also solved a very real health problem. Modesty and propriety kept many women from seeking medical care from male doctors. Even when they did, some doctors declined to perform physical examinations, particularly for gynecological issues, out of respect for the delicate sensibilities of their patients. Women could easily find themselves suffering from a dangerous or inappropriate treatment—or no treatment at all—without the benefit of a thorough analysis. But with female doctors, women could get the medical attention they needed. Next to teaching, medicine attracted more women than any other profession in the nineteenth century, the majority in irregular health systems.

Prejudice kept many African Americans out of organized medicine, both regular and irregular alike. While folk and herbal healers as well as midwives and other local healers were common in black communities, many medical schools and medical societies refused to admit black physicians, and many white doctors refused to treat black patients. Even so, David Jones Peck and Rebecca Lee Crumpler became the first African Americans in the United States to earn MD degrees, in 1847 and 1864 respectively, and eight black doctors served in the Army Medical Corps during the Civil War. But more common was the experience of Daniel Laing Jr., Martin Delany, and Isaac H. Snowden, who were expelled from Harvard Medical School in 1851 by Oliver Wendell Holmes in the face of intense pressure and opposition to their presence from white students. Even among otherwise liberal healers, discrimination was common. In 1870, homeopaths in Washington, DC, opposed admitting black candidates to the Washington Homeopathic Medical Society. Black medical schools and medical societies did form, but most were short-lived and underfunded. During the Civil War, the Freedman's Bureau began providing medical care to freed slaves and promoting education, but most African Americans faced intense racism and struggled to find and receive adequate medical care throughout the nineteenth century.[47]

By the 1830s, irregular systems had grown so numerous and successful that regular doctors increasingly found themselves facing a precarious and uncertain future. "Why are we sick? Why cannot the doctors cure us," asked health reformer Mary Gove Nichols. "We are tired of professions and promises."[48] Nichols was not the only one. Many Americans began asking themselves, and their doctors, the very same question.

The list of those who used and advocated for irregular health treatments, and likely contributed to their popularity, includes many of the nineteenth century's boldface names: Thomas Edison, Margaret Fuller, James Fenimore Cooper, Nathaniel Hawthorne, John D. Rockefeller, Mark Twain, Henry David Thoreau, Harriet Beecher Stowe, Edgar Allan Poe, P. T. Barnum, Abraham Lincoln, Susan B. Anthony, and Ralph Waldo Emerson. Some became outspoken supporters of one system, while others dabbled among the marvels on offer in the medical marketplace. Intrigued and hopeful, Americans, the famous and anonymous alike, came to irregular medicine seeking to make themselves happier, healthier, and more successful.

This is their story.

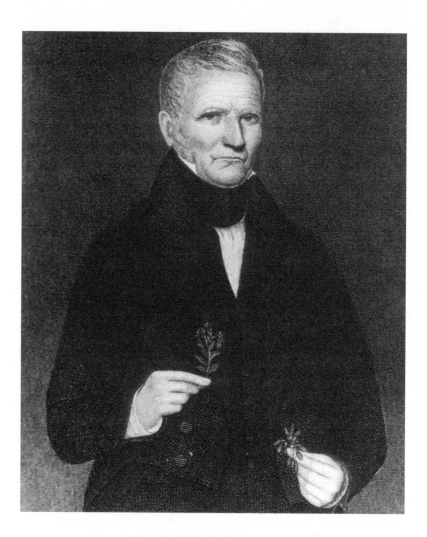

Samuel Thomson grew up with a love of herbs, experimenting as a boy with the plant remedies that would eventually form the foundation of his entire healing system. (National Library of Medicine, Bethesda, MD)

CHAPTER ONE

Every Man His Own Physician
Thomson's Botanic Medicine

Samuel Thomson believed poetry could heal. In 1812, he published his first medical poem, "Seamen's Directions," which combined ideological cheerleading with instructions for use of his remedies:

> Th' Emetic number ONE's design'd
> A gen'ral med'cine for mankind . . . Let number TWO be used
>   as bold,
> To clear the stomach of the cold;
> Next steep the coffee,
> number THREE,
> and keep as warm as you can be . . . My system's founded on
>   this truth,
> Man's Air and Water, Fire and Earth,
> And death is cold, and life is heat,
> These temper'd well, your health's complete.[1]

This mnemonic poem was one of dozens composed by Thomson and his followers, who urged patients and practitioners to memorize one or more of them for proper results.

Instructional poems were not the whole of Thomson's poetic offerings, though. He also used verse to deride the excesses of regular medicine and to celebrate the health benefits of herbs and other plants. One 1845 poem read:

They use [lobelia] in tincture, in powders and pills,
The patient it cures, but it never him kills;
It is first rate to cure in all cases of fevers,
But is hated and feared by the regular deceivers.[2]

Thomson's poetic fervor sometimes spread to his patients, too, who couldn't help but proclaim their devotion to Thomson and the healing power of his favorite remedy in couplets and quatrains.

Then LOBELIA, thou great Deliverer, come!
Purge from my eye this ochre hue ...
Make me benevolent and true ...
I'll own, O LOBELIA! My virtue is from you.[3]

Poetry was popular entertainment in the decades before the Civil War. People of all classes read poetry, composed their own verse, and entertained each other with recitations of favorite poems. Poems on love, marriage, courtship, death, passion, and piety, most of which were penned by women, appeared regularly in popular newspapers and magazines. Men wrote most Thomsonian poems, on the other hand, and they tended toward the instructional rather than the moral or flowery messages that characterized the era's other poetic outpourings. Thomson's medical poems did fit the literary and cultural flavor of the era, however, providing both amusement as well as a passionate argument for the reform of medicine.[4]

Samuel Thomson's medical system, known variously as Thomsonism and Thomsonianism, posed one of the first serious threats to regular medicine. Unlike many of the irregular systems that would follow him, Thomson's was fully homegrown, an American invention in a field of medical irregulars that often began in Europe before crossing the Atlantic. His system posited that the cure for every disease could be found growing in the hills, valleys, meadows, and woods of America. Rather than the painful and often toxic chemical and mineral compounds of regular medicine, Thomson whipped up tinctures and teas and concocted salves from herbs, leaves, and roots. He became so famous and well known for his botanic medical system in the early nineteenth century that he earned the nickname the "American Hippocrates," after the Greek physician widely regarded as the father of medicine. Thomson, perhaps, took the title a bit too seriously. His portrait in the frontispiece of his medical manual featured the barrel-chested founder with his high forehead and closely cropped hair be-decked in flowing Greek robes. Thomson brimmed with confidence in the rightness of his system and the horrors of regular medicine. He derided the arrogance of regular doctors and proclaimed that with his system, every man could be his own physician.[5]

Samuel Thomson claimed to have allied himself with nature from birth. Born in Alsted, New Hampshire, in 1769, Thomson learned about the healing power of plants as a child from family herbalist Mrs. Benton, who attended to nearly all his family's medical needs. Domestic and part-time folk healers like Mrs. Benton were common in early America, where a healer's reputation and authority came not from credentials but from his or her ability to make people feel better. Whomever people trusted with their lives and well-being earned the title "doctor." Herb doctors like Benton made no pretense of educa-tion or medical qualifications, but they were popular and respected in rural areas like Thomson's hometown, where the closest trained doctor was more than ten miles away: a potentially deadly distance depending on the severity of the illness.[6]

Benton's self-taught skills and knowledge of local plants left a deep and lasting impression on Thomson. She collected her remedies from the woods and fields near town, and she allowed the young Thomson to tag along. "The whole of her practice was with roots and herbs," recalled Thomson, noting with some awe at the time that they "always answered the purpose."[7] Like many young children, he put everything he found in his mouth, chewing pods, sucking on flower buds, and chomping leaves to discover, through firsthand experience both good and bad, the effect these had on his body. It was on one of these trips, when Thomson was only four years old, that he discovered *lobelia in-flata*, a plant he'd never seen before and one with a "taste and operation . . . so remarkable, that I never forgot it."[8] Large doses of lobelia taken internally cause people to vomit, an "operation" few could easily for-get. Thomson's experience with lobelia proved so memorable that it later became the foundation of the botanic medical system that would make Thomson a household name.[9]

Humans have cultivated and collected herbs, roots, and barks for medicinal purposes for thousands of years. In the fifteenth century, European exploration of North and South America introduced new plants to the herbal pharmacy, bolstering the use and importance of

botanical medicine and spurring on colonization. Ministers reinforced the value of discovery by preaching that God had provided
each region of the world with its own natural medicines. Christopher Columbus returned to Europe with cinchona bark (the source
of quinine), coca leaves (cocaine), sarsaparilla, and tobacco, among
other botanicals thought to have medical value. So important was
the search for medicinal plants that the British crown ordered the
seventeenth-century Virginia colony to cultivate gardens of native
plants for medical research and experimentation. In 1620, the Virginia
Company noted that its colony had great quantities of "Sweet Gums,
Roots, Woods, Berries for dies and Drugs" and asked colonists to
"send of all sorts as much as you can."[10] American Indians supplied a
rich source of advice and information to colonists with their extensive
knowledge of the New World's botanical drugs. Indians knew plants
that induced vomiting, reduced bleeding, stimulated sweating, and diminished fevers, all therapies common to regular European medicine
but achieved through other means.[11]

Guides to botanic medicine became popular in the sixteenth
century, and colonists brought many of their favorites with them to
America. A New World filled with new plants required new guides,
though, and in 1751, Benjamin Franklin published an American edition of the popular English herbal *Short's Medica Britannica* with an
appendix describing plants unique to North America. Early settlers
tended to use drugs imported from Europe when they could afford
them, and supplemented with native botanicals when they could not.
Many people planted medicinal plants in their kitchen gardens or
gathered them from the wild because medicine, like nearly everything
else in the American colonies, had to be made from scratch at home.
Among the most common botanicals in the colonial medical cabinet
were catnip, dandelion, skunk cabbage, pumpkin seed, and mustard,
few of which are used as such today. Some, like spearmint, pepper-
mint, and wintergreen, were transformed from active ingredients to
flavorings and scents in modern times. Almanacs and newspapers
featured recipes for medicines, while other remedies were passed on
through families. Plants still play an important part in modern medicine: nearly a quarter of pharmaceutical drugs are derived from botanical sources.[12]

Not every regular doctor welcomed the use of indigenous American plants, however. Some questioned the effectiveness of these rela-

tive unknowns compared with more familiar European medicines. But with European medicines often too expensive or unavailable, especially in frontier areas, nature cures became an essential piece of the colonial medical landscape.[13]

By the late eighteenth century, botanic medicine had increasingly found its way from home use to the therapeutic practices of regular medicine. Botany served the practical purpose of expanding the number of remedies available to regular doctors while also decreasing the costs of importing medicines and ingredients. Self-taught colonial botanist John Bartram spent much of his life collecting and studying plants and introduced one hundred new medicinal species to the European pharmacopia. In 1813, Benjamin Rush urged the trustees of the University of Pennsylvania to plant a botanical garden at the medical school in Philadelphia for the further study of American healing plants.[14] Although herbal medicine never comprised a large part of the practice of regular medicine, most regular doctors possessed at least a basic familiarity with the centuries-old practice. It was Thomson who took herbal medicine to new heights.

Although Thomson discovered the emetic power of lobelia as a child, he didn't put his discovery to beneficial use until two decades later. In the meantime, he amused himself, as children do, by urging others to try the plant and laughing as they discovered its unwelcome effects. In small doses, lobelia had a taste similar to tobacco and produced a euphoric effect that earned it the name "Indian tobacco" among the American pioneers. Overuse, though, caused the vomiting that so pleased the youthful Thomson. Lobelia's physical power over the human body enthralled as much as it entertained Thomson, though, and he spent much of his early life experimenting with plants, learning from local healers, and advising his neighbors on his finds. In later years, Thomson rarely tired of relating his personal story of discovery and self-education among the plants of his hometown.[15]

The limitations of regular medicine's healing powers became painfully clear to the twenty-one-year-old Thomson when his mother succumbed to tuberculosis. Witnessing the effects of mercury, opium, and other heroic dosages on her weakened system, Thomson developed an intense hatred of regular doctors and their drugs. He believed they inflicted unnecessary and gratuitous suffering in the name of healing with remedies he considered ineffective based on his observations. While he had yet to reach any conclusions about correct medical practice, Thomson believed that plants could do better and at less physical cost than heroic drugs. Any lingering doubts he may have had about the efficacy of the drugs of regular medicine disappeared several years later when his two-year-old daughter came down with scarlet fever. Intent on helping her recover without the standard treatments that had killed his mother, Thomson tried to cure her himself. He placed a pan of hot coals in water and vinegar beneath a chair and sat with his daughter wrapped in a blanket on his lap. He hoped the heat would eliminate her fever by raising her body temperature and inducing sweating. Her fever eventually broke and she made a full recovery. Regular doctors sometimes sweated patients too, but most did so with drugs containing opium and ipecac rather than through natural methods of heat and steam. Convinced that he had discovered the true source of healing in nature's apothecary, Thomson renounced the drugs of regular medicine and dedicated himself to the practice of herbal medicine.[16]

Word of Thomson's healing skills spread rapidly through his community, and by 1805, requests for his advice and medical assistance became so consuming that he gave up farming to practice medicine full-time. More than just a business move, though he had not been an enthusiastic farmer, his was a calling. "Every man is made and capacitated for some particular pursuit in life," declared Thomson. "I am convinced myself that I possess a gift in healing the sick, because of the extraordinary success I have met with, and the protection and support Providence has afforded me."[17] To meet the demand for his services, Thomson opened medical offices in New Hampshire, Maine, northeastern Massachusetts, and later in Boston. He traveled continuously, treating patients and proselytizing the benefits of nature.[18]

Itinerant healers like Thomson were common in the early years of the United States. Thomson was part of a new generation of independent Americans who disdained authority and elitism and who staked a path to success marked by perseverance, hard work, entrepreneurship, and often a life on the road. In his travels, he likely shared the road with any number of bonesetters, mesmerists, Indian healers, and medical device and potion peddlers who passed through the inns, theaters, and public houses of the Atlantic coast.[19]

Thomson covered thousands of miles speaking the language of common sense and promoting a simple self-help system he claimed was as comprehensible and accessible as nature itself. He announced his arrival in town by issuing invitations to a public lecture where he explained his system of medicine. Taking to the stage or even just the corner of a room, depending on the location, Thomson announced his intention to release patients from the tyranny of regular medicine by offering cheap and gentle remedies that could be found growing all around them. He decried university-trained regular doctors who shrouded medicine in Greek and Latin terms that served only to protect the monetary interest of the doctor and not the health of the patient struggling to be well and understand his sickness. "There can be no good reason why all the medical works are kept in a dead language, except it be to deceive and keep the world ignorant of their doings, that they may the better impose upon the credulity of the people," cried Thomson, "for if it was to be written in our own language every body would understand it, and judge for themselves."[20] The words were not the only problem. Thomson claimed that medical school itself prevented doctors from acquiring the experience necessary to effectively heal. "Their heads are filled with the theory, but all that is most important in the removal of disorder, they have to learn by practice," which, Thomson declared, they never received in formal training.[21]

The truth of Thomson's message lay in his own personal tale of woe and redemption. He began with his own family's struggles with illness and the terrors brought on them by regular doctors, and then proceeded to his valiant and ultimately successful efforts to save their lives with herbal remedies. He closed the dramatic story with his decision to submit himself and his life to his healing gift, asserting that knowledge gained through life experience exceeded that gained in any kind of medical school. Finally, he offered to demonstrate on willing—and usually purchasing—audience members. It was a performance that would find an easy home on late-night television today.[22]

As he traveled, Thomson continued to test and refine his methods and remedies. In 1806, Thomson effectively treated several people, including himself, for yellow fever during outbreaks in Boston and New York City. Traveling with only a few remedies on hand, Thomson first swallowed a half cup of salt dissolved in a pint of vinegar. His strength returned for a time, but he soon found himself so weak that he could barely walk the few yards to his New York City boardinghouse. He immediately took cayenne and then bayberry, each steeped in hot water, followed by a dose of bitters, each ingredients that would soon find their way into his healing system. "I soon recovered my strength and was able to be about," wrote Thomson. His successful experiments led Thomson to conclude that he had formed "a correct idea," as his method restored nature "to her empire."[23]

Thomson prided himself on finding a therapy that cured everything. Like many of his contemporaries, he viewed disease as a single entity. As such, every disease had essentially the same treatment. Thomson may have developed his theory in vocal opposition to regular medicine, but he reverted to ancient medical ideas to explain how it worked. Echoing thousands of years of medical belief, Thomson believed that the human body consisted of four basic elements that he called earth, air, fire, and water. Earth and water constituted the solid physicality of the body while fire and air gave that body life and motion. A vital power different from all of these gave humans life. This same idea underlay the humoral system of regular medicine as well as other vitalist medical systems. Thomson speculated that an imbalance in these elements, usually from some kind of obstruction, caused the body to lose the heat (the fire) necessary for health and life. To restore the body's heat, Thomson proposed clearing the body of any obstructions through sweating, purging, and vomiting; cleansing with appropriate remedies; and finally reinvigorating the body through stimulant plants. Doing all of this with natural remedies, rather than the harmful poisons of regular medicine, became the goal of Thomson's system.[24]

Thomson was not the first to associate cold with disease. Think only of the most universal of sicknesses, the common cold, likely named in the sixteenth century for symptoms that resembled those of exposure to cold weather. Ever since, cold weather and cold viruses have been associated, even if most doctors today do not believe that cold temperatures cause colds.[25]

In the beginning, Thomson relied almost exclusively on lobelia and capsicum (chili pepper, which caused an obvious feeling of heat) to heal, but with time, his system expanded to six primary botanicals. To these were added an additional seventy herbs and plants culled from folk remedies that could be found in most of the popular American and English herbal guides. He picked plants that stimulated rather than depleted patients as heroic measures tended to do because he believed that the purpose of medicine was to overcome any weakness brought on by the lack of internal heat. Thomson also sweated and purged patients like regular doctors, but he followed this up with invigorating herbs to restore patients from the weakening effects of these treatments; depletion without some means of renewal would only make the disease worse. Nearly all Thomson's remedies had known medicinal uses before him, though he claimed to have pioneered the use of lobelia and to have expanded the medical applications of capsicum. Thomson kept the names of his six core medicines secret, untroubled by the inconsistency between his own practice and his vehement criticisms of the opacity of regular medicine. Numbered one through six, these medicines became the method of his cure.[26]

Thomson's Number One medicine was lobelia, used to cleanse the stomach, promote perspiration, and create natural heat with its stimulating properties, though not enough heat to restore the body to balance on its own. That's what Thomson's Number Two began to do. Comprised of cayenne pepper, ginger, or black pepper, it roused the body and maintained the stomach's heat until the system could be cleared of obstructions. At this stage, Thomson sometimes advised steam baths, particularly in cases of high fever that had not yet broken, to induce the sweating that would eliminate any remaining obstructions.[27]

These steam baths were followed by medicines to clear the stomach and bowels. Thomson's Number Three remedy scoured the system with bayberry, the inner bark of young hemlock, the root of marsh rosemary, sumac, the leaves of witch hazel, or white pond lily. To further cleanse the intestines and lower bowels, Thomson often prescribed frequent enemas of bitterroot and bayberry, a mixture Thomsonians called "coffee." The name likely came from the mixture's dark color, though it could have come from the almost certain eye-widening jolt to the system that resulted from its use.[28]

After a successful cleanse, Thomson's next three remedies helped to calm the body down and return it to proper function. Thomson's Number Four restored the debilitated organs to their proper functions with various kinds of bitters steeped for tea. These bitter herbs and roots, like barberry and poplar bark, bitterroot, and golden seal, relaxed patients, stimulated their appetite, and restored the body's natural digestion. Number Five strengthened the stomach and bowels and returned proper digestion with tonic plants like poplar bark and the meats of peaches and cherrystones mixed with sugar and brandy. Finally, Thomson's Number Six, a mixture of gum myrrh and cayenne prepared with wine or brandy, which he also called Rheumatic Drops, eliminated any lingering pain and promoted natural heat. Number Six could also be applied externally when mixed with turpentine or gum camphor to pacify the nerves, relieve pain, and prime the body for its release from sickness.[29]

With the numbering of the remedies, patients had only to recall the instructions and count to six. To make the instructions even easier to remember, Thomson and his followers devised poems that served as simplified explanations of his system, as well as powerful polemics against regular medicine:

> When sick, we for the doctor send;
> He says, there is no chance to live,
> Unless I deadly poison give
> When this is done, the sick grow worse,
> Which takes the money from their purse;
> He says, "I've great regard for you,"
> But money is the most in view.[30]

At times the poems, particularly those written by Thomson himself, ranted on without reasoned argument. But overall, the Thomsonian poems covered a full range of emotion and prose style, from rage to joy and from sonnet to song. Dr. D. L. Terry's "The Botanic's Song of Liberty" had rousing lines meant to be sung:

> Merrily every bosom boundeth, merrily oh! Merrily oh!
> Where the name of Thomson soundeth, merrily oh! Merrily oh!
> There the bloom of health sheds more splendor,
> There the maidens' charms shine more tender;
> Every joy the land surroundeth, merrily oh! Merrily oh![31]

Memorizing these verses allowed followers to apply remedies without, Thomson claimed, knowing a single letter of the alphabet. The poems also provided rallying cries for practitioners forging ahead to remake medicine.[32]

Perhaps to bolster the case for the ease and simplicity of his system, Thomson professed to be illiterate in his early years on the road.

This was likely a tough claim to make and maintain since his system spread in significant measure by the written word, much of it written by Thomson himself. Although he had never attended school in a formal sense, Thomson was far from illiterate. He later dropped this charade—and released a flood of articles, poems, and books—but the story never completely died. In 1841, near the end of his life, Thomson's son John described his father as an "illiterate New Hampshire farmer" who nonetheless created a system that rapidly spread around the world, a reflection, perhaps, of the continued value many Americans placed on personal experience and self-education over a formal, classical education.[33]

Thomson's success was due in large measure to his tireless promotion and democratic rhetoric that resonated with popular prejudices against regular medicine—it almost certainly wasn't because of the treatment itself. The Thomsonian regimen could be incredibly tough with its courses of vomiting, sweating, and enemas: nothing about Thomson's system implied moderation. One Virginia woman endured six months of treatment that included three hundred sweats and sixty-six full scouring and heating courses of Numbers One through Six. The method essentially mirrored many of the therapies of regular medicine but used botanicals instead of chemicals to similar effect. Thomson's treatment was perhaps slightly better than bleeding and calomel but not by much.[34] Thomson also willfully ignored the fact that many of the drugs prescribed by regulars, such as opium, also came from plants. In his mind, medicine could be divided into two opposing categories that Thomson correlated with regular and irregular healers: mineral and vegetable. Thomson assured people that his remedies were safe because they came from nature, but critics loved to point out that nature could be deadly, too. Nicotine and strychnine, for instance, were deadlier than many minerals. "To speak of the mineral medicines as being exclusively poisons and of the vegetable ones as being always harmless, when the merest tyro [beginner] in botany or materia medica knows it to be otherwise, is indeed passing strange," asserted the Boston Medical and Surgical Journal in 1839.[35]

Like regular medicine, Thomson's treatments caused immediately visible effects on patients. People could feel lobelia's internal scrub on their organs and could hardly doubt the heat added to the body after a cayenne enema.[36] Sweating, vomiting, and stinging pain commonly accompanied even the most natural of remedies in Thomson's system. Patients expected medicine to hurt to know that it was working. Discomfort was part of the healing process, whether Thomsonian or regular medicine, at least until homeopathy began challenging that notion later in the century.

Thomson did not go unnoticed by the regular medical community. Regulars viewed Thomson with skeptical curiosity at first, but that quickly turned sour as he bashed their methods and claimed to have cured seemingly hopeless cases. Thomson treated patients for mercury poisoning, rheumatism, burns, and consumption. He found particular renown for his success in cases of dysentery spread through contaminated water and food. Regular doctors frequently treated sufferers with opiates that caused constipation and potentially harmed more than they helped by trapping the germs inside the body—not that anyone, regular doctors or Thomson alike, knew the true cause of the disease. Thomson's treatments, on the other hand, purged and cleansed the body, which may have helped to pass the infection out of the system more quickly, or at the very least, the vomiting kept patients from ingesting more contaminated food and water.[37]

The name Thomsonism was applied to his system early in his travels. Regular doctors had their own names for Thomson's cures, however "steamers," "pukers," and "despicable steam and pepper grinders" were among the most popular references to aspects of his treatment method. Practitioners themselves preferred Thomsonism, but such details mattered little to most advocates.[38]

Thomson's growing reputation in the Northeast infuriated many regular doctors, but this animosity tended to work to Thomson's advantage by clearly separating him from a profession that had already lost the confidence of many Americans. Historically, many of the people who had used the folk practice and self-care that Thomson built his system around could not afford professional medical attention and often didn't trust doctors. Public dissatisfaction among this group and other Americans made regular doctors attractive and easy targets for Thomson's promotional literature. He proclaimed that regular doctors knew nothing about healing except "how much poison [could] be given without causing death."[39] For many Americans, Thomson became a champion for the common man.

Thomsonism fit perfectly with the egalitarian spirit of Jacksonian America in the 1820s and 1830s. Like other medical irregulars, Thomsonians tended to attract people involved in other social reform movements. Thomson's followers viewed their struggle against the dominance of the medical professional as a struggle against all forms of domination and control. Echoing the evangelical revivals that sought to elevate the moral condition of the nation, Thomson promised to improve its physical condition by providing the tools to democratize medicine and make "every man his own physician." He encouraged people to engage directly with their health to be the agents of their own recovery. His books and periodicals dripped with folksy language as he sought to demystify medicine and call diseases by colloquial rather than Latin names. Thomson lashed out at regulars who attacked him and refused to even "stoop to examine a system on the ground of its intrinsic merit." Rather than be hoodwinked by medical science cloaked in jargon and doctors out to make a buck, Thomson invited people to embrace his simple and natural system.[40]

Thomson's faith that all people could be their own physicians clashed with the prevailing views of regular doctors, who thought little of their patients' abilities to comprehend even the most basic aspects of medicine. The ever-skeptical Oliver Wendell Holmes believed the general public "hopelessly ignorant" of medicine, demonstrating a record of perfect "incompetence to form opinions on medical subjects."[41] Georgia physician J. Dickson Smith wondered, "If each man is to be 'his own doctor,' to cast aside his books, and act upon his own idea of the case, what becomes of the science? . . . [A]ccording to this logic any ten year old boy can practice medicine 'scientifically.'"[42]

Thomson sold his method to patients through a prepayment system that operated something like a franchise. For twenty dollars (about $350 in today's dollars), buyers earned the right to practice Thomson's system on themselves and their immediate families. It was a steep price for the "common man" whom Thomson sought to win to his system. In 1830, the average male factory worker earned less than a dollar a day.[43] The system could quickly pay for itself, though, with the average cost of one doctor-delivered baby running from twelve to twenty dollars. The franchise plan, known as "Family Rights," proved extremely practical for Thomson's fledgling business. Thomson, like most doctors, was vulnerable to the whims of patients who anxiously sought a doctor's attention when sick but proved far less eager to pay for the service when well. Rather than keep track of a patient's bills over his sprawling practice, Thomson secured payment in advance of sickness, like a health savings account for use when needed. As he lectured, Thomson provided only a partial explanation of his system prior to purchase; the rest came with payment.[44]

As the number of purchasers grew, Thomson encouraged his rights holders to form Friendly Botanic Societies to encourage the sharing of ideas and information. These groups received half the profits from the local sale of family rights, and they published their own Thomsonian medical journals and articles. Thomson's societies represented the nation's first effort to turn what had been a largely home-based, independent practice into an organized medical system.[45]

Perhaps more essential to the spread of Thomson's system, these societies constituted a network of political activists committed to Thomson's cause and willing to lobby and challenge medical laws on his behalf. Medical licensing laws invoked the particular wrath of Thomsonians, who believed they stifled freedom and oppressed honest and talented men who healed without the legal advantage of a diploma. Arguing his case against licensure, Thomson tarred regular doctors as parasites and exploiters of the masses who used licensing laws to gain elite privileges over common people. The Thomsonian arguments proved incredibly persuasive. Thomson's own sons, John and Cyrus, both devoted botanic practitioners, pushed a wheelbarrow carrying a petition more than ninety feet long to the capitol at Albany, New York. During the debate that followed, one senator declared, "The people of this state have been bled long enough in their bodies and pockets, and it [is] time they should do as the men of the Revolution did: resolve to set down and enjoy the freedom for which they bled."[46] Thomson's relationship with his sons later disintegrated after the New York State Thomsonian Medical Society, with John as president and Cyrus as treasurer, ratified a constitution that allowed certain qualified individuals to operate general botanic practices with the society's approval. Furious at this imposition on his control over his own system, Thomson declared that only he had the power to grant this right.[47] At a Hagerstown, Maryland, hotel in May of 1839, members of the Thomsonian Society of Washington County gathered to celebrate the passage of laws allowing them to practice legally with a formal dinner and toasts to Thomson and to John Wharton, the lawyer who worked on their behalf. They also passed a set of resolutions praising the wisdom of Thomson and his system. "Resolved, That Dr. Samuel Thomson's trials and success have eventuated in the establishment of a theory supported by facts and experiments," read

Hagerstown grocer and president of the society Daniel Witmer to the assembled members. "That Thomson's cause is the cause of humanity, that he has a claim upon the confidence and gratitude of the world, courts of law have decided in his favor . . . and the god of nature and providence has elevated him to a place in the temple of fame."[48] Maryland wasn't alone. Between 1833 and 1844, thanks in large measure to the efforts of Thomsonians, nearly every state repealed or reduced the penalties for unlicensed practitioners, leaving it to the marketplace to sort out the true healers from the quacks.

As Thomsonism grew, Thomson designated "agents" to help him spread his system even further. Agents could sell additional family rights and prepare medicines while sharing in the profits of the sales. Many of these agents did whatever they could to sell as many rights as possible—and thus make as much money as possible—even to the point of exaggerating and misrepresenting Thomson's system. A few agents took their role as franchisers to mean that they could set up infirmaries where they administered medicines and treated people reluctant to treat themselves. These agents became, in essence, practicing doctors, actions that won the harsh condemnation of Thomson for directly opposing the intent of his system. Some of these facilities had beds for inpatients, and one infirmary in Norfolk, Virginia, treated more than six hundred people in its first year. "It has generally been the case, with those I have appointed as agents, that as soon as they have been sufficiently instructed to attend to the practice with success," declared Thomson, "[they] have attempted to get the lead of the practice into their own hands, and deprive me of the credit and profits of my own discovery."[49] Thomson also registered his disappointment with his agents in verse:

> As Doctor Thomson's Agent—he
> A bond had sign'd, to faithful be
> Unto the Doctor's views;
> His med'cines all, both wet and dry,
> Agreed of Thomson for to buy,
> And not his trust abuse.[50]

To protect his proprietary information from misrepresentation, Thomson patented his system in 1813. It had simply spread too far for him to meet with every rights holder personally. His success had also spawned a legion of copycats making claims similar to his own. Thomson's decision to patent his medical system was unusual but not unique. Before Thomson, Dr. Peter Davidson had received copyright protection from the state of New York for his proprietary cancer plaster, a paste that inflamed, swelled, and then supposedly destroyed the cancer, and Dr. Elisha Perkins patented his electric tractors, three-inch brass and iron rods with healing powers. With his patent in hand, Thomson spent the rest of his life tenaciously and a bit pompously guarding his system from imposters.[51]

Thomson turned to Benjamin Smith Barton and Benjamin Rush for advice on how to publicize and win support for his newly patented system. The busy Dr. Rush had little time for Thomson, but Barton advised him to seek celebrity endorsement for maximum success: "[M]ake friends of some celebrated doctors and let them try the medicine and give the public such recommendation of it as they should deem correct."[52] Thomson appreciated the advice but feared that some unscrupulous doctors might claim his system as their own and deprive him of the credit he so eagerly sought. He trusted Barton, though, and convinced him to try Thomson's system on himself and give his own recommendation. Unfortunately for Thomson, Barton died—not from a Thomsonian treatment—before he could render judgment.[53]

Thomson announced his newly patented system in newspapers and soon began appointing more and more agents to sell family rights to practice and distribute his medicines. Authorized agents often received notice in newspaper ads. "Dr. Samuel Thomson . . . now has the pleasure to recommend to the people of Boston and vicinity, Dr. JOHN LOCKE, who has had long experience in the practice and is well-qualified to administer relief to the sick," announced the *Columbian Centinel American Federalist*, followed by an address for Locke's office and an invitation to visit.[54] Thomson moved his own office to Boston in 1818 to better manage and centralize his business affairs in a larger, more accessible city. By 1833, Thomson had 167 agents operating in twenty-two states and territories.[55] Agents could sell rights to anyone who would pay. The right to practice on oneself and one's immediate family still cost twenty dollars, but now buyers had the option of paying one hundred dollars to start a mini-practice for non-family members. Thomson and his agents made buyers swear never to share the secrets of the system, nor could they ever resell it, subject to a sixty-five-dollar fine for each transgression.[56]

Even with his patent, Thomson still faced the difficult task of protecting his enterprise and his name. The patent gave him some legal protection against those who tried to steal his system, but Thomson became so paranoid about his property that it became a source of contention and division among his followers. Thomson soon came to regard many of his agents not as allies and friends but as enemies out to steal his profits for themselves.

Thomson's loose system of agents and rights holders made cohesion and unity challenging if not impossible, and made even more so by Thomson's demanding nature. Thomson fought to maintain tight control over his system throughout his life. He insisted that it was incapable of amendment or improvement by anyone but him, and he dismissed any competing or new ideas as illegitimate and treasonous. He sarcastically accused one agent of palming his "literary pillage upon the world as a book of reformation, new discoveries, and wonderful improvements," and called the efforts of other agents an attempt to "mislead and confuse enquiring minds."[57] Thomson's annual letter to his agents became predictable for its recitation of enemies, unfaithful agents, and "pretended friends" who had tried to change his system, insulted his character, and stolen profits from the sale of family rights. Some successful agents established their own regional reputations and broke with Thomson to start their own more lenient and inclusive botanical medical practices.[58]

Thomson filed suit against many of his own agents, as well as unaffiliated pretenders, to defend what he believed to be protected by federal law. Many of his claims were successful, but not every case went Thomson's way. With these losses, he could only print announcements listing the agents authorized to sell his system and denouncing everyone else as a botanic faker and quack, likely much to the amusement of regular doctors who saw them all, Thomson included, as quacks.[59]

Despite his admonitions against book learning, Thomson published his own book in an attempt to police the boundaries of his theory and to keep his system within reach of every agent and rights holder. In 1822, he published two lengthy works, often packaged together, the *New Guide to Health: Or Botanic Family Physician*,

Containing a Complete System of Practice on a Plan Entirely New and *A Narrative of the Life and Medical Discoveries of the Author*, the latter an autobiographical account of his conversion to botanicals. The books used plain and direct language to craft stories of the patients Thomson had cured, including many who had found no relief in regular medicine. Thomson claimed to have taken on some of these cases reluctantly, worried that his method may not work on people who had suffered for so long. One woman in Portsmouth, New Hampshire, came to Thomson for relief from a venereal disease she had suffered from for more than five years. Her doctors had "filled her with mercury to kill the disorder" and then "left her to linger out a miserable existence," Thomson wrote, adding, "I felt very unwilling to undertake with her, apprehending that it would be very uncertain whether a cure could be effected, [her illness] having been of so longstanding." But she insisted, and after three weeks of treatment with his numbered system along with sweats and purges, "her health was restored, and she returned home well."[60]

These types of stories filled the pages of Thomson's *New Guide to Health*, providing illustrations of the many types of people and cases that he could effectively treat as well as the kinds of people he hoped to attract to his system. In contrast to the sometimes fantastical and inflated language contained in the literature of other medical irregulars, Thomson described his system frankly and without ornament, as though to emphasize the intuitive rather than miraculous nature of his cures that he hoped would appeal to commonsense Americans.[61] Always careful of giving out too much information, though, Thomson did not include full instructions for his course of medicines. He continued to reserve this information for agents and rights purchasers.[62]

Thomson used his books to draw particular attention to the democratic character of his system. At a time ripe with distrust of professionalism and formal education, Thomson worked hard to portray himself as a friend and champion of the people. He explained how regular doctors wasted several years in school learning theories that had little relevance to daily practice when experience had long been shown to be the best teacher.[63]

Copies of the *New Guide to Health* appeared virtually everywhere in North America, going through twenty-one editions between 1822 and 1851.[64] Thomson may have prided himself on creating a medical system that any illiterate person could use, but his own book clocked in at nearly four hundred pages, suggesting a well-educated following.[65] The book spawned an array of imitators, including several from within his own ranks, just as Thomson had long feared. Some of Thomson's agents sold unauthorized copies of *A New Guide to Health* while others, such as Elias Smith, who was, for a time, Thomson's right-hand man, published their own botanic medicine books at a discounted price to cut into Thomson's business.[66] Thomson offered a reward to anyone who provided information on those who attempted to sell his system under any name other than his own.[67]

By the 1830s, Thomson claimed that more than a million people in a country of nearly thirteen million practiced his medicine, a number even regular doctors admitted was probably accurate. The proliferation of Thomson's books and other literature attracted followers and provided cohesion to a movement that might otherwise have fallen apart in the consumer marketplace. Just a few years later, in 1835, the Thomsonians bombastically proclaimed that one-sixth of the American population practiced only botanic medicine, and that in some states, particularly in the West and South, the number was closer to one-third.[68] "The people, the *common* people, have been found capable of examining, judging, and deciding correctly," declared the *Thomsonian Recorder.* "Give them the facts, the whole facts, and nothing but the facts. By them, we conquer!"[69] The governor of Mississippi corroborated these claims, announcing in 1835 that half the citizens of his state were Thomsonians.[70] It was true that Thomson found his greatest success in frontier regions of the country, where trained regular doctors were virtually nonexistent and many people relied on home medical care by necessity. A simple system that promised to cure everything with natural remedies at a low cost held undeniable appeal.

Like the other irregular systems that followed, Thomsonism was particularly welcoming to women. In fact, Thomson was the first to recognize women as legitimate medical practitioners on par with men in an organized system in the United States. Thomson's message that the family rather than the infirmary should be the primary forum for medical care proved a natural match for women, who had long acted as healers in their homes and communities. Thomson hailed the introduction and education to the plant world he had received from Mrs. Beaton. "All the valuable instruction I ever received was from a woman in the town where I lived, who had practiced as a midwife for twenty years," wrote Thomson, saying "she gave me more useful instruction than all I ever gained from any other source."[71] Not only could women practice Thomsonism, but their special role within the family as moral arbiters and caretakers made them uniquely qualified to provide medical care. Women could purchase the right to practice Thomson's system, just as any man could, and women were encouraged to buy and read medical guides, to establish Friendly Botanic Societies, and to act as agents. Thomsonian books often included information on female anatomy, conception, pregnancy, and birth at a time when women's health was rarely included in health texts, much less discussed in medical practice. Thomson, for instance, advised women to drink raspberry leaf tea for birthing pains, which many pregnant women continue to swear by to this day. Chemicals in the plant may help relax blood vessels and the muscles involved in contractions. He also became an early proponent of the continued use of female midwives over regular male doctors for obstetrical care at a time when regular medicine had become increasingly wary of anyone but trained regular doctors attending to women's care. "Thirty years ago the practice of midwifery was principally in the hands of experienced women, who had no difficulty," asserted Thomson. "The practice of midwifery at this time, appears to be altogether a matter of speculation with the medical faculty," depriving families "of their wives and children, by such ignorant and unnatural practice."[72] Thomson and his followers criticized the inexperience of male regulars delivering babies, their use of invasive techniques like forceps, and the high fees they charged for a service that women performed better.[73]

Among those to adopt Thomson's method were regular doctors, though not everyone came by choice. Thomsonism became so popular in some areas of the country that many regular doctors couldn't maintain their practices without publicly disdaining heroic drugs and bloodletting. Others offered patients a choice of botanic or heroic treatments.[74]

Ever suspicious, Thomson was seldom convinced that regular doctors had honestly made the switch to his system. He distrusted regulars who purchased rights or who appeared to embrace his system. Friendly Botanic Societies carefully examined the case of any regular doctor intending to switch, and Thomson directed agents to obtain a doctor's written pledge to follow Thomson's principles and to abandon mineral drugs, blistering, and bleeding. Regular doctors also had to pay more for the right to practice, up to five hundred dollars on a case-by-case basis.[75]

Thomson's distrust of the intentions of regular doctors was not completely misplaced. His success had attracted the animosity and criticism of many regulars, who denounced his system and looked for every opportunity to ridicule, punish, and accuse him of murder. The *New York Courier* reported that a Thomsonian had "steamed" one patient "into a corpse." A Mr. Jackson was "stewed in hot and drenched in cold water, crammed with lobelia and cayenne pepper until the stomach of the victim was literally scalded" to the point that he "became delirious, convulsed and apoplectic and died."[76] The case, however, never went to trial. Thomson's belief that healing required no special training particularly incensed regulars. Physician Daniel Drake labeled Thomson a "demagogue" who posed as "one of the *people*" and accused regular doctors of being "not *of* the *people*, but arrayed against the *people*, and bent on killing them off."[77] Many Thomsonians "openly abuse learning and its advocates; yet they prate about nature's laws," remarked a Mr. Sanborn in the *Boston Medical and Surgical Journal*. "They pretend 'to assist nature' in the cure of diseases. How can they assist nature unless they know how nature acts? They are quite as likely to contravene the laws of nature as to co-operate with her, unless they have thoroughly studied physiology and anatomy."[78] Regular doctors pointed out the errors in his theory and his course of medicine, though Thomson's basic approach of cleansing and restoring balance to the system was strikingly similar to that of regular medicine. Regular doctors were not interested in finding common ground, though. In 1808, Thomson was accused of sweating two children to death, and a year later of killing one Captain Trickey. Although the charges proved false, Thomson fumed over the "fashionable educated doctor [who] may lose one half his patients without being blamed; but if I lose one out of several hundred of the most desperate cases . . . it is called murder."[79]

Among the regular doctors who attacked Thomson was Dr. French of Salisbury, New Hampshire, whose successful indictment of Thomson for the 1808 death of Ezra Lovett came to haunt Thomson for decades. Thomson treated Lovett for typhus fever over several days and left him with strict instructions to stay indoors as he attended another patient. Lovett did not follow Thomson's orders, however. Instead, feeling better, he left home, caught a chill, and suffered a relapse that forced him to seek the care of a regular doctor. Lovett died a few days later. Learning of the case, French had Thomson indicted and imprisoned in November 1809 for "willful murder" with lobelia. Thomson spent forty days in jail before being brought to trial before the Massachusetts Supreme Judicial Court, where he pled not guilty. The jury promptly acquitted him, needing only five minutes of deliberation to conclude that Thomson had acted in good faith to cure the patient with no intended malice. The trial only complicated Thomson's life, however, as regulars in several states continuously pressured state legislatures for stricter laws to outlaw unlicensed doctors. They also routinely called for and supported coroner's inquests into the deaths of patients under the care of Thomsonians.[80]

Despite Thomson's suspicion toward regulars, his system benefited from those doctors willing to challenge orthodoxy and express doubt about the efficacy of heroic treatments. Among Thomson's most prominent supporters was well-known American regular Dr. Benjamin Waterhouse, who became the first to test the smallpox vaccine in the United States. Waterhouse was a vocal supporter of Thomson throughout his life, hailing Thomson's medical use of lobelia and vapor-bath processes as "valuable *improvement[s]* in our practice, if conducted by persons as experienced and sagacious as is the *Patriarch Thomson*." South Carolina physician Robert D. Montgomery praised Thomsonism for its simplicity and for holding out a "helping hand" to the "illiterate and untutored part of the human family" by "snatch[ing] them from pain and death."[81] The Thomsonians even counted the skeptical Oliver Wendell Holmes as an ally, a remarkable claim given Holmes's antipathy toward nearly every other irregular system, and one that likely surprised Holmes himself. The *Thomsonian Recorder* published several of Holmes's letters, where he described the beneficial use of vapor baths and expressed his appreciation for the healing powers of nature. Botanic remedies, wrote Holmes, were "in perfect harmony with life."[82] It should be remembered, though, that regular medicine included some herbal remedies and vegetable-based drugs by the nineteenth century, and many regular doctors praised the power of nature as a complement to, rather than a wholesale replacement for, heroic treatments. Even so, Thomsonians tended to seize on any mention of nature and botanicals among regular doctors as positive affirmations of their method and their system's ascent to dominance.

Even as Thomsonism grew in popularity, various fault lines had already begun to appear among its practitioners. Many of Thomson's agents and followers began to push for medical schools and associations to train the next generation of practitioners and to elevate the professional status of the Thomsonian system. While it had been fine to empower the common man in its early years, they argued, a level of professionalization was necessary for Thomsonism to truly compete with regular medicine. An official Thomsonian school of medicine would help to codify the methods and provide some stability to the loose network of botanic healers spread around the country who had otherwise few binding ties save for a twenty-dollar investment in a set of instructions. Thomson, however, adamantly opposed these institutions, believing them instruments of privilege and monopoly that destroyed the democratic character of his system. His stated purpose was to enable common people to care for themselves, and those that sought professional Thomsonian care instead would "not see the importance of trying to obtain the knowledge for themselves."[83] Thomson did not want to subject people to domination by any kind of professional, even professionals he agreed with. Nevertheless, at the 1833 national convention of rights holders, the Thomsonians voted to create a national infirmary, and two years later, in 1835, to establish a medical school.[84]

Tension over these issues was exacerbated by Thomson's difficult and uncompromising personality. Not even poetry could save Thomson from himself. His near-constant paranoid battle against his perceived enemies, even his own agents and partners, and his bombastic lack of modesty embarrassed and angered his followers. Any ideas to change or improve the system were met with scorn and charges of disloyalty, even when those modifications might have strengthened Thomson's position in the marketplace. While most botanic healers sympathized with the tough course that Thomson had traveled and the persecution he'd faced developing his system, many now felt that Thomson had no more reason to complain. "What more does he covet?" asked J. P. Shepherd in the *Botanico-Medical Recorder*. "He cannot expect to monopolize the plants which grow on Nature's bounteous bosom for all who choose to pluck them." Shepherd contended that having purchased a family right, "I avail myself of the contents ... as I deem proper."[85] Thomson's suspicious nature and powder-keg approach to leadership stunted the growth of his movement and forced followers to choose between staying loyal to their founder or breaking with him.[86] It was a division that quickly tore the botanical system apart.

Thomson's agents largely led the drive to reform Thomsonism, with each of the major botanical splits fostered by one of his agents. As early as 1832, Ohio agent Horton Howard led the first major defection with the publication of his *Improved System of Botanic Medicine Founded Upon Current Physiological Principles*. Howard added forty-two botanicals to Thomson's approved list of herbs and set about promoting his updated system in a medical journal devoted to "improved botanics." Unsurprisingly, Thomson threatened legal action to stop him, but Howard succumbed to cholera the following year and his improved system along with him.[87]

Thomson's own death in 1843 only sped up the fragmentation of his botanical system. Dozens of groups that used nearly every possible combination of "botanic," "reformed," "improved," and "independent" formed. More intent on attacking each other than presenting a serious challenge to regular medicine, most of these splinter groups disappeared by the Civil War. American interest in botanic remedies, though, only continued to gain ground.[88]

Alva Curtis led a more enduring offshoot. A former Thomson agent and editor of the *Thomsonian Recorder*, Curtis believed that the science of botanical medicine was too complicated to trust to self-discovery and independent learning. While he appreciated Thomsonism's appeal and popularity among those in rural areas or those lacking formal education, Curtis also saw how its informality hampered its recognition as a serious medical contender among educated Americans in urban areas. The only way to compete successfully with regular doctors, argued Curtis, was for the Thomsonians to become more like doctors themselves. He had urged Thomson to open a school because he knew many patent holders did not understand how to use Thomson's method the way its founder had intended, which had the potential to turn patients back to regular medicine.[89]

"If you could travel through the country and see what bungling work they make of your practice, you would cheerfully subscribe to the establishment of schools to teach the application of that practice and the meaning of your precepts," Curtis had tried to explain to Thomson.[90] Teaching people how to use the system properly would help the movement grow and stem the tide of those turned off by their own misunderstanding of the directions. Thomson, however, true to form, had refused to bend, promising to do everything he could "to prevent his system of practice from being swallowed up in the vortex of literature and science."[91]

So in 1836, Curtis had broken with Thomson and opened the Botanico-Medical College and Infirmary in Columbus, Ohio. Three years later, the school received a state charter, giving it legal status with regular medical schools and making it the first chartered Thomsonian medical college in the country. The school soon moved to Cincinnati and went through a number of name changes before permanently settling on the Physio-Medical College in 1850, a name it retained until it closed in 1880. A dozen other physio-medical colleges opened around the country before the last shut its doors in 1911.[92]

At the same time, another botanical healing group with no direct ties to Thomson rose to prominence. Like Thomson, Wooster Beach studied with a local botanic healer and wrote a popular book on domestic medicine. Unlike Thomson, Beach graduated from a regular medical school in 1825. Suspicious about the safety of regular medicine, though, Beach opened a school in New York City in 1827 to educate students on botanical remedies. Unable to receive a state charter in New York, Beach accepted an offer from Worthington College (today's Kenyon College) in Worthington, Ohio, to open a medical department. In 1829, the Reformed Medical College opened not far from where Curtis would open his school in 1836, becoming the first irregular medical school chartered in the United States.[93]

Although Beach's followers insisted that Beach, and not Thomson, had introduced the nation's first scientific botanical medical practice, most Americans could not tell the difference between the two systems, at least in their early years. As time passed, however, Beach's botanic medical system enlarged, and his followers became known as "eclectics" for their pragmatic approach to healing. The name also associated the movement with American common sense rather than the "pathies" of the other healing methods to come, including homeopathy, hydropathy, and allopathy, homeopathy's name for regular medicine.[94] "Use anything that works" was eclectic medicine's only principle, a stark contrast to the hard line that Thomson drew around his system. The eclectics alone among the nineteenth-century irregular medical systems made no attempt to devise a theoretical framework to explain their system. They distinguished themselves only by their reliance on botanical drugs and their rejection of bloodletting: any other therapeutic treatment was fair game, be it hydropathy, homeopathy, or something else that offered relief. The considerable latitude given to followers allowed eclectic medicine to adapt far more easily to new medical discoveries and made it a popular alternative to regular medicine. The *Medical and Surgical Reporter* commented, "The Eclectics keep themselves alive by swallowing everything which happens to turn up."[95] More than sixty journals and twenty schools were established before eclecticism as an organized movement finally faded from the scene in the 1930s.[96]

Besides the schools founded by Curtis and Beach, thirteen other colleges were founded on Thomsonian principles between 1836 and 1911. Instruction followed Thomson's basic idea of restoring the body's heat with natural ingredients. They relied on Thomson's basic remedies—lobelia, capsicum, and steam baths—but purposely expanded the number and variety of botanic remedies.[97]

By the mid-nineteenth century, Thomsonism in its original form had mostly disappeared, eclipsed by the panoply of botanic splinter groups as well as by the rise of other irregular medical systems such as homeopathy, mesmerism, and hydropathy. Thomson's contentious attitude ultimately led to the disintegration of the movement he worked so hard to forge and undermined his appeals to the common man. Thomson welcomed every American to use his healing method but only if they did so on his terms—his devotion to democratic inclusiveness only went so far. He was unable and unwilling to compromise and, as a result, found himself forever engaged in quarrels, even with those like Curtis, who sought to elevate and improve botanic medicine to the point where it could vanquish regular medicine. Both men wanted the same things but profoundly disagreed on the path to achieve it.

For all his failings, though, Thomson's anti-elitist and entrepreneurial spirit had satisfied the needs of many like-minded Americans. He effectively articulated the problems that many people had with regular medicine and provided the folksy language and democratic rationale that many other irregular healers would take up in the fight against regular medicine. More than just disagreeing, though, Thomson offered an alternative, presenting a theory and therapeutic solution in simple and direct language that anyone could—and millions did—understand. At his height, Thomson claimed to have converted more than three million Americans to his natural healing method. Although he probably exaggerated his influence, Thomson still achieved a high level of support that few Americans, particularly not those practicing regular medicine, could fail to ignore.[98]

Thomson hit on the marketing gold of selling natural ingredients for superior health nearly two centuries before it became commonplace. References to "nature," "natural," and following nature's plan appear throughout Thomson's *New Guide to Health*. He decried regular medicine's use of drugs like mercury and arsenic as "directly opposed to nature," and replaced them with plants and herbs that produced nearly identical results. "There cannot be the least doubt but there is medicine enough grows in our country, to answer all the purposes necessary in curing every disease," wrote Thomson. The "common people are kept back from a knowledge of what is of the utmost importance for them to know" by the power and profit motive of regular doctors. Thomson marketed his system as harmonious with nature and proclaimed his ingredients as pure, familiar, and as harmless as the trees and flowers growing around his followers' homes. All of the ingredients in his products were relatively pronounceable and recognizable, made by nature because nature knew best. Thomson's promotion of locally sourced, natural ingredients would scarcely seem out of place today.[99]

Thomson also used highly innovative administrative and organizational skills to sell his system. Thomson was exceptionally energetic and diligent in patenting and commercially distributing his methods throughout the country. His medical patent, a strategic move, was rare even in an era where patent medicines had becoming increasingly common. The number of valid patents granted by the federal government for medicines was small; many just used the term "patent medicine" to mean "secret" or "proprietary" without having secured exclusive rights from the government for production and sale of their products. This business and institutional savvy sharply differentiated Thomson from the mass of itinerant healers roaming the country's back roads and gave him a leg up in his attacks on the dominance of regular medicine.

Perhaps the most impressive and groundbreaking of all of Thomson's tactics, though, was his system of distribution. More than a century before McDonald's, Thomson established his own medical franchise system. In theory, visits with any Thomson agent were roughly equivalent, whether in Ohio, South Carolina, or Maine. This franchise system was perhaps the most American thing about Thomson, as he seized on the possibilities of the nineteenth-century capitalist marketplace to create an effective and efficient business model for selling medicine.

In 1838, five years before his death, Thomson agreed to have his head "read" by the famous American phrenologist Orson Squire Fowler. For a man with little praise for medical theory, not to mention regard for any idea that differed from his own, Thomson's willingness to submit to a reading is one measure of phrenology's growing popularity and influence; Thomsonism was no longer the only, nor even the most popular irregular medical system in the country. Consumers had more options. New irregular systems offered people an expanded range of medical alternatives. Premade medicines had become increasingly available and affordable, first in urban areas and then slowly moving out to the frontier. Fewer people needed, much less wanted, to make their own remedies at home.

Examining Thomson, Fowler found the sixty-nine-year-old's head "very uneven," suggesting a strong personality that "would make some noise in the world." His cranial organs suggested that he "courted opposition" and angered quickly. "To say that he was obstinate, even to mulishness," wrote Fowler, "is strictly correct." Thomson considered no challenge too great, and he found difficulties stimulating rather than dispiriting. His social organs suggested a polarizing personality that inspired either fierce love or extreme hatred. Fowler concluded that Thomson had little regard for the "old or the sacred" and that the "general, cast, tone, and tenor of [Thomson's] genius, was that of a plain, practical, common-sense man."[100]

Whether Fowler determined Thomson's true character from his meticulous head reading or from what he already knew of Thomson did not much matter. Thomson, the "American Hippocrates," had left his mark on both American health and the business of medicine, paving the way for irregular systems that would continue to revolutionize the way Americans thought about health and wellness, and giving notice to regular medicine that something had to change.

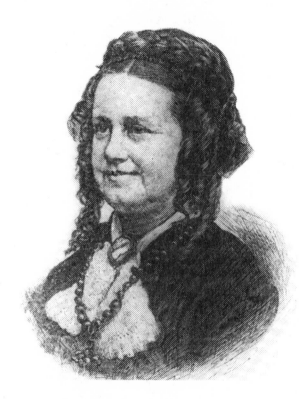

Only the second woman to receive a medical degree in the United States, Lydia Folger devoted her life to improving women's health through teaching, writing, and lecturing on the benefits and uses of phrenology. Her marriage to renowned phrenologist Lorenzo Fowler in 1844 gave this intelligent and well-spoken woman a larger platform for her work. (National Library of Medicine, Bethesda, MD)

CHAPTER TWO

The Only True Science of the Mind
Phrenology

Lorenzo Fowler knew he'd found the woman for him after feeling the bumps on the head of Lydia Folger. The two first met just weeks before, in March of 1844, when Fowler examined the head of Folger's uncle Walter, a man known to his neighbors as something of an eccentric, as "odd as huckleberry chowder," as some put it.[1]

Less than a month later, Fowler was back to take a reading of the woman who had caught his eye on his first trip, perhaps concerned that fools might run in the family. With Lydia Folger, he had nothing to fear. Nearly eleven years Fowler's junior, Folger was well spoken, intelligent, and charming with a commanding presence even in her early twenties. Her scholarly and scientific interests would later lead her to become a lecturer, writer, educator, and only the second woman to receive a medical degree in the United States. But first she had to submit to a head reading, one that served as both a personality test and courtship ritual.[2]

Fowler passed his fingertips over her skull and adjusted his craniometer, a caliper-like device that spanned the head. His instruments allowed him to construct a topographical map of Folger's head, capable of revealing her intelligence, personality, and character. He found Folger's brain to be of "full size" and her mind agile and active. Not merely book smart, Folger learned "from everything she sees, hears, or read." She wasn't all brains: she also had all the makings of a good wife, with "strongly developed" social and domestic natures and "strong parental feelings." Fortunately for Fowler, he also discovered that she was unable to "enjoy herself without mate or companion."[3]

The reading complete, Fowler must have made a good impression on Folger as well. The two married less than six months later on Nantucket. In Folger, Fowler found a phrenologically suitable wife—a not unimportant factor in the "head conscious" 1840s—as well as a mate whose intelligence and skill would prove vital to his family's effort to build and sustain phrenology's popularity in the United States.

To anyone who has ever shaved his or her head and been horrified by the lumps and dents hidden beneath, the idea that those bumps said anything about a person's character might be unsettling. But for millions of Americans in the nineteenth century, phrenology provided comfort and insight, a way to know and understand behavior and personality with seemingly scientific precision. Why do we act the way we do? What determines the patterns of our behavior? How can we be better people? Every generation seeks answers to these questions, and in the mid-nineteenth century, phrenology provided one incredibly popular and influential explanation.

With phrenology, doctors could easily determine not only that someone thought, felt, and coped with life in a particular way, but *why*. Its advocates hoped phrenology would become a new diagnostic tool for mental health and a way to understand the brain and its function. But phrenology quickly spread beyond the doctor's office to become a whole cultural and social system largely divorced from its roots.

Physician Franz Joseph Gall first developed his theories on the anatomy and function of the brain in eighteenth-century Vienna, where Sigmund Freud would later foster another science of the mind, psychoanalysis, in the late nineteenth century. Born in Tiefenbrunn, Germany, in 1758, Gall grew fascinated by the physical structure of the body as a medical student, first in Strasbourg and then Vienna. As a physician, he became a skilled anatomist who learned to dissect the brain to show the origins and pathways of cranial nerves. Gall's initial question came from something he'd observed in childhood: classmates who excelled at memorization also tended to have large protruding eyes. Theorizing about the connection, Gall suggested that the part of the brain located behind the eyes must be associated with verbal memory. Since all those bulging eyes indicated a shared talent for memorization, Gall supposed that that part of the brain must be more developed, which caused the eyes to bug out. This anecdotal observation and his later anatomical work on the structure of the brain led Gall to formulate his new science of the mind.[4]

Gall conceived of the brain not as a single organ, as most believed at the time, but as a mosaic of many specialized organs that each governed a particular mental or emotional function—an idea now thought to be mostly correct. He certainly wasn't the first to try to locate personality in body organs. For centuries, philosophers and scientists had proposed locations for the source of human emotions and character traits. Aristotle, for instance, had suggested that anger came from the liver, a belief still common today in traditional Chinese medicine. Plato took a sunnier view of the liver, describing it as the source of joy and desire while placing anger in the heart. During Gall's time, prevailing theory held that the brain was the center of immediate mental processes but that feeling and personality came from the soul. Gall was one of the first to hypothesize that all mental and emotional activity occurred in the brain.[5]

Through his study, Gall came to believe that the brain was the organ of the mind, and its shape a reflection of the mental composition of its owner. He also asserted that the shape of the skull matched the shape of the brain within it, so that studying the bumps and indentations of the skull could reveal information about the size, structure, and function of the brain areas beneath it. A large brain organ correlated with a bump on the skull, and vice versa. At the time, before X-rays and CT scans, observing head shape presented the only way to study the living brain.[6] While head size could indicate overall mental power, Gall didn't believe that its overall size revealed anything about how the mind was actually organized and functioned, the idea that became the heart of phrenology. That knowledge could only come by studying the individual parts of the skull.[7]

Gall tested his theory on the heads of psychiatric patients, artists, and criminals—people with extreme character traits he hoped to find written on their skulls. Even better than just examining heads, Gall also liked to collect skulls for further study and demonstrations. Gall's friendship with the deputy chief of police in Vienna helped to enrich his collection as the officer likely had easier access to the criminal minds Gall sought. For those heads still in use by their owners,

Gall made plaster casts. By 1792, on the basis of hundreds of these head studies, Gall concluded that there were twenty-seven innate human faculties (Gall's word for mental or emotional traits or abilities) located in the brain.[8]

The size and development of these areas implied a greater or lesser amount of each trait. These faculties included everything from reproduction and affection to vanity and musical ability. Each was associated with a discrete part of the brain, which Gall called organs, and a detectable bump on the skull. Not all traits were positive. Gall classified murder and thievery as "evil" and "bad." Other traits, such as the sexual instinct, were only beneficial in moderation. Gall believed that knowledge of these immoral traits would help individuals keep them suppressed. Of these twenty-seven traits, humans shared nineteen with animals, including reproductive instincts and a sense of sound. Some of Gall's critics found this animal/human convergence to be particularly offensive. They did not see any connection between the mental and emotional worlds of animals and humans. Gall located all of the specifically human functions, which included religiosity, wit, and moral sense, in the cerebral cortex because he knew from his work in comparative anatomy that it was noticeably larger in humans than animals.[9]

Although Gall gets most of the credit, he was not the first to suggest that the brain, and particularly the cerebral cortex, might not be a single organ. In the fourth century BCE, Hippocrates noted that injuries to one side of the head often resulted in weakness on the opposite side of the body, a significant insight, though one that psychologist and historian Stanley Finger cautions should be read with the understanding that physicians of the time knew almost nothing about how the brain worked. Hippocrates was less concerned with determining brain function than with elevating the status of the brain to the body's primary motor and emotional organ, a major shift from existing beliefs of a ruling heart.[10]

Several centuries after Hippocrates and nearly a century before Gall, Swede Emanuel Swedenborg suggested that different parts of the brain may control various physical and mental functions. Born in Stockholm in 1688, Swedenborg came to medicine from a background in mathematics, astronomy, and mining. He grew so entranced with decoding the mysteries of the human body that in 1736, he left his job as the director of Swedish mines to devote himself to medicine and the study of the relationship between the body and the soul. He immersed himself in his studies as a purely intellectual pursuit with no interest in actually becoming a practicing doctor. He visited medical centers in France, Italy, and the Netherlands to shadow doctors and learn about the brain and the nervous system. From these experiences, Swedenborg theorized that the brain must be broken into areas with different purposes, because how else could humans function without mixing up their senses, such as the ability to see, taste, touch, and hear? As evidence of his theory, he noted that injuries to the brain did not affect all abilities equally. A head injury could cause visual loss while not affecting the sense of smell or hearing. Swedenborg's pioneering conjectures on the brain remained largely unknown, though, overshadowed by the mystical visions he reported experiencing in the 1740s that found him communing with Christ, spirits, demons, and angels. Scientists had a hard time taking seriously the ideas and observations of someone who also claimed to see things unseen. These visions led Swedenborg to abandon medicine for theology, a course on which he never looked back, and one that inspired and influenced such people as poet William Blake, writer Ralph Waldo Emerson, and nurseryman and folk legend Johnny "Appleseed" Chapman. Swedenborg's theories on the brain were not discovered until 1868 and not translated for decades more. So Gall came to lead the movement toward the theory of a functionally divided brain.[11]

Even without the mystical issues that relegated Swedenborg to the fringe, Gall struggled for acceptance in the scientific community. Much of the criticism focused on the validity of his research methods. Gall avidly collected heads and skulls for study but quickly threw out any that didn't fit his hypotheses. Worse, he sometimes contradicted himself to include particular examples that he liked. Gall's detractors also disparaged his focus on society's extremes: criminals and the insane on one end, and the most famous and intellectually gifted writers, thinkers, and artists on the other. Gall visited prisons and asylums to observe and collect material, studying the heads of five hundred robbers and murderers and attributing their misdeeds to enlarged organs of acquisitiveness and destructiveness, as well as a small organ for love. He did not just confine his observations to humans. He also looked out for unusual animals, collecting the skulls of dogs that ate only stolen food or those that managed to navigate themselves home from great distances. Gall defended himself by claiming that the relationship between the body and brain could be more easily determined in these outlier cases. He was so sure of his belief that the cranium was an accurate cast of the brain that he stuck almost exclusively to skull shapes in making his pronouncements. By 1802, Gall had collected more than three hundred skulls from people with well-documented mental traits, ranging from the literary to the murderous.[12]

An excellent speaker and self-promoter, Gall took his theories on brains, heads, and personality on the road, lecturing widely throughout Europe in the early 1800s. His talks were something of a scientific circus. He traveled with a collection of human and animal skulls and cranial casts, as well as wax models of the brain and, for good measure if unclear reasons, two monkeys. Gall illustrated his theories with skulls and live dissections of the spinal cord where he traced the path of nerves. Though he considered himself a serious scientist, Gall availed himself of the same tricks used by patent-medicine sellers of the time, who often used music, drama, and other theatrics on their tours to attract an audience. Gall's lectures and writings made him a European celebrity.[13]

Yet it was his disciple, German physician Johann Spurzheim, who made phrenology a household word in the United States. Spurzheim first met Gall at one of his lectures in 1800, and the two began collaborating in 1804 after Spurzheim finished his medical training. Spurzheim even coined the name "phrenology" for the new science. The name combined two Greek words, *phren*, meaning mind, and *logos* for study or discourse, making phrenology literally a "discourse of the mind." Gall never called it that, however. He preferred *cranioscopy* instead because phrenology seemed to focus on the mind, where he cared most about the brain. But Gall's name never caught on, and phrenology became the popular term for it, with Spurzheim its top marketer and public face.[14]

With Spurzheim's assistance, Gall published his monumental four-volume *Anatomy and Physiology of the Nervous System in General and the Cerebrum in Particular* between 1810 and 1820. This tome detailed his entire doctrine, which was, in part, a rebuttal of criticisms made by France's Académie des Sciences. Gall and Spurzheim had hoped to win the académie's approval as a mark of their standing in the world of science, but it was not to be. The commission assigned to review his work rejected Gall's application and downplayed his ana-tomical contributions to medical science.[15]

Spurzheim and Gall soon found themselves at odds with each other, too. The disagreement over the name of their science was only a surface mark of a much deeper tension over the meaning and use of phrenology. Gall saw himself as a scientist, who defined phrenology specifically and narrowly as a science of the mind resting on dissec-tion and anatomical research. Spurzheim, on the other hand, though trained as a physician, saw himself as a philosopher and reformer. Like many of his contemporaries, Spurzheim viewed the poverty, violence, and vice that had accompanied industrialization and urban-ization with concern. He wanted to use phrenology to solve social problems and to empower individuals toward self-improvement.

Spurzheim didn't disagree with Gall's main premise that the shape of the skull reflected the development of the brain organs respon-sible for specific functions. Where he differed was in the moral value given to functions of the brain. Gall's classification of some faculties as evil did not fit with Spurzheim's evolving ideas of a basic human benevolence. He did not believe that any faculties were by necessity good or bad; it was simply an imbalance of these attributes that led to sinful words and actions. Spurzheim further argued that naming faculties after a single mode of conduct, as Gall had done, failed to en-compass all of the behaviors that each could produce. Seeking greater latitude for the kinds of activities governed by a particular attribute, Spurzheim renamed several of the functions with more neutral titles. Murder, for example, became destructiveness to illustrate the variety of manifestations violent tendencies could take. Others, like cunning, religion, and poetry, were given suffixes like "-ive" or "-ness" to suggest a range of possible outcomes. In Spurzheim's scheme, writing a poem was only one possible result of having a large organ for poetic-ness. Spurzheim also added new organs, including hope and moral sense, increasing Gall's original twenty-seven faculties to thirty-three.[16]

Perhaps more important for phrenology's growth, Spurzheim believed that people could change. It was this potential for indi-vidual betterment that intrigued him the most about phrenology. Through training and education, Spurzheim argued that people could strengthen their positive brain organs. Like weightlifting builds muscle mass, the brain was an organ to be exercised. The phrenolo-gist acted as the brain's personal trainer, advising patients on the best course of activity based on their cranial reading. Spurzheim's views starkly contrasted with those of Gall, who was less optimistic about human nature and potential for improvement. Seeing depravity all around him, Gall attributed evil acts to the very makeup of humans. He argued that traits, good or bad, were inherited and therefore somewhat fixed. Spurzheim, however, believed that phrenology offered the tools people needed to learn about themselves and to apply that knowledge to make the world a better place.[17] Here was a "practical system of mental philosophy," he claimed, that would improve the education of children, the reformation of criminals, and the treatment of the insane.[18] Eloquent and dashing, with sideburns that zigzagged down his cheeks from his upswept brown hair, Spurzheim and his message of hope, self-knowledge, and social improvement proved to be exactly what Americans wanted, and packed lecture halls greeted him on his 1832 tour of New England.

This wasn't the first time phrenology had come to the United States. American physicians John Warren, John Bell, and Charles Caldwell had learned about phrenology in Europe in the 1820s and returned home eager to spread the word. Caldwell became one of phrenology's most ardent and well-known advocates in American medicine. Known as the "American Spurzheim," he went on to write the first American book on the subject.[19] Regular doctors responded favorably to phrenology at first because they hoped that it would open up the mysteries of the mind, transforming what had long been abstract concepts into something concrete that might aid in diagnosis. But throughout the 1820s, phrenology remained primarily an academic pursuit, followed by some regular doctors but not many others outside of medicine and science. Spurzheim's lecture tour brought phrenology to the masses in the 1830s.[20]

While phrenology became very popular in Europe, it was in the United States that it found its most devoted audience. One reason phrenology attracted so many followers was that it seemed to provide the toolbox for the American dream. No matter how humble your beginning, anyone could learn about him- or herself using phrenological principles and then use that knowledge to strengthen desired qualities through personal initiative and perseverance. Phrenology affirmed core nineteenth-century American values about an individual's unlimited potential for growth and development. The prospect of consulting science for answers rather than the traditional received wisdom of religious and political leaders appealed to an American society with a strong anti-authoritarian and anti-elitist bent. People could reach their highest potential simply by paying close attention to their physical and mental attributes and those of their potential mates. Phrenology seemed to provide what the strict Calvinist religion of Puritanical America had not: a way to better what God gave you, empowering individuals to help shape their own future, and making man the master of his own mind.

Spurzheim's whirlwind lecture tour triggered phrenology's explosive growth in North America—unfortunately, it also killed him six months later, when he caught a cold and died a short time later. Spurzheim remained committed to his cause until the end, though, claiming only the desire "to live as long as I can for the good of science." Fittingly for his chosen field, Spurzheim's brain and skull became part of a phrenological collection, given first to the Boston Athenaeum and then to the Boston Phrenological Society.[21] The man who prepared Spurzheim's skull for display declared it "conspicuous, with its ideal facial angle as an example of a highly cultivated and intellectual type." Several years later, in 1840, Spurzheim's skull was joined by that of James Roberton, an admirer who asked to be displayed alongside his hero forever, a request largely honored to this day as both reside in the Warren Museum Exhibition Gallery at Harvard University.[22]

Thousands came out to watch Spurzheim's funeral procession to Boston's Mount Auburn Cemetery, including the entire medical faculty of Harvard and all of the members of the Boston Medical Association. The service included a stirring performance of "Ode to Spurzheim," composed after his sudden death by poet John Pierrepont and sung by the city's Handel and Haydn Society. "For the stores of science brought us, / For the charm thy goodness gave, / To the lessons thou has taught us, / Can we give thee but the grave?" implored one stanza.[23] That Spurzheim's funeral attracted such a wide and distinguished audience attests to the great interest and credibility given phrenology by Americans in its early days. His was hardly the funeral of someone thought a quack.

The *New England Magazine* reported soon after his death that Spurzheim had remarkable success in attracting converts to phrenology, "not only from among mere lecture-goers and literary triflers, but from the most scientific and learned in various professions: Physicians, Surgeons, and Lawyers, of great present eminence."[24] The Massachusetts Medical Association proclaimed his death "a calamity to mankind." English writer Harriet Martineau, who visited the United States the same year as Spurzheim, reported that "the great mass of Americans became phrenologists in a day." Ralph Waldo Emerson hailed him as one of the greatest minds in the world, while the *American Journal of Medical Sciences* declared, "[T]he prophet is gone."[25]

With Spurzheim's death, phrenological authority passed to Scotsman George Combe. A lawyer by training, Combe was far more interested in human psychology than legal wrangling. He had first met Spurzheim in Edinburgh in 1816, and though skeptical of phrenology at first, Combe soon found himself drawn to Spurzheim's optimistic vision of the mind. In 1820, Combe and his brother founded the Edinburgh Phrenological Society, the first of its kind in the world. Most of its members, primarily young middle-class professional men, had been converted to phrenology at the hand of Spurzheim himself.[26]

Combe simplified the scholarly theories of Gall and Spurzheim to make them more accessible to regular people. He shared many of Spurzheim's optimistic beliefs but added a few of his own in accordance with the philosophies of natural law and secular society popular in Europe. Like Spurzheim, Combe did not believe that humans were flawed by design; instead, evil resulted from violations of natural laws through either ignorance or willful disobedience. Everyone could attain happiness by living morally and personally believing in God—which put him squarely in the camp of other nineteenth-century reformers of all stripes, from temperance advocates to abolitionists. Combe also delved more deeply into physiology and used phrenology to advocate for the health of the rest of the body and its environment. He claimed that the size of the faculties wasn't the sole means of assessing mental capacity: the health and condition of the whole person had to be considered as well. Anything that reduced what he called "natural vitality"—from coffee and alcohol to tight corsets and urban living—was potentially harmful to overall health.

Combe was particularly interested in using phrenology to improve education, his interest driven in part by his own childhood. Born in 1788 and one of twelve children raised in a small house at the foot of Edinburgh Castle, Combe remembered enduring lessons that consisted solely of memorizing and translating Latin texts. Forced to sit for hours, Combe found no outlet for his childhood energy, nor did he find the mental stimulation he craved. Any restless movement drew fierce punishment. His teacher, Mr. Fraser, kept order with "The Rod of Correction," a knotted riding whip that produced brutal welts and sometimes drew blood when cracked over students' arms and legs. From these experiences, Combe came to believe that education should prepare students to become rational future citizens by nurturing their physical, moral, and intellectual capacities. Focusing on dead languages only left the child ignorant "of the constitution of the social system in which he is destined to move." How could students successfully navigate the world if all they knew were the words and texts of societies long since past? Above all, said Combe, learning should be pleasurable. The interests of students should be encouraged and classroom activities designed to dovetail with each student's natural talents and proclivities as discovered through phrenology. He suggested lessons that taught students to ask questions and to learn through discovery and hands-on investigation rather than the standard course of memorization and passive listening.[27]

Combe published his theories, philosophies, and advice for living as *The Constitution of Man* in 1828, a book not completely devoted to phrenology but one that helped to cement phrenology's association with the Protestant ethic of progress, hard work, and self-improvement. In addition to the educational applications of phrenology, Combe proposed that marriage should be based on the pairing of the best-developed brains, and that criminals should be kept in solitary confinement to break their evil thoughts and desires and replace them with new moral influences. Combe's book became a phenomenal success. More than 100,000 copies sold in the United States and Britain, and Ralph Waldo Emerson called it "the best sermon I have read for some time." It was said that only the Bible and John Bunyan's *Pilgrim's Progress* were more likely to be found on the shelves of English-speaking homes in the 1830s.[28]

By the time Combe arrived in the United States for his own lecture tour in 1838, phrenology had all but ceased to be strictly a medical science. It had instead come to resemble a social movement with its patchwork of scientific, religious, and moral components. Practitioners and followers had spread its message to the far corners of the nation. Phrenological charts began appearing in the pages of popular magazines. The Boston-based *Ladies' Magazine* published diagrams of the head from three angles along with detailed listings of each faculty, its location on the head, the qualities associated with it, and some general comments on each faculty's prevalence in the general population. Readers learned that "conscientiousness" tended to be larger in children than in adults, which the author saw as a "poor reflection" on the state of American manners.[29]

Americans from all classes of society found much to admire in phrenology. The upper classes liked it because it reassured them that the social hierarchy that placed them on top was "natural"; the emerging middle class and working classes liked it because its meritocratic message confirmed their hope of advancement through personal striving and self-improvement.[30] Phrenology seemed to provide answers for all kinds of questions, only a handful of them medical, which led to both its explosive growth and its near divorce from its purely scientific origins. Moreover, phrenology also became commercialized in the United States, in large part due to the efforts of the remarkable Fowler family.

The Fowler brothers, Lorenzo Niles and Orson Squire, turned their interest in phrenology into a substantial business based in New York City in the 1830s. The eldest brother, Orson Squire Fowler, hadn't set out to be a phrenologist. The son of a farmer and church deacon from upstate New York, Orson first pursued the ministry but found his true calling in Spurzheim's theory. He began to lecture on the topic to his classmates at Amherst College in Massachusetts and offered head readings for two cents each.[31] His enthusiasm soon infected his younger brother, Lorenzo, along with the rest of the family, including younger sister Charlotte; her husband, Samuel Wells; and Lorenzo's wife, the attractively headed Lydia Folger. After graduation, the brothers put aside their plans for a life in the church for another kind of missionary work: "Phrenologize Our Nation, for thereby it will Reform the World!"[32]

The phrenology preached by the Fowlers had a particularly American spin. Taking Combe's programs of physical and mental hygiene, the Fowlers translated phrenology into a doctrine of perfectionism, a set plan designed to create a perfect social and moral system. This idea of perfection fit the millennial ideas so common among many kinds of reformers in the nineteenth century. The Fowlers also added new faculties to Spurzheim's thirty-three, including conjugality (attachment to one's partner), vitativeness (love of life), and bibativeness (fondness for liquor), though they had to stop after a few additions because there were limits to how much the fingers could plausibly "read" on the head. The Fowlers' version of phrenology was an attempt to bring together all the strands of science capable of improving the mind or benefiting mankind, which they believed would herald a new and better world.[33] And like all true-blooded nineteenth-century American entrepreneurs, they also just happened to sell all the phrenological gear and accessories needed to make this happen.

The Fowlers aimed their commercial phrenology at regular people through their lecture tours and popular literature, promoting themselves with the ancient Greek aphorism "Know thyself." Their missionary fervor was matched by a shrewd business sense and theatrical flair. Appearing in theaters and lecture halls across the eastern United States beginning in 1834, the Fowlers explained the basics of phrenology and offered hands-on analyses of volunteers' heads. The lectures were free (though the examinations were not) and drew large crowds as well as a few celebrities.[34] Few could resist sales pitches that promised to

> point out, and show how to obviate, at least one fault, and cultivate one virtue, besides reinvigorating health—the value of which ASTOR'S MILLIONS can not equal! Shall, then, the trifling examination fee prevent what is thus INFINITELY valuable? Will you allow this to intercept your MENTAL progress, especially if just starting in life? In no other way can you even obtain for your self, at such a trifle, as much good—as great a luxury.[35]

The following year, in 1835, they set up an office in Clinton Hall, at the corner of Nassau and Beekman streets, in New York City.

After her marriage to Lorenzo Fowler in 1844, Lydia Folger began lecturing on phrenology, physiology, anatomy, and hygiene to largely female audiences. Having a female phrenologist on board was a tremendous boon to the Fowlers' business, as many women were uncomfortable attending lectures on health given by men. In 1849, when she was only twenty-seven years old, Lydia enrolled in the newly established Central Medical College of Syracuse and Rochester, New York. The curriculum of Central Medical College, an "eclectic" medical school, consisted of plant remedies, diet, and hygiene. Lydia received her medical degree a year later, only the second woman in the United States to do so (the first, Elizabeth Blackwell, graduated from New York's Geneva Medical College in 1849). In 1850 she became principal of the "female department" at her alma mater, becoming the first female professor of medicine in the United States. She also established her own medical practice in New York City, specializing in the health of women and children, while continuing to write and lecture on phrenology with her husband.[36]

Many women practiced phrenology, though fewer became recognized leaders like Lydia than in other forms of irregular medicine. In part, this was because phrenology lacked organizational structure and cohesion. There was no national phrenological association, and most patients had a one-time encounter with a phrenologist rather than an ongoing relationship. Phrenology was largely an individual pursuit. Most phrenologists supported women's rights, adopting the phrenological view of women as full human beings endowed with human potential. Many phrenologists used the science to argue for the mental equality of the sexes while others found evidence of particular strength in faculties traditionally associated with women like morality, benevolence, and religiosity. Female phrenologists like Lydia and Charlotte Fowler examined and lectured before audiences of women almost exclusively. The same was true in nearly all medical fields, regular or irregular, as modesty and social propriety tended to keep women and men separated, particularly in matters of the human body. But while it was rare for a woman phrenologist to give a head reading to a man, female patients could and did receive readings from practitioners of either sex.[37]

In 1838, the Fowlers began publishing the *American Phrenological Journal*, which quickly became one of the most widely read magazines in the nation and remained in circulation until 1911. They also published a library's worth of inexpensive books on health and reform topics. These publications advised readers on the best daily regimens of diet, work, and play for proper mental functioning. Others, many penned by Lydia, offered advice on marriage and on conceiving and raising children. By the mid-nineteenth century, the Fowlers' publications could be found all over the country, and phrenological ideas had become a part of everyday conversation.

The Fowlers' New York City offices, known as the Phrenological

Cabinet, became one of the most visited places in town. Combining the attractions and oddities of P. T. Barnum's American Museum, a carnival sideshow, and a scientific curiosity cabinet, the museum easily provided visitors a full day of entertainment. Busts, mummies, and paintings from around the world covered the walls and filled display cases. Visitors could look at the heads of murderers and pirates, as well as those of famous leaders like President John Quincy Adams and Julius Caesar. The Fowlers also had casts made from George Combe's extensive skull collection. The busts were particularly important, being one of the chief tools of the phrenologists' trade. The Fowlers also instructed others how to make their own head casts, though they recommended that followers first practice on an apple to get the hang of it before attempting a human head.[38] These busts provided a road map of the head, demarcating all of the organs of the mind with clearly marked boundaries on a smooth-crowned model of the skull.[39]

Visitors could test their ability to judge character by viewing the collection that represented "racial types," skulls of people from different races, and "persons of eminence in talent and virtue, and . . . those who were notorious for crime."[40] The idea that a man's character could be read led some to attempt to make determinations of the moral, intellectual, and social development of different human races based on the shape of their heads and jaws. After Charles Darwin popularized the idea that humans descended from apes, some saw different facial features like the protruding jaw and sloped forehead as signs of lower development and thus a closer relationship to primitive man, which became the basis of racial stereotyping. Classes were offered to teach phrenology to anyone who wanted to learn. The youngest Fowler, Charlotte, taught classes geared specifically toward women. Since admission was free, visitors came in hordes.[41]

Tourists could take a piece of their visit to the Phrenological Cabinet home with a stroll through the museum's extensive gift shop. The Fowlers offered a set of seventy phrenological watercolors for thirty-five cents and phrenological busts, the particular specialty of Lorenzo, for sale as souvenirs. These "high quality" busts, "showing the exact location of all the Organs of the Brain," sold for $1.25 and could be sent by freight or express for those who couldn't make the trip to New York.[42] Lorenzo's original design can still be found for sale in novelty stores today.

As with many other irregulars, phrenology wasn't the Fowlers' only interest, and their office became a meeting place for all kinds of reformers. This wasn't surprising, as the idea of perfectibility that imbued phrenology could also be found in the rhetoric of other popular social reform movements. The Fowlers championed vegetarianism, mesmerism, temperance, and even architectural reform. Of architecture, Orson Fowler believed that octagonal houses, in particular, were more healthful because the eight walls formed wider angles than the typical ninety degrees, allowing for the freer circulation of fresh air. The cost and space efficiency of the design also made the houses accessible to the rich and poor alike. Lydia Fowler and her sister-in-law Charlotte also campaigned for women's rights out of their offices, seeing phrenology as scientific evidence of women's equal mental capacity and thus their ability to work, vote, and certainly lead. "Reform, *Reform*, REFORM, is emphatically the watchword of the age," declared Orson Fowler.[43]

In the early 1840s, the Fowlers attacked the inadequacies of the American educational system, particularly condemning the lack of rights afforded to children. Of course, one of the rights that the Fowlers believed all children should be entitled to was that of having a phrenologically based education on the model first proposed by Combe. It must have thrilled them to read that noted school reformer Horace Mann proclaimed himself "more indebted to Phrenology than to all the metaphysical works I ever read."[44] Mann had been greatly influenced by Combe's theories. He adopted *The Constitution of Man* as a text for the normal schools of Massachusetts, and even named his son George Combe Mann for his phrenological hero. The Fowlers only hoped that other educators would prove so enlightened.[45]

Although they became the most well known, the Fowlers weren't the only ones selling and promoting phrenology in the United States. By the late 1830s, itinerant phrenologists crisscrossed the country giving head exams and handing out periodicals and other information. More than twenty thousand traveling phrenologists plied their trade throughout the nineteenth century, many using it as a first step out of their childhood home and into adulthood. Reading heads gave young men a way to get off the farm and make a good living before settling down and marrying.[46] There was probably not a community in the nation that did not entertain at least one visit from an itinerant phrenologist. These traveling phrenologists also benefited from the demonstrative nature of examining heads. Americans did not just want to read about scientific advances, but to engage with science directly. Phrenology offered that chance and made Americans head-conscious in a way they had never been before.

Phrenologists often took head readings using a device called a craniometer. Gall had invented the device based on his knowledge of the anatomy of the brain. He believed that the ridges of the brain gathered behind the ears and radiated outward, so he created a tool that rested in the ears like the points of a compass. Rotating the device over the skull, a phrenologist could measure the size of each organ using the phrenological chart as a starting place.[47] Do-it-yourself guides offered instruction and tips for finding each organ. Draw a line from "the outer angle of the eye, to the top of the ears, and extend it straight backward an inch and a half to an inch and three quarters, and you are on Combativeness," counseled *The Illustrated Self-Instructor in Phrenology and Physiology*. "This organ starts about midway to the back part of the ears, and runs upward and backward toward the crown of the head. To ascertain its relative size, steady the head with one hand, say the left, and place the balls of your right fingers upon the point just specified letting your elbow be somewhat below the subject's head, which will bring your fingers directly across the organ." Once in the right position, the phrenologist felt for the fullness and sharpness of the organ.[48] Skilled phrenologists—as well as those out to make a quick buck—could complete readings in about thirty minutes.

Head readings tended to be flattering, or at least so vague as to not be insulting, since bad feelings could hurt repeat business. Readings tended to shore up prevailing attitudes and reflected contemporary beliefs about the appropriate roles of men and women. Women's skulls usually exhibited strong parental feelings and large organs of "Benevolence" and "Inhabitiveness," just the areas needed to keep women at home with the kids.[49] As William James noted in his *Principles of Psychology* in the late nineteenth century, "Phrenology hardly does more than restate the problem. . . . To answer the question, 'Why do I like children?' by saying, 'Because you have a large organ of philoprogenitiveness,' but renames the phenomenon to be explained."[50] Nevertheless, confirmation was what many people wanted, and it brought crowds of supporters to the phrenologist's doors.

Many of these itinerant phrenologists were eminently practical, recognizing the value of providing actionable, concrete advice. This kind of counsel was in great demand as America became a nation of increasing geographic and social mobility. It was also quite a different tack than that taken by Spurzheim and Combe, who were far more theoretically oriented and had little to offer people looking for tangible answers to life's basic questions. Practical phrenologists, on the other hand, functioned more like psychics, determining career aptitudes or marriage prospects with declarative prognostication. Unlike psychics, though, phrenologists appeared to have science on their side, a considerable attraction in post-Enlightenment nineteenth-century America.[51]

The Fowlers, too, were highly practical in their phrenology, offering what they called vocational guidance and employment counseling. They were so successful at it that some employers required job applicants to bring a recommendation of their abilities from the Fowlers. For those in search of a calling, the Fowlers had a list of "developments" that would lead to success in particular careers, almost like a career aptitude test, but one that measured your head rather than your demonstrable skills. Lawyers, for instance, required a large area of "Eventuality" to recall cases, while the perceptive faculties should dominate the medical profession. The mechanic needed a sizable zone of "Constructiveness." For those wanting to follow in the Fowlers' footsteps, a good phrenologist needed a "first-rate head" marked by good perception, an excellent memory, strong "Comparison and Human Nature," "Constructiveness," and "Ideality."[52] Once people knew what line of work they wished to pursue, they needed only to cultivate the faculties necessary for success in that particular calling.

Phrenology could work against employment as well. In 1867, the New York Times reported that a Montreal postmaster had fired several employees after a phrenologist found them deficient in skills he deemed essential to the job. "The moral and intellectual bumps were found deficient, so much so that it was impossible to retain those gentleman any longer as public servants," claimed the phrenologically devoted postmaster.[53] Heads did not lie. Unless, of course, they did. A decade earlier, Godey's Lady's Book, the most popular and highest-circulation women's magazine of the nineteenth century, proclaimed that women had an advantage over men in potentially deceiving the phrenologist. All they had to do was adjust their hair. "Upon most of the betraying prominences, complete disguise may be put, and those which are creditable and beautiful may be greatly thrown into relief, heightened and made to tell upon expression. An inch forward or backward in the placing the knot of the hair, gives the head (the most common observer sees, without knowing why) a very different character," stated the author. A woman could "make her head show, phrenologically, for pretty much what she pleases."[54]

Work wasn't the only area for which the Fowlers offered advice: they also counseled on love. The Fowlers declared that love, like all areas of life, was governed by exact scientific rules; you needed only to consult a phrenologist to learn how to apply them. Using guidelines dictated by temperament and phrenological development, the Fowlers created charts that would help clients choose "congenial companions for life." Generally, their advice was straightforward and not unlike that found in modern advice columns. Persons of the same temperament, especially if on the extreme end of that temperament, should not be married. The same held true for those of opposite temperaments. Instead, people should aim to find mates with compatible and complementary traits. "Suppose your very large Benevolence fastens upon *doing good* as your highest duty," wrote Orson Fowler, "how can your feelings in other respects harmonize with a selfish companion, whose god is gain, and who turns coldly from suffering humanity, refusing to bestow charity, and contending with you for casting in your mite." Some of their advice was less predictable, though. Those with "bright red hair should marry jet black" and the curly haired should never marry another with curly hair, the style and coloring of hair presumably indicating character traits that would clash.[55] *Godey's Lady's Book* declared phrenology would do away "with all doubt and misgiving" in love as potential mates could now "woo by the book."[56]

Countless public figures had their heads examined by the Fowlers, whether out of curiosity, hope, or belief, and the results were often published in the Fowlers' *American Phrenological Journal*. Showman P. T. Barnum, abolitionist John Brown, newspaperman Horace Greeley, future president James Garfield, and poet Walt Whitman all offered their heads for examination. Statesman Daniel Webster received the flattering report that his skull was to ordinary heads "what the great dome of St. Peter's is to the small cupolas at its side."[57] Women's rights advocate Susan B. Anthony was, at first, rather obliquely described as "an original character" but the reading went on to praise her: "those who look for a passive and submissive spirit will not find it here; but they will find a brave, resolute, vigorous, and willing worker." Clara Barton, the founder of the American Red Cross, was said to have picked her career based on a reading by Lorenzo Fowler. He examined her head in the mid-1830s and advised her mother to "throw responsibility" upon the then-fifteen-year-old Barton, for she had the mind of a great teacher.[58] Lorenzo also read the head of the then-unknown Allan Pinkerton and declared he "would make a capital detective; he would smell a rogue three miles [away]." Pinkerton later went on to found the Pinkerton National Detective Agency, which became one of the most famous agencies of its kind, in part for foiling an assassination attempt against President Lincoln in 1861.[59] Legend has it that President Ulysses S. Grant also chose his military career based on a head reading.[60]

Phrenological ideas traveled far and wide and through every profession in the United States, including politics. After an 1842 visit to Washington, DC, writer Charles Dickens reported that he was asked his impression of the nation's political heads. They didn't mean "their chiefs and leaders," wrote Dickens in wonderment, "but literally their individual and personal heads, whereon their hair grew, and whereby the phrenological character of each legislator was expressed."[61] Phrenology offered politicians a powerful means to affirm the quality of their character or, in other instances, to redeem reputations gone awry. After Vice President Andrew Johnson gave a drunken speech to the Senate at President Lincoln's inauguration in March of 1865 (suffering from typhoid fever, Johnson consumed several glasses of whiskey to give him strength before the event), Johnson had been dogged by accusations that he was a drunkard and unfit for political office. In 1866, the *New York Times* published a profile of Johnson that included his phrenology. He's "a man of warm impulses, indomitable will and courage, upright and philosophical, patriotic," and most important of all, "strictly temperate." The writer concluded that the rumors of Johnson's drinking habits could not possibly be true based on his healthy appearance and upstanding head bumps.[62]

Writers seized on phrenology as a creative decoder for revealing knowledge about themselves and their characters. Phrenology as psychology was taken seriously and permeated the literature and novels of the day. Louisa May Alcott, William Cullen Bryant, Stephen Crane, William Dean Howells, Henry Wadsworth Longfellow, and James Russell Lowell were among the many writers to submit to phrenological exams to understand themselves better. Other writers incorporated phrenology into their stories. Edgar Allan Poe used phrenology as a tool to analyze human nature in short stories such as "The Imp of the Perverse," "The Business Man," and "The Fall of the House of Usher." In a short story titled "A.D. 3000," by an unnamed author in *Harper's New Monthly Magazine*, a Rip Van Winkle-esque man awakes to find himself in a future where a State Phrenological Commission examines the heads of fifteen-month-old babies to determine their future vocation. On leaving the room, "each infant has a ticket pasted on its person, bearing the name of the trade or profession to which it is destined."[63] Even the white whale in *Moby Dick* cannot escape having his head read, or, more accurately, his spine, since his brain is too small to be "adequately charted." A thorough reading of the facial bumps and vertebrae of the whale leads Ishmael to aptly conclude that the whale has an unusually large "organ of firmness or indomitableness." Melville also compares Queequeg's head favorably with that of George Washington, though Queequeg "was George Washington cannibalistically developed."[64] Phrenology also made frequent appearances both serious and satirical in the Editor's Drawer column of *Harper's*.

Among the countless books, pamphlets, and other written material churned out by the Fowlers was the debut work of Walt Whitman, *Leaves of Grass*. Whitman published the first edition himself, but the Fowlers' office was one of only two retail outlets for the book. The second edition came out under the Fowlers' publishing imprint. Whitman had first developed a strong interest in the field in 1846, reading and commenting on phrenological articles in newspapers and journals and writing positive reviews of phrenological manuals. In 1849, Whitman received what he considered a highly favorable reading from Lorenzo Fowler. The analysis described a man who chooses to "fight with tongue and pen rather than with your fist," who was "too open at times," and without "enough restraint in speech." "You are independent, not wishing to be a slave yourself or to enslave others," dictated Lorenzo. "You have your own opinions and think for your-self." Whitman was a man who could "compare. illustrate. discrimi-nate. and criticize with much ability."[65] The picture of the future poet, or "Printer" as Lorenzo noted of his occupation, was just what Whit-man hoped to see in himself, an aspiring, individualistic poet. He credited phrenology with giving him the conceptual basis for *Leaves of Grass*, claiming to have used "phrenological methods for the interpre-tation of character" as he wrote. Many of his poems exemplified phre-nological principles of individualism, optimism, self-improvement, and worship of the body. His many references to facial features, in-cluding his own, indicated the importance he placed on physiognomy as both a guide to living and an artistic source. He wrote honestly on taboo topics, including sex, because he shared the Fowlers' faith in the aphorism "know thyself" and their belief that any fear could be overcome through open discussion. Whitman's understanding of phrenology shaped his thinking on a variety of reform subjects, in-cluding education, women's rights, religion, and health. Believing, like the Fowlers, that a healthy body housed a healthy soul, he thought that perfection was attainable when the two merged on equal terms. Whitman quoted sections of his reading—"large hope and compari-son"—time and again in his writings and published his phrenological chart in at least five publications, as if seeking to prove to readers that he was living up to his phrenological potential.[66]

The national obsession with head size and shape also infected daily conversation. Many modern phrases trace their roots to phrenology, including "highbrow" and "lowbrow," "well rounded," and "shrink" (as in "shrinking" certain undesirable qualities). "Getting your head exam-ined" also has phrenological roots. Though generally considered an insult today, in the past, it was just what most people wanted.[67]

Phrenology had its skeptics, of course, and not least among them was Mark Twain. Twain's mock horror at the "humorless" hole found in his head by Lorenzo Fowler was but one example of the phreno-logical terms and concepts he wove into his stories. In a somewhat malicious character sketch of an acquaintance known as "Jul'us Cae-sar," Twain writes that he "was a phrenological curiosity: his head was one vast lump of Approbativeness [vanity]; and though he was as ig-norant and as void of intellect as a Hottentot, yet the great leveler and equalizer, Self Conceit, made him believe himself fully talented, learned and handsome as it is possible for a human being to be."[68] But

Twain took phrenology more seriously in his own life, investigating its claims of character detection and psychological guidance and continually submitting to head exams.[69]

For some, though, Twain's humorous skepticism did not go far enough. From its earliest days in Europe, phrenology faced plenty of criticism, mostly from doctors, scientists, religious leaders, and politicians. The Austrian government ordered Gall to stop lecturing in 1801 for fear that his talks would cause people to "lose their heads" and become materialists, believing only in the truths written on their skulls rather than those of God. Gall soon fled Vienna for France, but there, too, he faced a backlash that threatened his credibility. French scientist Marie-Jean-Pierre Flourens became one of Gall's most powerful adversaries. Flourens systematically tested Gall's theories on animals, removing portions of the brains of dogs, rabbits, and birds to examine how the remaining sections functioned. His experiments led him to conclude that Gall was wrong, that the brain acted as a whole unit and not as discrete parts. Damage to one area caused other parts to take over and perform the same function. He published his findings in two explosive exposés. The battle over the truth of phrenology didn't just occur in the lab. Flourens also tried to paint Gall as a crazed lunatic so driven to collect skulls that "every body in Vienna was trembling for his head, and fearing that after his death it would be put in requisition to enrich Dr. Gall's cabinet."[70]

The backlash wasn't just confined to Europe. In Washington, DC, Professor Thomas Sewell rejected phrenology as a method for understanding the brain. He argued that brain injuries rarely affected bodily function in the way predicted by phrenology. Moreover, Sewell argued that the brain couldn't possibly be measured from the skull alone. Oliver Wendell Holmes took a similar line of criticism, though in typical Holmes form, it was far more snappy and clever than the others. He compared the skull to a safe that enclosed contents—the brain—unknowable from the outside:

> The walls of the head are double, with a great air-chamber
> between them, over the smallest and most closely crowded
> "organs." Can you tell how much money there is in a safe, which
> also has thick double walls, by kneading its knobs with your
> fingers? So when a man fumbles about my forehead, and talks
> about the organs of Individuality, Size, etc., I trust him as much

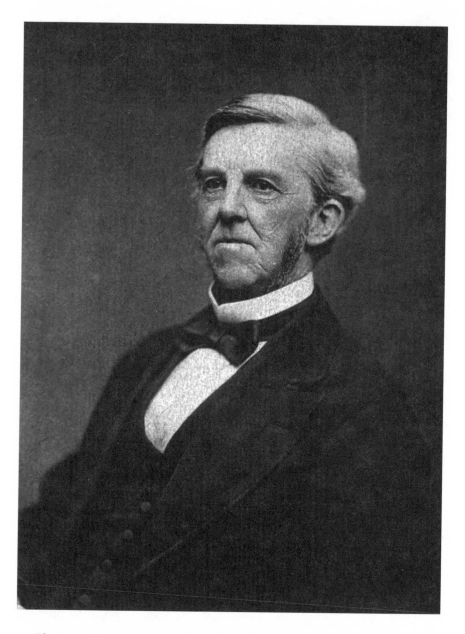

Physician Oliver Wendell Holmes was critical of
all irregular health systems, including homeopathy
and phrenology. (National Library of Medicine)

as I should if he felt the outside of my strongbox and told me that there was a five-dollar or a ten-dollar bill under this or that particular rivet.[71]

Holmes did not state outright that phrenology was wrong, but rather that there was no way to prove that it was right either, which made its status as a true science questionable.

Phrenology also floundered as a viable academic pursuit. The *American Journal of Phrenology* flopped as a magazine for professional phrenological researchers soon after it began. Many American doctors who had once praised phrenology denied ever having supported it when it became equated with other laughable "sciences" like astrology, Thomsonism, and palmistry in the late 1840s and 1850s. It didn't help phrenology's reputation that the Fowlers, no matter how much they claimed to truly believe in the science, had created a highly profitable venture for themselves. Their museum, promotional campaigns, and product line made them appear no different than those hawking mystical potions in the eyes of many regular doctors. American doctors Warren, Bell, and Caldwell, who had eagerly brought news of phrenology home with them from Europe in the 1820s, died with no mention of phrenology in their obituaries, even though Caldwell had written a landmark book on the subject. Phrenology had clearly passed beyond medical respectability by the mid-nineteenth century, dismissed entirely by many of its early proponents.[72]

The Fowlers' popularity invited special abuse from scientists, ministers, and even other phrenologists angling for business. By the 1840s, they were labeled quacks and their business denigrated as a humbug. Rival phrenologists often advertised themselves as superior to the Fowlers, while one took to impersonating Lorenzo and called himself L. N. Fowler. Orson Fowler fought back, especially against those practitioners whom he believed tainted the field by using phrenology as a swindle. The Fowlers never claimed to be doctors or scientists, only reformers who truly believed in their cause and its benefits to humanity.[73]

Even as phrenology fell out of favor in academic circles in the 1840s, it remained wildly popular and influential in American culture until late in the nineteenth century. More than perhaps any other nineteenth-century medical alternative, phrenology came to be about far more than just health and disease. In the absence of clear proof of how the brain really functioned, phrenology's detractors struggled to expel it from the realm of science. It was much easier to say something was a legitimate science, as phrenology's proponents did, than to prove it was not. Phrenologists cited Isaac Newton, Galileo, and William Harvey as examples of scientists who challenged common ways of thinking and were rebuked in their own time before finding wide acceptance. Phrenologists urged people to observe and decide for themselves the truth of phrenology, and to not simply accept uncritically what they were told. That anyone could learn to do phrenology meant that anyone could also decide what was true or not true about it. The openness of phrenology's vision and practice proved vital to its spread and staying power. Popular attention only began to shift away from phrenology as other health movements rose to prominence and as new scientific discoveries captured the American imagination in the 1850s and 1860s.[74]

By the twentieth century, phrenology had mostly lost its scientific authority and much of its popular appeal. A few diehards, among them the children and grandchildren of the Fowlers, still practiced. The progress of medical science offered new and better tools for understanding the brain. To many Americans, phrenology now seemed old-fashioned and ridiculous.

That's not to say that the phrenologists hadn't gotten some things right. Gall placed the brain at the center of all cognitive and emotional functions at a time when some physicians still located some of the "passions" elsewhere, such as the heart and liver. Although he wasn't the first to suggest it, Gall made the brain the foundation of his system, which brought increased attention to the theory.

Gall based his conjectures on his expert anatomical observations. From his work in comparative anatomy, Gall knew that the nervous systems in many lower animals consisted essentially of a spinal cord without much of a brain. More sophisticated animals, however, had larger, more developed brains, particularly the cerebral cortex. From these observations, Gall suggested that the cortex must be the highest-functioning part of the nervous system and that more sophisticated animals developed larger brains. This view of the nervous system was relatively new at the time, as most contemporary anatomists thought of the spinal cord as simply the "tail" of the brain. Gall also suggested functional differences between gray and white matter in the brain and described a host of features of the cranial nerves, concepts foundational to modern neuroscience.[75]

Gall's fundamental idea of a brain composed of faculties with different specializations ultimately proved correct, though the direction in which phrenology went with this insight was not. Gall was the first to make the strong case for the possibility of brain function emerging from spatial organization. Although Flourens's findings and smear campaign worked to marginalize Gall in scientific circles, localization resurfaced again and again throughout the nineteenth century. In 1861, French surgeon and anthropologist Paul Broca showed that damage to one area of the brain can make a person unable to speak coherently without affecting the ability to understand others. His findings seemed to vindicate the brain localization idea behind phrenology, but because phrenology had fallen into such disrepute, Broca was careful to draw distinctions between his work and Gall's. Holding phrenology at arm's length, Broca described his own theory of cortical localization in the part of the brain that came to be called "Broca's area" as different from the cranial localization of Gall. It seems fair to think of Gall as a visionary with the right idea but faulty logic and a flawed methodology. His chief antagonist, Flourens, on the other hand, used a more scientific method to test phrenology but reached the wrong conclusion. Later in the nineteenth century, British neurologist David Ferrier created maps of the motor and sensory functions in the cerebral cortex that owed a clear debt to phrenology.[76] More recently, in 2002, scientists in the Brain Mapping Division at the University of California, Los Angeles, announced the creation of a "large-scale computational brain atlas" to "visualize" brain structure and function, and to store "information on individual variations in the brain structure and their inheritability." Gall could have made a similar announcement two centuries earlier, though with far more primitive tools.[77]

The nineteenth-century fascination with the brain isn't all that far removed from our modern obsession with the mind. We have once again elevated the brain to cultish status, celebrating and perhaps even aggrandizing its power and purpose to shape the world. Everything and every field now seems to have a "neuro" component, from neuromarketing to neuroeconomics, a transmutation of language strikingly similar to that which occurred in the nineteenth century as phrenological terms passed from the laboratory to daily conversation. Brain science often seems less a hard science than a means of fortune-telling. Colorful and detailed PET and fMRI images of the brain appear in magazines and newspapers, on television and online, encouraging us to think of almost everything through its effect on the brain. These images have become the modern equivalent of the phrenological charts that adorned the walls of pharmacies and general stores and were featured in the pages of magazines and books. Many of us continue to hope, as the phrenologists did, that mapping the brain will reveal the secrets of human nature that, once known, will allow for its manipulation and transformation, and ultimately for personal improvement. Popular neuroscience seems to suggest that concentrated efforts to improve the brain will make us smarter, faster, and more efficient, and maybe even lead to perfection. Headlines and book titles like *Super Brain Power, Brainfit, Use Your Brain to Change Your Age, Coaching with the Brain in Mind*, and *Rewire Your Brain for Love* scream that the key to life—a better job, better health, better love, better children, better looks—is the brain, no matter the improvement sought and regardless of how little we actually know about how the brain works. It's the phrenology of the twenty-first century, and Americans are as ravenous for it today as they were in the nineteenth century.[78]

The Fowlers remained dedicated to phrenology for the rest of their lives, and continued to live colorful lives despite phrenology's declining status. Orson Fowler continued to offer phrenological exams but left the family business in the 1850s to concentrate on publishing and on promoting radical reforms in the areas of marriage, parenting, and sex. His publications on sex shattered his reputation in the straitlaced Victorian era, and he died in relative obscurity in 1887. Lorenzo and Lydia Fowler moved to England in 1863 and opened a branch of their firm on London's Fleet Street, near Ludgate Circus, bringing phrenology back to the home country of their mentor, George Combe. The Fowler Phrenological Institute flourished abroad, offering classes on phrenology, displaying casts and busts, and selling publications. Their lectures led to the creation of new phrenological societies just like those that tours by Spurzheim and Combe had inspired decades earlier. Lorenzo founded the British Phrenological Society, the last organization to form in the movement, in 1886, and it continued to meet and promote phrenological ideas, with only limited interruptions, until 1967.[79] Never ones to stand on the sidelines, the Fowlers also advocated for other forms of healing, entranced by the ever-flowing stream of exciting new medical theories. In the late 1840s, they added the official periodical of hydropathy, the *Water-Cure Journal*, to their stable of publications. They believed that hydropathy was destined to "not only surpass, but to swallow up or *wash away*, every other medical system now existing among men," releasing humanity from its dependence on the "drugopathic system."[80]

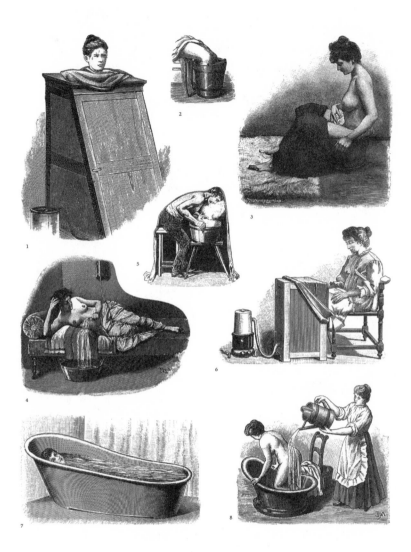

The water cure advised patients to take water in a variety of ways, from steam baths and full tubs to showers and foot and sitz baths. Each application served a specific purpose in the hydropathic regimen and was specially prescribed depending on the patient's particular ailment and her ability to endure treatment. (*Anatomical and Medical Illustrations*, ed. Jim Harter, Dover Publications, 1991)

CHAPTER THREE

Quenching Thirst, Healing Pain
Hydropathy

Announcing the November 1850 birth of his daughter in the pages of the *Water-Cure Journal*, Thomas Nichols declared that childbirth could be both easy and nearly pain free for women. His wasn't the smug and unknowing opinion of a man standing idly by while his wife labored for hours in another room. His wife, in fact, fully agreed with him.

Mary Gove Nichols achieved her miraculous birth with a strict daily regimen. She avoided alcohol, caffeine, dirt, and all medicines. She exercised regularly, ate healthy foods, wore comfortable clothes, and took daily baths in cold water—and it hadn't worked just for her. As a midwife to others, Mary described the pain experienced by women under her care as "slight" and not the "pangs worse than those of death" experienced by most women. Throughout her own pregnancy, Mary published reams of advice on how to achieve pain-free childbirth that were hardly a guarantee, much less a panacea, despite her devotion.

Mary's secret was hydropathy, a system of healing that relied on the power of cold, pure water. Both husband and wife knew that water produced healthy pregnancies from Mary's own experience. She'd suffered the agony of four successive stillbirths before submitting to its rigorous but healthful routine. The efficacy of the water cure for pregnancy and childbirth "comes so near the miraculous, that I hardly expect to be believed," wrote Thomas.[1] But believe people did, especially since the advice came from the Nicholses, who went on to become two of the most influential and authoritative advocates of hydropathy in the nation.

Today, when it seems that most Americans carry a water bottle to drink their eight daily glasses, the importance of water to health seems obvious. But for hydropaths, water was more than just a sugar- and calorie-free drink: it was a social good able to cure nearly every disease as well as the social and cultural ills that threatened the health and stability of society. Drinking was not the only way to enjoy wa- ter's munificence, though; water was also to be experienced through elaborate rituals of bathing, showering, soaking, sweating, and wrap- ping. This diversity of baths, not to mention the idea of bathing itself, was highly unusual for most Americans. In 1835, a letter from a reader in the *Boston Moral Reformer* asked, "I have been in the habit during the past winter of taking a warm bath every three weeks. Is this too often to follow the year round?"[2] Hydropathy was not a medical sys- tem in the traditional sense of a doctor administering treatment to a sick patient. Instead, it functioned more as a water-based lifestyle plan with a vision of radically transforming the world through personal health achieved through nature's purest substance.

Hydropathy grew out of the observations and experiments of Vincent Priessnitz. A peasant born in 1799 on a farm in Silesian Austria, located in today's Czech Republic, Priessnitz noticed as a child how cold-water compresses could ease the pain of sprains and bruises. Water's potential as a cure-all revealed itself to him after an 1816 farm accident. One day while he was baling hay, a runaway horse and wagon trampled the teenaged Priessnitz, leaving him with several broken ribs and a bruised left arm. The doctor from a nearby town told him that the severity of his injuries made it unlikely he'd ever work again. Priessnitz, however, refused to accept this prognosis.[3]

Priessnitz began testing the power of water to ease what drugs and heroic therapies could not. He wrapped himself in wet cloths and ate very little while consuming large quantities of cold water. To reset his broken ribs, he pressed his abdomen against a chair and in- haled deeply, allowing the expansion of his chest to push his ribs back into place. Priessnitz eventually recovered from his injuries, and the success of his self-cure led him to broaden his investigation into the curing power of water. Similar to those of his irregular healing breth- ren, his story of discovery became an integral part of his developing system, a "personal revelation" about the failure of regular medicine and an awakening to the possibilities of a cold-water cure.[4]

As word of Priessnitz's success spread throughout his village, others came seeking his council. Priessnitz treated people with water internally and externally. He soon gained a notable reputation for his achievements. To care for all who came to him for help, Priessnitz opened the Grafenberg Water Cure, sometimes referred to as "Water University," in the mountains of Silesia in 1826. By 1829, he had perfected his method of water-based healing.[5]

Priessnitz treated patients with water in three ways: externally, by bath or shower; locally on certain parts of the body, through washing and soaking; and internally, through drinking or enemas. Nearly as important as the water, he stressed the importance of the doctor-patient relationship, and how clear communication and human touch contributed to wellness.

It's not clear if Priessnitz actually understood how his system worked. He made hazy reference to cold water's ability to relieve inflammation and to restore healthy fluids lost by disease. But mostly he fell back on perhaps the most intuitive and basic explanation for its efficacy based on his observations: water dissolved disease particles and carried them to the skin, where they could be washed away. Priessnitz believed that sickness resulted from some kind of contamination in the body that he called morbid matter, an idea common among both regular and irregular medical practitioners. Bleeding, vomiting, and drugging, the tools regular medicine used to eliminate disease, only weakened the body and ruined its natural systems, argued Priessnitz.[6] The process of expelling disease in his system caused a "crisis" in the body that produced visible results such as boils, rashes, diarrhea, sores, and sweating. All were signs that the treatment was working. Priessnitz prescribed cold baths, cold showers, cold compresses, and wet bandaging or blanketing to cleanse and open the pores, aid circulation, and invigorate the skin as it drew putrid matter out of the body. As if that wasn't enough water, he also ordered patients to drink a minimum of ten to twelve glasses of cold water per day. Taking Priessnitz perhaps a bit too literally, English doctor James Wilson claimed to have drunk thirty glasses of water before breakfast each day of the eight months he spent at Grafenberg.[7] He also took nearly one thousand baths and spent 480 combined hours wrapped in wet sheets during his stay.[8]

The idea of therapeutic bathing wasn't new. Humans have soaked in communal baths and natural mineral springs since antiquity. The ancient Romans, for instance, took bathing to elaborate heights, constructing ornate baths near mineral springs where the wealthy could "take the waters" while also indulging in other pleasures of the flesh. The Japanese have enjoyed hot springs known as *onsen* for at least a thousand years, and many European explorers noted the bathing rituals and sweat lodges used by some Native Americans in North America. Most of these early bathing practitioners did not attribute the health benefits to the water itself. Instead, the water was thought to have mystical qualities or to contain spirits released by the action of the water. Hydropaths, in contrast, viewed water as the cure in and of itself.[9]

Priessnitz's method also differed from the spa therapy that had accompanied regular medicine in Europe for centuries. Most noticeably, the waters at Grafenberg had no particular chemical distinction, unlike the famous spas of Bath in England and Karlsbad in Germany, where patients soaked in warm springs and drank the mineral waters. At these spas, water was administered in only two forms—drinking or dipping—and it was always warm and never cold. Regular physicians recommended spa therapy for only a small number of conditions, including rheumatism, gout, and bladder stones. Even at its height in the seventeenth and eighteenth centuries, spa therapy comprised only a tiny fraction of a doctor's regular practice, and water was never the sole therapeutic agent; water was simply one part of a treatment plan that usually involved the more common heroic therapies of bleeding and purging. Perhaps the biggest difference between spa therapy and hydropathy, though, was the atmosphere. Many people were drawn to the therapies at Bath Spa in England not for medical purposes but to enjoy the dancing, drinking, gambling, and seducing that occurred in and around these popular watering holes. Hydropathy, in contrast, focused almost exclusively on healthful activities, and its patients tended toward the earnest and somber. Merriment and debauchery would only distract them from their goal: the perfection of humanity through individual health.[10]

The medical benefits of cold water were not unknown to regular doctors. Despite the popularity of spas, many physicians criticized the value of warm mineral springs for fighting disease, not to mention the unhygienic conditions that existed inside many of the bathhouses.

These critiques led to countless books on the curative powers of cold water in the eighteenth century with titles like *Psychrolusia, or History of Cold-Bathing; The Curiosities of Cold Water;* and *An Essay on the External Use of Water.*[11] John Wesley's popular eighteenth-century medical manual, *Primitive Physick: Or, an Easy and Natural Method of Curing Most Diseases*, asserted that cold water could cure nearly every disease if properly administered.[12] These ideas were common in the United States, too. Benjamin Rush advocated the use of cold bathing to "wash off impurities from the skin."[13] Even with this attention to the medical benefits of water, cold water played only a small therapeutic role until Priessnitz popularized it as the one and only cure to all disease.

Washing disease away wasn't Priessnitz's only concern, however; he also sought to deny it entry into the body through a healthy lifestyle of diet and exercise. Hydropathy emphasized hygiene and healthy lifestyle choices far more than regular medicine and even more than other irregulars. Priessnitz argued that filth and poor diet gave disease easy access into the body. In *The Hydropathic Encyclopedia*, American hydropath Dr. Russell Trall explained that disease was "produced by bad air, improper light, impure food and drink, excessive or defective alimentation, indolence or over-exertion, [or] unregulated passion." For Trall, it all boiled down to "unphysiological voluntary habits."[14] In other words, sickness resulted from laziness, a lack of exercise, and junk food, the familiar chords of obesity debates to this day.

Believing hot food, like hot water, dangerous, Priessnitz recommended cold foods at mealtimes and a diet free from stimulants such as alcohol, coffee, and tea. He also took the flavor out of most meals by outlawing mustard, pepper, and most spices. Hydropathic food tended toward the coarse and heavy for a sound and fibrous internal cleansing. Priessnitz explained that the way to strengthen a "weakened stomach is to avoid all the causes that have contributed towards destroying its tone."[15]

Priessnitz also prescribed large amounts of exercise throughout the day. Working out, particularly after cold baths, helped to "stimulate the proper therapeutic reaction."[16] Walking outdoors became the most popular form of exercise, but in bad weather, patients could do gymnastics or even dance indoors. For some conditions, patients lifted weights or jumped rope. Others chopped wood. Women received the same prescriptions for physical activity as men; that women exercised and were highly encouraged to do so was very unusual at a time when frailty and fainting were prized feminine qualities.[17]

Priessnitz's water cure in Grafenberg became renowned throughout the Western Hemisphere. Thousands came to take the cure, including many European princes and princesses, barons, and counts. Visitors marveled at Priessnitz's ability to diagnose disease and devise a treatment plan simply by studying the quality and cast of a patient's skin. He never checked the pulse, looked at the tongue, or asked patients about their complaints, the standard methods of disease detection. One patient who made the trip to see Priessnitz was Elizabeth Blackwell. Although not a fan of irregular medicine generally, she came in 1850 seeking relief for an inflamed eye. Diet and exercise strengthened Blackwell's overall health, but her badly inflamed eye never cleared and eventually required removal. Even though his treatment failed Blackwell, Priessnitz's therapy proved effective for most ailments, and by 1840, nearly seventeen hundred patients per year sought treatment at Grafenberg.[18]

Priessnitz's success spurred countless imitators and admirers. Hydropathic institutes opened in England in the 1840s. Dr. James Wilson, of the thirty glasses of water before breakfast, opened his own water cure called Grafenberg House in Malvern, England, in 1842. Wilson gave each patient a Grafenberg flask so that they, too, could drink a few gallons of water before breakfast. Older health spas at Bath and Brighton refurbished and adopted Priessnitz's now fashionable regimen. These English water cures attracted all kinds of people, including Scottish historian and writer Thomas Carlyle, author Charles Dickens, scientist Charles Darwin, and poet Alfred (Lord) Tennyson. Of these, Darwin was perhaps the most enamored of hydropathy. He returned home from Malvern and constructed an outdoor shower and bath in his garden that he used daily for five years under the ministrations of his butler. He also bought a horse for exercise and limited his work to two and a half hours daily, which he reported renewed his strength.[19]

Not everyone was so taken with Priessnitz's successes, though. In the mid-1820s, physicians in the neighboring town of Friewaldau brought Priessnitz to court for practicing without a medical license. The court found Priessnitz not guilty, however. Because he used only water and no drugs of any kind, the judge determined that Priessnitz could not be said to be unlawfully practicing medicine. His acquittal won him and hydropathy even greater renown.[20]

Hydropaths trumpeted the ability of water to cure—or at the very least alleviate—all manner of acute and debilitating diseases that regular medicine had failed to treat. They emphasized water's ability to cleanse, purify, soothe, cool, relax, renew, and wash away ills. Even with hydropathy's sometimes hyperbolic praise of its power, water both gave and sustained life on earth, so critics struggled to deny its primacy and importance to health. Good health was natural, hydropaths argued, and it was the way God intended people to be. While hydropaths didn't tend to claim spiritual awakening or communion for those who took the cure, they also didn't deny these encounters if they happened to occur when someone was taking the waters.[21]

The first water cure in the United States opened its doors in 1843, followed by a second the next year. Both were in New York City and were operated by disillusioned regular doctors.[22] Even before they opened, Americans had some familiarity with hydropathy. Newspapers and medical journals had carried stories and reports on hydropathy in Europe throughout the 1830s. Medical journals tended to be critical of the practice, pointing out the dangers and shortcomings of a single-remedy system just as they had done with Thomsonism. Some Americans had even visited water cures while traveling in Europe, bringing back firsthand accounts of their experiences. Americans had examples of water cures closer to home, too. Travelers had long raved about the healing merits of Saratoga Springs in New York, White Sulphur Springs in West Virginia, and Hot Springs in Virginia.[23]

Hydropathy spread quickly throughout the United States, largely due to the efforts of physicians Joel Shew and Russell Thacher Trall. In 1843 Shew abandoned his regular medical practice to open the nation's first hydropathic institute. Tireless in his reform advocacy, Shew owned and operated several water cures over his life, partnered on others, and wrote books and articles extolling the power of water and the significance of the water cure to the history of medicine. Trall, another disaffected regular doctor, opened the country's second water cure in 1844 and transformed hydropathy into an all-inclusive and very American healing philosophy that emphasized self-improvement and reform. Merging his interests in hygiene, food reform, phrenology, temperance, and vegetarianism, Trall crafted a system that left virtually no aspect of life unregulated, from work to sleep to meals and morals. For patients suffering from mental ailments, including "ungovernable passions" like anxiety, jealousy, and narcissism as well as other ailments like depression and sleepwalking, he recommended "mental medication" of "pleasant, cheerful, and *sensible* company, with a light and easy, yet regular and steady business occupation." He suggested several options for sleep disturbances, including "Walking the room in a state of entire nudity," which Trall declared produced "remarkably quiet and refreshing sleep" among some of his patients. Besides disease, he also counseled on the proper age of marriage, claiming that children born of young parents "are more animal and less moral and intellectual than those born nearer the middle period of the life of the parents." He advised that the best marriages and the best children came from women aged twenty-two to twenty-five who married men between twenty-five and thirty years old.[24] Not content to trust his patients to understand his dietary advice, Trall even published a hydropathic cookbook filled with bland, spice-free, mostly vegetarian recipes for whole-grain breads, gruels, and boiled vegetables.[25] Trall based his theory on the laws of nature and made his hygienic system, with water as the central element, one that anyone could use, understand, and benefit from.[26]

Dissatisfied with the speculative nature of Priessnitz's system, some American hydropaths did try to come up with their own theories for how hydropathy worked. Those that had converted to the field from regular medicine used their knowledge of disease and physiology to imagine how various impurities could invade the body. Germs were still decades away from discovery. These hydropaths proposed theories far more complex and sophisticated than those of the peasant Priessnitz to explain how cold water could heal everything: it dissolved morbid accumulations in the system and ejected them through the skin, lungs, bowels, and kidneys; it stimulated stronger action in the capillaries; it invigorated nerves; or maybe it drew blood from a place of excess to a deficient part.[27]

The water-cure movement spread through word of mouth and patient testimonials, a process fostered in large part by the *Water-Cure Journal and the Herald of Reform* and similar publications. These publications reported hydropathic innovations and dramatically highlighted amazing water-cure successes as well as the horrible failures of regular medicine. The *Water-Cure Journal* enjoyed remarkable success from its founding in 1845, acquiring more than fifty thousand subscribers by 1850, and surviving, under various names, until 1897.[28] Some of that success may be attributable to phrenologists Orson and Lorenzo Fowler, who took over publication of the journal in 1848. Master salesmen but also true believers in both phrenology and hydropathy, the Fowlers occasionally touted the benefits of the water cure in the pages of their other popular periodical, the *American Phrenological Journal*.[29] The mixing of these topics invited the criticism of the *Boston Medical and Surgical Journal* in 1846, for combining the "false schemes" of hydropathy with the "noble and lofty views which are the characteristics of Mr. Fowler's [phrenological] philosophy."[30]

Despite its generally low regard in many regular medical circles, hydropathy became incredibly popular among the American public. Hydropaths claimed their system aided rather than interfered with nature in its fight against disease, a popular position also claimed by Thomson and his botanics. Its natural curing agent and simple theory of disease offered a welcome and comprehensible alternative to the harsh drugs and the inaccessible language of regular medicine. Relying on the application and drinking of pure water rather than special mineral waters also allowed hydropathy to be easily adaptable to home use, which held particular appeal in a nation that expanded faster than it could produce trained doctors of any kind. Perhaps most appealing of all, though, was hydropathy's new concept of healthful living: the promise of personal perfection through the adoption of the water cure. The system's rules for eating, drinking, exercise, and sleeping provided a sense of meaning and order to followers while also giving them the autonomy to treat themselves: it was personal freedom within tightly controlled strictures. Many hydropaths set themselves up as lifestyle coaches, offering advice and answering questions on nearly every aspect of life. Hydropathy's moral earnestness—many followers also advocated for temperance, vegetarianism, and even abolition—appealed strongly to lower- and middle-class Americans looking to improve their social and economic status.[31]

Hydropaths strongly believed, like many other kinds of nineteenth-century reformers, that improving the habits of the individual would uplift all of American culture if not the whole of humanity. They shared their generation's boundless optimism in human potential and a romantic notion that Americans could achieve greatness through an act of individual will. Unlike other reformers, though,

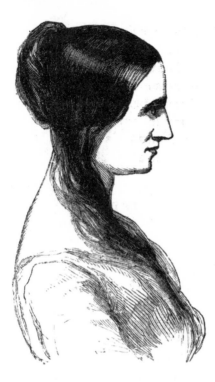

Mary Gove Nichols was
a prolific writer and vocal
advocate for the benefits of
the water cure and of women
understanding the workings
of their own bodies.
(Sarah J. Hale, ed.,
Woman's Record [1853])

hydropaths avoided organized and formal political involvement. For
the hydropaths, the clearest and best path to improvement lay in personal health. They painted a compelling vision of the good life and
supplied the entire system by which they believed it could be achieved.
"We labor for the Physical Regeneration of the Race, well knowing
that only through this can we successfully promote the Intellectual
and Moral Elevation of our fellow-men," proclaimed the *Water-Cure
Journal*. "We ask all who have brothers and sisters of the Human Family, to aid in this work, by becoming Co-Workers with us in the great
cause of HUMAN HEALTH."[32] Hydropathy seemed to promise that if
every person followed its method, humans could eliminate not only
disease but all human suffering. The harmonious and moral society
that would result would allow everyone to create and control his or
her own future. Hydropaths were realistic, though. They realized that
not every person would achieve their vision of perfection, but they
applauded those who strove to reach it anyway.[33]

At the same time that Shew and Trall expanded hydropathy's

reach and theoretical underpinnings, it was Mary Gove Nichols and her husband, Thomas, who made hydropathy famous, even before they began flaunting the pain-free birth of their daughter. Born in Goffstown, New Hampshire, in 1810, Mary Sargeant Neal was the precocious daughter of a freethinking father who encouraged her active and curious mind. She started school at age two, and by age six, she had read all of Plutarch. After her family moved to Vermont, her formal schooling became more sporadic, but she continued her self-education by reading everything she could get her hands on. As a teenager, she pored over the pages of the books her medical student brother brought home, fascinated by the workings of the human body but perhaps also wondering why she could find so little information on the health of women like herself.

An unhappy marriage in 1831 to Hiram Gove, who disdained her reading and creative writing, helped turn Mary into a champion of women's rights and a prominent health reformer. Trained as a hatter, Hiram lacked the skills to support his family, so Mary taught, sewed, and published stories and poems to sustain them, all the while enduring his contempt of her writing and personal correspondence. Marriage without love made each hour "an eternity of misery," she wrote. Despite her unhappiness, Hiram refused her a divorce. To ease her mental and physical suffering, Mary defied her husband and turned back to the medical books that had so enthralled her as a child. She discovered Sylvester Graham, an early advocate of dietary reform, vegetarianism, and hygienic reform and determined that women's well-being and happiness depended on the freedom achieved through personal health.[34] Excited by her newfound knowledge, Mary wanted to share her message with others. She particularly wanted to tell other women of the salvation that could be found in knowing about and taking charge of their own bodies. Her husband's disapproval of her activities, even as he benefited from the money she earned from her advocacy, only fueled her "burning zeal to save women from the miseries she saw, and from some that she endured."[35]

In 1838, Mary Gove made a name for herself lecturing (a scandal in and of itself for a woman) on the shocking topics of women's health, anatomy, and physiology. Women's health was a topic rarely, if ever, discussed at the time, much less in public. With no women regular doctors, many women ignored their own health problems and endured in silence to avoid being seen by male doctors, which many deemed improper. An often sickly woman herself, much of it brought on by the stress of her terrible marriage, Mary made it her mission to relieve other women of the crushing burden of physical and mental suffering. Hundreds packed lecture halls to see the thin, dark-haired woman with an open and intelligent face and exuberant brown eyes discuss the healthy female body.[36]

In the summer of 1845, finally free of her husband after leaving him and returning to her parents' home in 1841, Mary traveled to Brattleboro, Vermont, to investigate the water cure recently opened there by Priessnitz disciple Dr. Robert Wesselhoeft. Hydropathy wasn't new to her; she'd been reading about it and advocating many of its principles in her lectures and writing for several years, but she lacked formal training in its tenets and use. Impressed by what she saw, she began training as a water-cure physician, offering physiology lessons to patients in exchange for her education.

The town of Brattleboro sat on the Connecticut River where it met Whetstone Brook and the West River in southeastern Vermont. Surrounded by mountains, forests, meadows, gorges, and waterfalls, the area offered plenty of outdoor recreational opportunities for patients taking the cure. "A more suitable spot for such an undertaking could not well have been chosen," proclaimed one patient.[37] Although Shew and Trall had opened urban water cures, most institutions operated in rural areas along rivers, streams, and lakes. Hundreds opened around the country in the 1840s and 1850s, some operating only a few months while others lasted more than a century. Most people who went to a water cure suffered from chronic diseases like asthma, dyspepsia, or gout. Visits tended to last one to three months. Nestled in bucolic settings, these facilities sold hydropathy but also the beauty and tranquility of the surroundings as a respite from the ills of a hectic urban life. The Elmira Water Cure in New York boasted of its sweeping hills and woods, "overlooking the entire city, the river and valley of the Chemung, and the hills around, giving miles of the most varied and beautiful scenery. Our elevation gives us dry and bracing air, so necessary in the cure of Catarrah, Throat and Lung diseases, Rheumatism, Neuralgia, and Scrofula."[38] Many of the larger water cures had sleeping quarters, a dining hall, a bathing area, and an exercise hall. To protect women's modesty, most cures had separate bathing facilities for men and women as well as female bath attendants, nurses, and even doctors.[39]

Water cures often aimed their services at a particular clientele—women, teachers, weary ministers, or people suffering from certain illnesses—but they also serviced a variety of patients who made their choice based on the scenery or attractions offered rather than on medical specifics. Round Hill House in Massachusetts recruited healthy people to come "for a season of recreation from the cares of business, where pure air, pure water, lovely walks and rides, and captivating scenery, may be enjoyed, without 'stint or measure.'"[40] Round Hill was one of any number of water cures attempting to attract those less interested in medical care than in recreation and social opportunities. Mark Twain found his visit to a European cure so pleasant he quipped, "If I hadn't had a disease I would have borrowed one just to have a pretext for going on."[41]

Wesselhoeft's Brattleboro Hydropathic Institution was one of the most exclusive and expensive water cures in the United States. Initially welcoming eighteen patients, it eventually grew to accommodate two hundred at a time, among them some of the nation's leading politicians, social reformers, and writers, including President Martin Van Buren and writer Harriet Beecher Stowe. Wesselhoeft had carefully examined several other springs before determining Brattleboro's to be of superior quality and purity for the institution he planned. It also helped that the town was only a one day's journey by train from Boston, New York, and Albany, major population centers that would provide clients to his fledgling business. Located on a quiet street away from Brattleboro's main business district, the institute's main buildings formed a square enclosing a courtyard with an elaborate fountain. Covered verandas offered areas for exercise in bad weather and cool breezes in the summer. Cold running water pumped into the separate buildings for men and women, each equipped with a variety of baths, as well as single and double rooms for sleeping. A "dancing saloon and parlor" connected the men's and women's buildings. Fresh water from springs located in the hills surrounding the town flowed continually into the plunge baths, twenty-five feet long and fifteen feet wide. In the nearby woods, patients found showers, twelve sitz baths (a waist-high bath used to treat lower-body ailments), an eye bath, an ear bath, and a river shower. Further on, a wave bath fed by the flume of a small millpond was located on the high bank of the Whetstone Brook.

Coaches met patients at the Brattleboro train station and brought them directly to the institute. One week's stay cost eleven dollars in the winter and ten in the summer. The difference in price reflected the hydropathic insistence that cooler temperatures, like cooler water, made for more effective and comfortable cures; "even the severe cold of winter is no real obstacle to [the cure's] continuance."[42] The price didn't include the hefty supply of sheets and other equipment patients were expected to bring. Each patient was instructed to supply at least two large woolen blankets, a feather bed or three comforters, a course linen sheet for cutting into bandages, two course cotton sheets, six towels, and one injection instrument for enemas. Supplies could also be purchased on site. To save money, patients could also stay at a boardinghouse in Brattleboro and use the outdoor baths for the discounted rate of five dollars per week.[43] Nonetheless, few Americans could afford the indulgence of a trip to Brattleboro at a time when the average wage of a male factory worker in the 1850s hovered around one dollar daily.[44]

Water treatment protocols differed from practitioner to practitioner and from patient to patient, but most hydropaths followed the pattern set by Shew's first New York City cure. The wet sheet became the usual and most popular mode of application because it "cools febrile action, excites the action of the skin, equalizes the circulation, removes obstructions, brings out eruptive diseases, controls spasms, and relieves pain like a charm." While the icy coldness of the fabric could be shocking at first, Thomas Low Nichols described a near immediate "pleasant glow, a calm, and usually a profound sleep" that quickly followed.[45] While Priessnitz's original system called for water to be used both internally and externally, most American hydropaths believed that water worked best when applied gradually through the skin. The wet sheet became the standard method of application. First, the attendant would dip a sheet of cotton or linen in cold water and spread it on several thick wool blankets. The patient would then be wound up in the sheet and blankets by the attendant and secured with pins or tape. Once wrapped, patients would shiver and then lie sweating on feather beds for anywhere from twenty-five minutes to several hours depending on the seriousness of the illness. After they worked up a good sweat, the attendant unwrapped them and plunged them in a cold bath followed by a brisk drying. For severely debilitated patients, the wet-sheet treatment could be too much, so an alternative known as the wet dress was used instead. A loose-fitting, nightgown-like garment, the wet dress allowed patients to dispense with the services of an attendant and to walk comfortably while also soaking up water. Most wet-dress patients also went to bed in the outfit, a damp and presumably clammy night of sleep.[46]

The wet dress soon found a following outside the water cure as well, influencing the mid-nineteenth-century Bloomer costume for women, the semiofficial dress of women's liberation. The loose gown with wide sleeves and a skirt falling over baggy trousers seemed the perfect outfit for healthy women who sought comfort and freedom from the strictures of standard women's wear. Popular fashion of the time called for tightly laced corsets, layers of petticoats, and floor-length dresses. Some women dragged fifty pounds of clothing around with them, making walking, not to mention breathing, challenging. Female water-cure patients reveled in the freedom of the wet dress, and they often took that freedom one step further and cut their long hair short for easy drying.[47]

Fed up with their restrictive clothing, many women—along with many progressive men—began advocating for dress reform as one part of a whole package of rights and freedoms for women. Elizabeth Smith introduced her modified-for-street-wear wet dress to the fashion world in 1851 after sharing her new style with her cousin and women's rights leader, Elizabeth Cady Stanton. Journalist Amelia Bloomer discovered it when Stanton came for a visit and showed off the new style. Bloomer soon began writing enthusiastically about it in the *Lily*, the nation's first reform newspaper for women. So great was Bloomer's fervor that her name became indelibly linked with the style, though Bloomer and her fellow wearers suffered merciless ridicule for their fashion choice. Bloomer abandoned the style in 1859 but not her desire for more reasonable clothes as she continued to advocate for sensible women's clothing throughout her life.[48]

The wet sheet and dress were but one tool in an intense regimen of bathing, soaking, walking, and showering. Educator Catharine Beecher was an early and active promoter of hydropathy, and she came to Brattleboro in the summer of 1846 seeking ways to improve her health. Rarely sick as a child, Beecher claimed that it was only once she had to earn a living as a teacher, confined indoors all day, that she suffered her first nervous breakdown.[49] Packed into a wet sheet at 4 a.m., Beecher remained wrapped like a waterlogged mummy for hours. As her body heat warmed the sheet, she began to sweat profusely beneath her tight wrappings. Beecher was then unwrapped and immersed in a cold plunge bath. This morning soak was only the beginning of her day. She was then sent outdoors to walk as far as she could, drinking five or six tumblers of cold water to stay hydrated before and after her exercise. Many patients walked to Cold Spring, a beautiful pure water stream running down from the mountains. Another path meandered from Elliot Street, where the institute was located, past a woolen mill, along shaded roads and trout streams, to Centerville and back. Returning from her walk, Beecher stood under an eighteen-foot-tall cold-water shower for ten minutes. After this she walked and drank some more. At 3 p.m., Beecher sat in a sitz bath filled with cold water for thirty minutes. She then walked and drank again. At 9 p.m., she sat for thirty minutes with her feet resting in a bucket of cold water. Beecher ended her day as it began nearly seventeen hours earlier, wrapped in wet bandages. She repeated this experience every day of her three-month stay. Her experience and those of others she'd observed convinced her that water cures should be "multiplied all over the land, as the safest and surest methods of relieving debilitated constitutions and curing chronic ailments." "Without exception," declared Beecher, "*all* are improved in general health, [and] . . . *none* are injured."[50]

Methods varied depending on the nature of the complaint. In 1849, a thirty-two-year-old woman with dark hair, gray eyes, and a ruddy complexion came to Dr. Wesselhoeft seeking relief for dyspepsia (indigestion), back pain, and fatigue. She'd tried everything, from pills, powders, herbs, and teas to Thomsonism with no relief. She estimated she'd been bled at least twenty times. Wesselhoeft examined her and determined that her dyspepsia was long gone, replaced by sickness generated from all of the medicines and treatments she'd tried. He first had her bathe before he wrapped wet bandages around her stomach and abdomen. She drank water and received several enemas. He then wrapped her in a wet sheet until boils appeared, "sure that all would go on well." The boils healed but the patient only felt worse. The next day, she began to "vomit large quantities of bile and—worms! Yes! This was her disease!" Wesselhoeft instructed her to drink sixteen tumblers of water and an attendant gave her four water enemas daily. She was told to eat nothing but peas, beans, and coarse bread, fiber to help the worms pass through her system. Finally, she endured three days of diarrhea, evacuating most of the worms and much of her strength in the process. Exhausted and weak from her ordeal, the woman then underwent a rehabilitation process that Wesselhoeft began to "return her to health." He kept her wrapped in wet bandages, removing them each day as they grew brown and crusty as the disease left her body. More than a month later, the woman claimed her health at long last restored.[51] Intestinal worms can cause vomiting and diarrhea, though it's unlikely that this woman actually vomited worms. Most intestinal parasites come from contaminated food or water or from contact with larva-infested soil. Fibrous foods can help them pass out of the body through the bowels, so Wesselhoeft's treatment may have aided this patient's natural body process of eliminating the worms. Hydropathy's hygiene regimen perhaps helped to prevent reinfection and rehabilitated her with whole foods and water.

Wesselhoeft taught his students, Mary Gove among them, the art of individual prescription, adapting cures to each patient's symptoms, stamina, and age. "The same treatment that would cure one might fail entirely with another," she later noted.[52] Hydropathy was very physical work for the physicians and attendants, too, requiring great strength to rub patients, lift blankets drenched with water, and to assist people in getting in and out of their beds, baths, and wraps. Mary left Brattleboro with a profound respect for the healing power of pure, cold water to cure nearly all disease given the appropriate skill, time, and dedication.[53]

After three months in Brattleboro, Mary became the resident physician at the New Lebanon Springs Water Cure in New York. But the rigorous physical demands of the work proved too much for her. She moved to New York City in 1846 and began giving lectures and writing articles and books on health and hydropathy. Twenty women signed up for her first series of twenty two-hour lectures on the structure and function of the body. That same year, 1846, her *Lectures to Ladies on Anatomy and Physiology*, first published in 1842, earned a second and much wider printing, as well as a positive review from the poet Walt Whitman and even the regular medicine periodical the *Boston Medical and Surgical Journal*. Edgar Allan Poe, writing in *Godey's Lady's Book*, praised her enthusiasm and speaking skills, proclaiming her "in many respects a very interesting woman." Mary's evident charms and reformist impulses attracted a variety of writers, philosophers, musicians, and artists to her home, including Poe, who recited "The Raven" in her living room, but also social reformer Albert Brisbane. Mary Gove's clear and rational writing greatly enhanced the popularity of the water cure, and her references to the medical works of Hippocrates, Galen, and French physiologist Francois Magendie inspired reader confidence in her breadth of medical knowledge. Rather than adopting inaccessible medical jargon, she followed in the path of her fellow hydropaths and medical irregulars like Thomson. She appealed to the intelligence of her readers and spoke plainly to educate patients and practitioners. Mary continued to treat patients, many of whom traveled across the country seeking her services and advice. Though she'd never attended medical school, by the late 1840s, she led a doctor's life and had earned a reputation as a trustworthy medical expert.[54]

Things were looking up in her personal life, too. Mary's husband, Hiram Gove, finally consented to a divorce in 1847. That same year on Christmas Eve, she met a young writer named Thomas Low Nichols, whose writing and progressive views on women she admired. The two married the following July. Inspired by his new wife's work in hydropathy, Thomas enrolled in medical school to study "the very errors and absurdities" of regular medicine, graduating from New York University with a medical degree in 1850.[55]

While residential water cures and the personalized services of practicing hydropaths like Nichols did attract the wealthy and famous like Mark Twain, Brigham Young, Susan B. Anthony, and Catharine Beecher, hydropaths consistently emphasized the importance of keeping their cures affordable. Yet, in the mid-nineteenth century, the average cost of a visit to a water cure ranged from five to fifteen dollars a week with additional charges for other services. Some institutions offered discounted rates to those patients who brought their own food and washed their own clothes. Even so, a visit to a water cure remained out of reach for many Americans, who could ill afford to miss work and spend half a month's wages on a week's worth of care. Most of those who could afford to visit a cure could also afford other kinds of health care, including regular medicine, so both regulars and hydropaths competed, at some level, for patients of a similar socioeconomic class.[56]

But, unlike regulars, hydropaths also made a philosophical commitment to accessibility and stressed the value of home care. Like the Thomsonians, hydropaths strongly believed that everyone should have access to health care and medical knowledge. They also recognized the pragmatic benefits of domestic hydropathy in spreading the water cure as widely as possible. Many hydropaths published home medical manuals and guides for self-doctoring that detailed the kinds, timing, frequency, and duration of baths required for particular illnesses, as well as information on exercise and diet.[57]

Hydropathy translated well to home use because of the responsibility it placed on patients for affecting their own cure. Passivity had no place in hydropathy. Patient cooperation and dedication to the process was essential, no matter where treatment occurred. Unlike regular medicine, hydropaths deemphasized the authority of the physician in favor of creating independent patients able to diagnose and care for themselves. Patients thus had a substantial responsibility for their own outcomes. "If a patient thoroughly understands his or her disease, and has the requisite energy to accomplish a cure," wrote Mary Gove Nichols, "it may be done almost anywhere, and with very meager advantages." She recounted stories of female patients who managed to heal themselves even while weak with disease through their own "indomitable energy."[58] Hydropaths believed that hygienic habits were best mastered through willpower and self-control, an ideology that mirrored wider societal beliefs about personal responsibility and social improvement. While this had the potential to render ill health a personal and moral failing, adherence to a system placed some but not all responsibility for healing on the efficacy of the system itself. Self-care allowed everyone to participate in hydropathy, and the success of the treatments, whether achieved at home or at a water cure, were widely publicized and given equal treatment in hydropathic journals.[59]

Empowering people to care for themselves went hand in hand with hydropathy's rejection of university training as a prerequisite for practicing. Hydropathy was far less hierarchical than regular medicine and even other nineteenth-century irregular systems like homeopathy, in part because hydropaths never sought professional medical status. Anyone could practice hydropathy and find success, including the self-taught. While some debate arose in the 1850s over whether to establish uniform credentials and standards, proponents arguing that it would improve care and patient outcomes, hydropaths never seriously acted on the issue and it did not come up again in an organized fashion. Most hydropaths believed that the only qualifications necessary should be a personal commitment to the principles of hydropathy and a willingness and ability to practice them responsibly.[60] Clearly, these principles and hygienic living were intended to eliminate the need for drugs and heroic therapies, and many hydropaths did insist that water cure and regular medicine shared no common ground or interests. But rather than compete directly with regular medicine, hydropaths instead believed that regular medicine would naturally fade away as it became increasingly irrelevant in the face of rising universal health and social harmony.[61]

Despite the egalitarian views of many hydropathic practitioners, in 1851, Mary Gove Nichols and her new husband, Thomas Nichols, opened the nation's first hydropathic medical school, the American Hydropathic Institute, in New York City. Concerned about the dangers of the misapplication of cold water, not to mention charlatans masquerading as hydropaths for profit, the Nicholses believed that the potency of water required expert guidance. They hoped their school would make water-cure training more formal and respectable—a more professional alternative to regular medicine. Similar efforts continued among some hydropaths until well after the Civil War, most notably in New York City, where Russell Trall opened his New York Hydropathic School, later the Hygeio-Therapeutic College, in 1853. The Nicholses' school offered a full medical course in anatomy, physiology, chemistry, surgery, and obstetrics and had all the necessary plumbing for a complete hydropathic education. Students could also visit hospitals, clinics, anatomical museums, and medical libraries in the city for additional learning opportunities. More than teaching about water, though, Nichols wanted to provide a medical education for women to meet the national demand for female doctors.[62]

With few exceptions, most of the nation's medical schools refused to admit women. Elizabeth Blackwell had only been admitted to New York's Geneva Medical College on a technicality after faculty passed the decision of whether to allow her admission on to the all-male student body. As a joke, they voted yes, and Blackwell matriculated despite the opposition of most of the students and faculty to her presence.[63] At the American Hydropathic Institute's inaugural ceremonies, Mary Nichols delivered an address entitled "Woman the Physician" that argued for the importance of female doctors. Rather than reject cultural assumptions about women's caring nature, she claimed women's innate talents uniquely qualified them for the profession. "Women are peculiarly fitted to practice the art of healing . . . [because of the] tenderer love, the sublimer devotion, the never to be wearied patience and kindness of woman," she proclaimed.[64] Thomas echoed his wife's sentiments, writing in the *Water-Cure Journal* that women's "diseases have been the subject of mercenary speculations, of mischievous medications, of torturing mechanical inventions, of nameless brutalities, and detestable charlatanism" with "little or no relief."[65] Enrollees in the American Hydropathic Institute understood from the start the reformist goals of its founders, and the Institute's first graduating class included nine women and eleven men.[66]

The Nicholses' progressive views of women aligned perfectly with hydropathy's expansive view of women and women's health. Hydropaths shared their era's belief in women's softer, more caring nature: they just did not see this as a justification for keeping women out of the medical profession. At the time, regular medicine tended to regard being female as a disease in and of itself. Ruled by reproduction, women were deemed irrational, intellectually inferior, and emotional, and their biological processes treated as illnesses in need of containment. Physician Edward Johnson, who used hydropathy alongside heroic therapies, fumed that regular approaches to childbirth were "irrational, indefensible and most preposterously foolish" in treating birth as though "it were some formidable and dangerous malady."[67] Hydropathy took the radical step of naturalizing women's life stages. For hydropaths, puberty, menstruation, childbearing, and menopause were not dread diseases needing intervention but natural processes in a woman's life. Women did not become weak and ill because of their gender but because of some outside cause, just like men. Hydropaths celebrated women's nature and exalted rather than denied their historic role as family and community caretakers. They urged women to take an active role in their own health, and to maximize their health and happiness through diet, exercise, and other hygienic practices, all of which dramatically expanded women's power to determine and control their own lives within the hydropathic worldview.[68] As a result, hydropathy provided a refuge for progressive women, and many of America's first generation of women doctors came out of hydropathy.

Encouraging women to get involved in hydropathy contributed to the financial health of the nation's water cures as well. To attract women and their money, hydropaths needed female attendants and practitioners to serve them. Modesty and the intimate nature of the treatment demanded that women be treated and served only by other women. The large cures had at least one woman physician on staff, and most cures boasted of their male- and female-only bathing facilities in advertisements. A few cures had exclusively female staff and clients. It seemed to work. Women consistently outnumbered men in attendance at hydropathic institutes. It's not hard to imagine why.[69]

For many women, visiting a water cure was the first, and perhaps only, time their needs were put above those of their husbands and children. As Dr. Silas O. Gleason of the Elmira Water Cure explained, "[T]here was a large class of patients for whom physicians could do little in their home environment. They needed a change of scene, systematic and constant oversight and the most healthful of mental, moral and physical aid, free from the cares and despondency that came of a routine that had grown depressing."[70] Gleason operated his cure with his wife, Rachel Brooks Gleason, a respected doctor in her own right, who counted Mark Twain's wife, Olivia Langdon Clemens, among her patients.[71] Writer Harriet Beecher Stowe was among the women who relished the break from her husband, children, and housework when she took the cure at Brattleboro. "Not for years, have I enjoyed life as I have here," she admitted, "real keen enjoyment—everything agrees with me." She loved the daily exercise—a real change from simply running after her children—and the companionship of the other women at the cure, which included, for a time, her sister Catharine Beecher. Stowe's husband, Calvin, on the other hand, couldn't wait for her return, reminding her that it had been "almost 18 months since I have had a wife to sleep with me. It is enough to kill any man."[72]

Hydropathy's popularity and the glowing testimonials to its curative powers did not mean that taking the cure was always pleasant. Some treatments, especially cold-water enemas, were common practices that few hydropaths discussed openly. That's probably for good reason. For constipation or diarrhea, patients quickly drank at least two pints of water, enough to produce distension of the colon in some people. Sufferers of chronic or acute mucous discharges and other genital conditions received cold injections via a zinc wire straight into the vagina or urethra.[73] The wet sheet wasn't always a treat either. One Boston man reported that his sheet froze stiff in less than three minutes during a visit to a cure one winter. Even so, he still reported that it had done him good.[74]

Worse than the wet sheet was the shower for many patients. At a time when few people bathed regularly, let alone had ever experienced a shower, a cold hydropathic stream falling from a height of at least ten feet offered a rude introduction. Some patients shouted, struggled, and attempted to run away when the spray hit them. First-timers could be pounded flat by the force of the stream. One English patient recalled being knocked over "like a ninepin." Another woman tried to lessen the force of the water by standing on a chair to decrease the distance between her head and that of the shower, but the water felled them both. The shower became even more perilous in winter when icicles could form and fall like daggers on the patient below.[75]

Drinking too much water could be deadly, too. Ingesting more water than the kidneys can properly handle can dilute the concentration of salt in the blood necessary for proper functioning of the body, a condition known as hyponatremia. Left untreated, a patient may lapse into a coma that can lead to death. It takes a lot of water to cause hyponatremia, but James Wilson perhaps flirted with danger, though unknown at the time, by drinking so many glasses of water before breakfast.[76]

Hydropathy's critics delighted in recounting patients' tales of peril from the nation's water cures and heaped abuse on hydropaths. American medical journals did their best to discredit hydropathy by making frequent references to Jean-Jacques Rousseau's harrowing 1736 experience at a water cure, where, Rousseau claimed, the waters had "nearly relieved me, not only of my ills, but of my life." Few seemed to care that Rousseau's visit occurred a century before Priessnitz had developed his system. Cartoonists loved to depict water-cure patients so swollen with water that they exploded or, alternatively, patients so saturated that they needed wringing out.[77] After Catharine Beecher's ringing endorsement of hydropathy and her experiences at Brattleboro appeared in the pages of the *New York Observer*, the *Boston Medical and Surgical Journal* sarcastically rejoined, "Ah! Blessed era for the washerwomen! How should the hotel chamber-maids rejoice? There is no longer need of airing or drying sheets . . . the miserable wretches who have gone out of the world with pleurisy and rheumatism, from sleeping in these damp envelopes, were entirely mistaken; they were actually better for it, or would have been had they not stopped too soon."[78]

Not many irregular medical systems escaped the harsh gaze and withering critiques of Oliver Wendell Holmes, who traced the evolution of the water cure while critiquing another of his favorite targets, homeopathy, as yet another ridiculous and illogical system. Holmes characterized Dr. Wesselhoeft as one of many "empirics, ignorant barbers, and men of that sort . . . who announce themselves ready to relinquish all the accumulated treasure of our art, to trifle with life upon the strength of these fantastic theories."[79] Many other people, including some outside medicine, agreed with him. On a trip to Europe, American writer John W. DeForest visited Priessnitz's cure at Grafenberg. He complained not only of the treatment he received but also of the climate, the water regimen itself, and the food, which he called "an insult to the palate and an injury to the stomach."[80] Poet and writer John Townsend Trowbridge was more generous than Holmes and DeForest, praising the restful conditions he experienced while visiting a water cure even though the treatments provided him little relief from his so-called "nervous debility" that kept his mind constantly whirring and disrupted his sleep. He was less impressed with his fellow patients, however, whom he accused of being self-absorbed, concerned only with their invalidism, a topic of conversation he found "not cheeringly tonic."[81]

Although hydropathy continued to be widely popular, pessimistic reports on the validity of a single-cure system continued to appear through the mid-nineteenth century. The *Boston Medical and Surgical Journal* reported that water had proved unsuccessful at treating most illnesses. Many regular doctors were convinced that hydropathic patients got better not because of the treatment but because its very mildness let nature do its job.[82] And it was true that most patients who visited water cures got better. In part, it was because most patients had to travel to a water cure, which virtually excluded those with serious acute or critical conditions from the start. Even those who practiced at home had to have the strength and stamina to follow the routine. Most patients suffered mild or chronic complaints often brought on or aggravated by the stresses of modern urban living. To feel better, they needed only some rest and relaxation, which hydropathy usually provided. Some critics also pointed out that despite hydropaths' claims to the contrary, the water-cure regimen was just as rigorous and invasive as heroic medicine with its weeks of wraps, long walks, showers, enemas, injections, and demands to drink more than ten glasses of water a day. Maybe it was better to be bled once than to endure more than fifteen hours a day in treatment, even if it was only water.[83]

Hydropaths themselves struggled to stay loyal to water as a cure-all. Practitioners came to hydropathy with varying levels of qualifications, experience, and motivations for practicing. From the very beginning, some followers combined water cure with homeopathy, vegetarianism, medical gymnastics, and vapor baths. Sylvester Graham's hygiene program, especially its promotion of vegetarianism and exercise, formed a natural partnership with hydropathy, and the two often coexisted at water-cure institutions. Grahamites liked hydropathy because it was natural and did not involve drugs, which they, too, saw as unnecessary and harmful. Temperance advocates also found common cause with hydropaths, who shared their high regard for water as the only healthful beverage.[84]

All of these practices peaceably coexisted because unlike Samuel Thomson, hydropaths never enforced a dogmatic adherence to a strict theory and set of practices; all practitioners, more or less, agreed on the basics of the system but were free to carry them out however they saw fit. At Brattleboro, Dr. Wesselhoeft allowed small doses of regular medicine when used in combination with hydropathy. Mary Gove Nichols blended hydropathy with other theories and systems when treating patients. She allowed her patients to use homeopathy on occasion, figuring that dabbling in other irregular systems was always preferable to regular medicine. She herself had run a Grahamite boardinghouse in Boston before turning to hydropathy. While this flexibility allowed for much more personal interpretation and camaraderie among hydropaths and other reformers, it also undermined hydropathy in the end by minimizing the very things that made hydropathy unique as a healing system. A diversity of personalities and beliefs discouraged standardization and sometimes even led to practices that contradicted pure hydropathic theory.[85] This became increasingly true as overall health hygiene—clean drinking water, waste disposal, sanitary housing—began to supplant water as the primary healer in the mid-nineteenth century. Hydropaths came to place as much faith in diet and exercise as water as the century wore on, a shift that removed the distinctive healing properties attributed solely to water. They gave up their systematic approach to water without offering an alternative means of advancing their principles. Without water, hydropathy lost its core value as well as its rationale for wrapping, bathing, and other water-related treatments.[86]

The hydropathic embrace of other therapies and novel ideas had its limits, though: most hydropaths ignored new discoveries and innovations in regular medical therapies and research, such as vaccinations, which cost them in the end. Scientific advances in the second half of the nineteenth century elevated the hospital and the laboratory to prominence, relegating self-taught and untrained doctors to the periphery of the emerging professional and scientifically oriented medical field.[87] In a world that seemed increasingly complex, Americans began turning to experts to guide them. With hydropaths unwilling to distinguish between degree-trained practitioners and those who came to water cure by experience, they no longer appeared to be on the cutting edge of reform.[88]

Hydropathy also continued to resist national organizations and professional schools at the same time that regular medicine and even other irregulars were finding identity as cohesive and institutional powers. The Nicholses' drive toward a professional education for hydropaths with the opening of their American Hydropathic Institute failed to gain traction. They operated the school for three terms and then abandoned it. Trall's New York school suffered from low standards and a "woefully inadequate" staff, according to one chronicler.[89] Other hydropathic schools opened in New Jersey, Pennsylvania, Tennessee, and Minnesota, but most closed quickly. Moreover, rigorous standards and formal training were contrary to the democratic tenets of hydropathy, so these educational efforts were handicapped from the start.[90]

To ensure a more secure economic and social position for themselves, regular doctors established medical societies and legislative standards aimed at excluding hydropaths from participating in the growing field of public health. Medical councils, hospitals, and city boards of health banned hydropaths from serving even as the issues they often addressed, like sanitation and green spaces, were much the same hygienic measures promoted for decades by hydropaths for health and healing. Hydropaths tried to fight back by criticizing regular doctors for taking the power of choice away from patients in deciding who could and could not practice medicine.[91]

Despite regular medicine's refusal to recognize them as legitimate doctors, though, many of the hydropaths' principles and innovations slowly became incorporated into regular medicine over succeeding decades. Advances in the germ theory of disease in the 1860s and 1870s led to an appreciation of bathing and overall cleanliness among regular doctors, who began to adopt and endorse the lifestyle recommendations long advocated by hydropaths. Bathing and staying hydrated with water appeared in a range of late-nineteenth-century health literature authored not by hydropaths but by new self-proclaimed experts in hygiene and public health maintenance. Later, in the early twentieth century, medical scientists also joined with public health proponents to address many of the issues that hydropaths and other hygiene reformers had long fought for like sanitation, diet, and exercise.[92]

The nation's changing political and social culture also drowned hydropathy. The Civil War in particular brutalized hydropaths' dreams of achieving individual and cultural perfection and harmony through their tenets of self-control and good health. They found that their idealism could not stand up against the harsh realities of a war that pitted Americans against one another.

The upheavals of the Civil War sped along shifting tides in popular culture as well. Following the war, what made for a good citizen changed. The self-denial and self-control that marked the early nineteenth century gave way to a more self-indulgent, pleasure-seeking, and consumer-oriented American people. Restraint and moderation, hydropathy's unspoken mottos, were not the way to make a fortune in urban industrial America. Women also gained more public influence in other areas, eclipsing what had been a unique and empowering aspect of hydropathy. Many women joined a variety of social and political reform movements, including suffrage and labor activism, that invited the active participation of both men and women.[93]

Many water cures that survived the Civil War raised the temperature of their water and introduced gentler treatments to maintain their business. The increasing availability of in-home plumbing made the water cure less unique, so institutions added more non-water offerings to attract clients. Cures in Massachusetts and New York added billiards, dancing, vaudeville performances, and bowling. The cold-water cures also faced competition from luxurious resorts that catered to the conspicuous leisure of the wealthy and fostered a concept of health that was far more passive and recreation oriented— much more like the spas of old.[94]

Even with hydropathy's decline, Mary Gove Nichols never stopped working and advocating for the causes in which she believed. In the 1850s the Nicholses turned increasingly from treating women's illnesses to a more radical attack on what Mary believed to be the ultimate source of their troubles: marriage. Despite being happily married to Thomas, Mary never forgot the personal injury she suffered at the hands of her first husband. True marriage, she argued, came from love, not the legally binding strictures that largely left women powerless victims of their husbands. Thomas agreed. The idea of marriage as an institution outside the law was a real shocker in 1850s America, though, and earned the Nicholses branding as "free lovers." Not to be confused with the 1960s idea, free love in the 1850s was a movement opposed to marriage, at least as an institution regulated by government. Many advocates equated marriage with slavery for the wife. Even among hydropaths, the Nicholses' views on marriage were pretty far out there, driving them to the fringes of the main current of health reform. In 1861, at the outbreak of the Civil War, Mary and Thomas sailed to England and rode out the war abroad, publishing stories and articles that had little do with health, medicine, or hydropathy. After the war, they returned to health reform, operating a health resort in Malvern, England, the same town that hosted the institution of the water-guzzling James Wilson. They also wrote on medical topics, though without the overtones of free love that sank their reputation in the United States.[95]

At the end of her life, Mary joined the ranks of another health trend, mesmerism, and relied more on magnetic power than water to heal patients. She passed her hands over injuries and provided magnetized objects to patients that cured without physical contact. In 1882, Mary received a diagnosis of breast cancer and soon attempted to treat herself with the methods she had long advocated for others. Every morning and every evening she magnetized her body for ten minutes. Bathing remained integral to her routine, and she took almost daily baths for health. She also exercised regularly and maintained a Grahamite vegetarian diet. She practiced a little homeopathy. Through it all, Mary continued to see and treat patients until two weeks before her death on May 30, 1884, dedicated to the end to improving the health of humanity and the prospects of women—a truly visionary and progressive woman. Mary's frankness on the physiology of women's bodies and the constraints of marriage contrasted sharply with the prudery of her age.[96]

Hydropathy was not a complete failure: that Americans bathe regularly, drink lots of water, aspire to regular exercise, praise a low-fat and high-fiber diet, and wear nonconstricting clothing all reflect hydropathy's early influence. These preventative health measures theorized and practiced by hydropaths in the nineteenth century became the foundation of modern healthy living still practiced and advocated by many nutritionists and doctors today. Few gyms, health and beauty spas, or athletic training rooms fail to provide users with some form of hydropathic therapy, be it a whirlpool, steam room, sauna, or swimming pool. The entire industry that exists in spas, Jacuzzis, hot tubs, and swimming facilities hearkens back to hydropathy's insistence on the importance of water to human health. Water resorts, while no longer hydropathic, still promise vacationers relaxation and renewal, the same promises made by water cures. These destinations continue to attract visitors with their beautiful views, entertainment options, and flowing water.[97]

Perhaps hydropathy's most visible legacy is in the popularly held belief in drinking eight glasses of water a day. This notion was appropriated and echoed with increasing fervor in the late nineteenth century by the temperance movement. By the 1910s and 1920s, American newspapers and magazines were filled with exhortations to consume eight glasses of water for health on a daily basis. Although scientists and doctors continue to disagree over how much water is enough, the idea of drinking fluids regularly for health remains undisputed.[98]

Although hydropaths appear not to have called disease "toxins," their theory of using water to remove a disease-causing agent expressed this concept still very present in modern conversations about health. Today, many irregular therapies promise to flush toxins from the body through various methods, including water, in detox and cleansing diets and also advocate whole foods and exercise. The idea of flushing toxins likely predates hydropathy, but the system nonetheless provided a very clear articulation of an idea that became wildly popular and influential in irregular health.

Hydropathy also informed the reform movements that fought to clean up cities in the late nineteenth century. The emphasis of hydropaths on the importance of nature and fresh air in their treatments, and of renewal and possible perfection in the beautiful natural areas where they located their water cures, influenced the drive to create parks and green spaces in major cities. A visit to a park, like a stay at a water cure, was seen as the antidote to the ills of modern life. Efforts to improve city services for hygiene and to curb disease, particularly sewers and indoor plumbing, also have their antecedents in hydropathy.

Hydropathy lives on today as hydrotherapy and consists primarily of therapies performed in water, hot and cold packings for injuries, steam baths, foot baths, and wet compresses. Sebastian Kneipp, a German priest, is largely credited with reviving hydropathy in the late nineteenth century and transforming it into its modern form. Building on Priessnitz's work, Kneipp added various water temperatures and pressures to the therapy regimen. Kneipp water baths, mineral bath salts, and other bathing products are still sold today. Hydropathy also plays a large part in modern sports medicine, which emphasizes the importance of water as an anesthetic, sedative, energizer, and aid to muscular exertion. Athletes often soak in ice-filled tubs after exertion to improve recovery, though some studies have questioned the efficacy of this practice, while other people use hot baths to ease sore muscles.[99]

What has changed between hydropathy then and now is the value attached to diet, exercise, and water. Today, these practices are less of a universal social good and more of a personal choice. None of the current rhetoric around spas, exercise, and drinking water offers to perfect humanity in the process, but it remains a primary means of self-improvement. Both today and in the nineteenth century, Americans' near obsessive concern with physical fitness and health corresponded with a highly competitive, industrial life where fitness represented yet another asset with the potential to improve performance and individual advancement. This pursuit of fulfillment and meaning through health may represent an attempt at order and control in the midst of forces that seem large and unmanageable.[100]

So hydropathy's decline did not mean the end of its principles and ideas. Much of what had once seemed strange and highly irregular advice—to exercise, drink water, bathe regularly, to breathe in fresh air—had become more widely accepted as common sense by the late nineteenth century among a broad swath of Americans, including regular doctors. Some hydropaths continued to practice while still others became homeopaths, joining what had become an increasingly powerful and organized challenge to regular medicine by the time the Civil War broke out. Both hydropaths and homeopaths condemned heroic therapies and believed in more natural remedies and clean living, but homeopaths would take their system to more mystical ends. They also became more powerful. Homeopaths converted untold numbers of regular doctors, opened dozens of medical schools, formed local and national associations, and published journals that rivaled and even bested much of what regular medicine had to offer, earning homeopathy regular medicine's most vitriolic condemnation and the best chance of vanquishing heroic medicine.

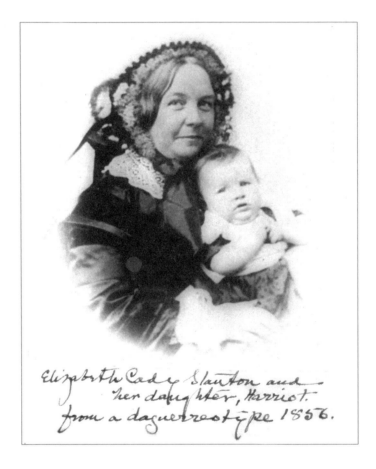

Elizabeth Cady Stanton and her daughter, Harriet. from a daguerreotype 1856.

Elizabeth Cady Stanton first learned about homeopathy in the 1830s, and she quickly became an enthusiastic convert and practitioner of the system, hailing the power it gave women over their health care and their bodies. (Wikimedia Commons)

CHAPTER FOUR

Dilutions of Health
Homeopathy

For Elizabeth Cady Stanton, homeopathy felt like nothing less than liberation. Even better: this freedom could be purchased through the mail. "Dear me, how much cruel bondage of mind and suffering of body poor woman will escape," wrote Stanton to her friend and fellow women's rights advocate Lucretia Mott, "when she takes the liberty of being her own physician of both body and soul."[1] Stanton had first heard about homeopathy from her brother-in-law Edward Bayard in the 1830s. Diagnosed with heart disease, Bayard had received a discouraging prognosis from his New York City doctor. Dismayed by the news, Bayard tried homeopathy at the urging of his wife. Bayard's recovery under the care of homeopath Augustus P. Biegler, using concoctions of diluted drug treatments, so astonished Bayard that he gave up his law practice to devote himself to the study of homeopathy.

Bayard's miraculous turnaround also convinced Stanton to give homeopathy a try. "I have seen wonders in Homeopathy," she reported to her cousin Elizabeth Smith (she of hydropathic wet-dress fame), and "I intend to commence life on Homeopathic principles."[2] She purchased a home homeopathy kit and began doctoring her family, friends, and neighbors in Seneca Falls, New York. Stanton found taking charge of her health incredibly powerful, and she expressed great pride in her self-reliance. She nursed her children through malaria, whooping cough, mumps, and broken limbs with homeopathic therapies. She described the 1852 homeopathic birth of her daughter as an "easy" fifteen-minute labor with a quick recovery. Practicing do-it-yourself homeopathy, Stanton joined the tens of thousands of lay practitioners who, along with formally trained homeopaths, made homeopathy a real and formidable contender to radically reform the practice of medicine.[3]

Despite its egalitarian leanings, homeopathy did not share the populist origins of Thomsonism and hydropathy. Instead, like phrenology, it began with a regular doctor. Homeopathy developed from the experimental pharmacology of disillusioned German physician and scholar Samuel Christian Frederick Hahnemann. Born in Meissen, Germany, in 1755, Hahnemann exhibited a remarkable aptitude for languages from a young age, mastering eight foreign tongues by the age of twenty-four. He used his language skills to finance his medical education in Leipzig, Vienna, and Erlangen, teaching German and French and translating medical, historical, and philosophical works. But by the time of his graduation from the University of Erlangen in 1779, Hahnemann had begun to question the effectiveness of the existing medical system. The medicine he had learned seemed to lack the scientific rigor found in other fields, founded more on superstition than reason.[4] A doctor trying to find a cure for intermittent fever, explained Hahnemann, would logically "turn his attention solely to learn what medicines the experience of bygone ages has discovered." He searches "and to his amazement discovers that an immense number of medicines have been celebrated in intermittent fever. Where is he to begin? Which medicine is he to give first; which next, and which last? He looks round for aid, but no directing angel appears." And even if one remedy did emerge as the clear favorite, Hahnemann complained that the same prescription sent to ten pharmacies resulted in ten different preparations. So the doctor "must hope for the best, and trust to good luck!" He examined common medical treatments for arsenic poisoning and psychiatric disorders and found them far from adequate. Contemporary medicine, declared an exasperated Hahnemann, was far too uncertain to be scientific, "founded upon *perhapses* and blind chance" rather than anything demonstrably provable.[5] Hahnemann became so appalled by the practice of medicine that he abandoned it completely in 1782 and turned to writing and translating scientific texts full-time. He also studied botany, pharmacology, and chemistry, searching for the answers that regular medicine had failed to provide him.[6]

One book seemed to offer a possibility. While translating Scottish physician William Cullen's *A Treatise on the Materia Medica* into German in 1790, Hahnemann became intrigued by Cullen's explanation of how cinchona bark healed malaria. The dried bark of a South American tree, cinchona contained quinine and had been used in Europe since the sixteenth century. It also had the rare distinction of being one of few drugs in common usage with an unquestioned and demonstrative therapeutic value. Cullen claimed that cinchona also strengthened the digestive system, but Hahnemann's own experiences taking cinchona had left him nauseated and sick. Skeptical of Cullen's claim and curious by nature, Hahnemann decided to experiment on himself. Hahnemann hoped his experiments might provide a scientific and rational explanation for how and why this particular drug worked for malaria, which he believed regular medicine sorely lacked.[7]

For several days, Hahnemann ingested large doses of cinchona, taking careful note of its effects on his stomach. The cinchona left him feeling chilled, feverish, weak, and without appetite. He reported that his "feet, finger ends, etc., at first became cold. I grew languid and drowsy; then my heart began to palpitate and my pulse grew hard and small, intolerable anxiety, trembling (but without cold rigour), prostration through all my limbs."[8] The once healthy Hahnemann now appeared to have all the symptoms of malaria. When he stopped his daily dose, the symptoms disappeared. His observations soon led him to conclude that "substances which excite a kind of fever . . . extinguish the types of intermittent fever."[9] Cure a fever with a fever, or like cures like. This epiphany led Hahnemann to articulate what he called the law of similars, or *Similia similibus curantur*. It became the first law of his new system, one that he and later his followers hoped would revolutionize medicine.[10]

An approach to healing based on similars was not new. Hahnemann himself likely knew about it already. Ancient Romans advised the consumption of a raw liver from a rabid dog to cure rabies, and colonial Americans used yellow mustard seeds to ward off yellow fever and jaundice. Even today, the "hair of the dog" after a night of hard drinking could be construed as a homeopathic remedy for a hangover.[11] Heroic medicine, however, saw no necessary correlation between disease and treatment. Most regulars treated fevers with bloodletting and laxatives that produced strong bouts of nausea. Rather than reproducing symptoms, regular therapy sought to eliminate—or, more often, change—the symptoms. Hahnemann argued that this "heterogenous" method attacked healthy organs and weakened the whole system rather than directly targeting and extinguishing the original disease with a similar one "in a prompt and rapid manner."[12] Mimicking the symptoms would cause the body to push out the original disease and substitute the artificial one.[13]

Although Hahnemann had first discovered his theory by swallowing large amounts of cinchona, he wondered if a smaller dose might actually be better. He worried that standard doses magnified a sick person's symptoms to a potentially life-threatening degree. "In illness the body is enormously more sensitive to drugs than in health," asserted Hahnemann.[14] Hahnemann began testing smaller and smaller doses and found that he could still emulate the disease but without aggravating symptoms. In fact, it seemed that the less he gave—even doses as small as a millionth of a gram—the better he could produce an artificial disease with curative effects.[15]

But doses this small could barely be seen much less handled. Hahnemann found a solution in dilutions, or what he later called the law of infinitesimals, in which he dissolved one grain of drug in ninety-nine parts water, alcohol, or lactose. This mixture would then be combined and mixed again, and then combined and mixed again, and so on to the thirtieth dilution, at which point the mixture theoretically contained only $1/10^{60}$ grain of the active substance.[16] Hahnemann believed that this small dose gave the body enough ammunition to reproduce the symptoms of disease but not so much that the body could not quickly rid itself of both the drug and the sickness.[17]

Hahnemann was not the only one to suggest the healing power of small doses. In 1796, English physician Edward Jenner demonstrated that a small amount of cowpox given to otherwise healthy people appeared to produce immunity to smallpox. Hahnemann praised Jenner's breakthrough as an excellent homeopathic example of how a similar disease could prove effective in destroying the original disease. Jenner's method was not exactly homeopathic since it had not undergone dilution and cowpox was a preventative measure rather than a cure for an active disease, but Hahnemann nonetheless saw smallpox vaccination as an affirmation of homeopathic ideas. Despite Hahnemann's approval of the practice, though, vaccination would later prove a divisive and controversial issue among homeopaths wary of the consequences of giving nondilute diseases to otherwise healthy people.[18]

Hahnemann published his initial findings and theory in "Essay on a New Principle for Ascertaining the Curative Power of Drugs, with a Few Glances at Those Hitherto Employed" in 1796. The paper clearly laid out his central idea: "In order to cure diseases, we must search for medicines that can excite a similar disease in the human body."[19] Hahnemann named his new system *homeopathy* from the Greek root *homoios* (like) to emphasize its focus on similars. He had a new name for regular medicine, too: *allopathy*, from the Greek root *allos*, meaning different. Nonhomeopathic irregulars soon adopted the name as well, and allopathy became the common irregular sobriquet for regular medicine.

Reflecting his insistence on scientific discipline, Hahnemann went to painstaking lengths to ensure that his findings and drug trials were rigorous. His procedures presage much of what is standard in clinical trials today. Rather than rely on the superficial comparisons of common origin or physical appearance (yellow mustard for yellow fever, for example) that had informed ancient healing practices based on similars, Hahnemann found matches between the drug and disease through extensive experiments that he called *provings*, from the German word *Prüfung*, for test. He chose the word carefully. Hahnemann wanted to be sure the name illustrated his care in providing the truth to patients. For homeopathy to work, the action of all medicines had to be determined, and the only way to do that, Hahnemann believed, was to test them on healthy people. Hahnemann moved from first testing remedies on himself to testing them on his neighbors. Only after he was absolutely sure of the effects of a substance did he use it on sick patients. This method is now standard in modern medical trials, where new treatments are first used on healthy people to evaluate safety and then the sick to evaluate efficacy. Every substance was tested singly because compounds of two or more ingredients made it impossible to know the effects of the individual substance.[20] To assist in the proving, Hahnemann recruited volunteers and required that they take careful and voluminous notes on every twitch, twinge, and change they experienced during the trials. He advised one of his provers testing *Helleborus niger* to take it "any day when you are well, and have no very urgent business, and have not eaten any medicinal substance (such as parsley) at dinner." He directed him to "take one drop of this to eight ounces of water, and a scruple of alcohol (to prevent its decomposition), shake it briskly, and take an ounce of it while fasting; and so every hour and a half or two hours another ounce, as long as you are not too severely affected by what you take."[21] Because every person was different, many individuals needed to test each remedy and record their symptoms—mental, emotional, and physical—to create a full and accurate proving of all possible effects. "Provers" had to stick to a moderate diet free of spices and alcohol, aside from the scruple used in mixing, and to avoid extreme physical or mental exertion. Each symptom received careful attention as to whether "eating, drinking, talking, coughing, sneezing, or some other bodily function" altered its form. Based on his initial experiments, cinchona became Hahnemann's first remedy.[22]

Testing remedies was an enormous task. Hahnemann and his followers ingested common herbs and minerals, plants, fungi, barks, and shellfish. They examined hops, toadstools, oyster shells, poison ivy, and ragweed. Nearly everything homeopaths added to their healing catalog had been known and used medically for centuries. In every case, they used small doses. Hahnemann came to believe that no substance was poisonous if taken in the proper—tiny—quantity.[23]

Hahnemann published the first compilation of his drug provings, listing medicines and symptoms caused by each, in his 1811 *Materia Medica Pura*. A Latin term, *materia medica* means the body of collected knowledge of substances used for healing—in homeopathy's case, all of the provings. While not specific to any one form of healing, the term is widely used in homeopathy to mean all of the homeopathic remedies. Even as he released the book, Hahnemann emphasized that the testing would never be finished. Hahnemann wanted the homeopathic medicine chest to continue to grow and improve with new discoveries and time. By the end of the nineteenth century, more than seven hundred remedies had been studied and catalogued.[24]

Many regular doctors saw homeopathy as nothing less than absurd. Some took issue with Hahnemann's provings. They claimed his results invalid because he did not compare the reactions of his provers with a control group not taking drugs. That no such tests likely existed for most if not all heroic therapies appears not to have bothered most regulars, who often demonstrated a hypocritical blindness to the unscientific and speculative nature of their own techniques. Regulars prescribed drugs and performed treatments without the kinds of detailed observations and studies done by homeopaths, and almost certainly did not employ control groups to determine the efficacy or benefit of their depletive methods. Hahnemann's precise methods of observations and exactness in accumulating data, while lacking the randomization and blinding of trials today, provided a level of testing virtually unheard of in eighteenth- and nineteenth-century medicine, and made homeopathy appear far more scientific than contemporary regular medicine.[25]

Others ridiculed the symptom lists in the *Materia Medica Pura* with its pages describing "yawning and stretching," "easily falls asleep when reading," and "an excessive liability to become pregnant." Other remedies seemed to produce contradictory results. What was a doctor to do when faced with several drugs causing both constipation and diarrhea, impotence and excessive sexual desire? The extraordinary detail given to each symptom required an almost superhuman degree of self-awareness. Not to mention that not all provers reported the same symptoms from the same substances. The flowering plant aconite, also known as monkshood, for instance, could produce headaches that felt like your eyes might fall out or ones that felt like your brain was being moved by burning water—both headaches but with very different feelings that could be difficult to identify. It also caused "distraction of the attention when reading and writing," and "dryness of the upper eye lids." Each remedy produced a staggering number of symptoms, from ninety-seven on the low end to more than a thousand on the other extreme. To Hahnemann, though, the details that regulars found so ridiculous distinguished the homeopathic approach and provided the keys to its efficacy. Regular medicine was far too general to be helpful, he argued, lacking the crucial details that made each sick person's case unique and ultimately, treatable.[26]

If the symptoms struck regular doctors as ridiculous, the homeopathic dilutions made them virtually apoplectic. They argued that dilutions of these magnitudes made it statistically improbable that any of the original substance even remained in the dilution. The law of infinitesimals seemed to defy Avogadro's number, which set the point in the dilution process where a molecule in any given substance could no longer theoretically exist.[27] "Either Hahnemann is right, in which case our science and the basis of our thinking is nonsense, or he is wrong, in which case this teaching is nonsense," declared German physician T. Jurgensen.[28] It comes as no surprise that the astute Oliver Wendell Holmes questioned the rationality of anyone who believed that a man with a mortar and pestle could "take a little speck of some substance which nobody ever thought to have any smell at all, as, for instance, a grain of chalk or of charcoal, and that he will, after an hour or two of rubbing and scraping, develop in a portion of it an odor, which, if the whole grain were used, would be capable of pervading an apartment, a house, a village, a province, an empire, nay the entire atmosphere of this broad planet upon which we tread." Those who subscribed to such views, Holmes declared, were simply "incapable of reasoning."[29] Regular physician Eli Geddings was a little more generous, expressing his skepticism that small doses would work but concluding that homeopathy could prove a blessing for lessening upset stomachs.[30]

Small doses also jarred against a culture that expected a big effect from drugs. Regulars frequently prescribed drugs by the spoonful, not by the fraction of a gram. If patients didn't bleed, vomit, or blister, how would they know they were getting better? Hahnemann and his followers took the radical position of arguing that healing didn't have to hurt. They advocated for treatments that gave patients little or no feeling of physiological or physical change because healing, they argued, had nothing to do with the physical material of the remedy. Nor was disease a physical entity.[31]

Homeopathy, like many other eighteenth- and nineteenth-century medical theories, including regular medicine, was a vitalist system. Advocates believed that disease resulted from an imbalance or blockage of the body's invisible but powerful life force. Symptoms were "the product of the disease itself," but they were not themselves the actual disease. "There does not exist a single disease that can have a material principle for its cause," wrote Hahnemann. "On the contrary, all of them are solely and always the special result of an actual and dynamic derangement in the state of health."[32]

Hahnemann did not believe that the body could defeat disease and restore its balance on its own. He, like many of his regular contemporaries, discounted the body's natural healing power, believing it crude and imperfect. Setting aside nature, Hahnemann claimed that the body's "native army" could only defeat the "enemy" with the firepower of the homeopathic remedy he called the "auxiliary troops." "It is the organic vital force of our bodies which itself cures natural diseases of all kinds," declared Hahnemann, "whenever, by means of the proper homeopathic medicines, it is placed in a position to conquer, which, indeed, it never could do without the auxiliary force." In other words, the homeopathic remedy gave the vital spirit the firepower to defeat illness. Small doses, Hahnemann argued, so small the material substance may not have even existed anymore, did not matter. What mattered was the remedy's spirit-like dynamic energy that bolstered, mingled, and restored the body's own invisible vital force, this energy being the most effective means of reaching and acting on the energy of the body.

Dilution alone could not activate a remedy's energy. Hahnemann's experiments led him to conclude that a medication must be shaken, rubbed, and banged against a leather pad to transform from its crude form to one energized by its "inner medicinal essence." Only then would it be ready to work with the body's vital force. Hahnemann referred to this process of dilution and strengthening as "dynamization." So even as the effectiveness of the diluted remedies seemed to defy logic, homeopaths believed that the solution "remembered" its former self, which gave it a liquid potency that made healing possible.[33] Hahnemann's firm belief in the unlikely power of small doses led him to call these extreme dilutions "high potencies."[34]

Patients could not sit idly by and wait for homeopathy to marshal the body's native army alone. Hahnemann expected patients to be familiar with homeopathic theory and to have read his 1810 homeopathic manual *Organon of the Rational Art of Healing*. Composed in 271 aphorisms, the book fully laid out his principles and theories, gave directions for use, and offered guidance for doctors on how to detail their cases. Proper homeopathic prescribing relied on patients' awareness and articulation of their illness experiences, including their emotions. For many women, this attention during their exam was the first time medicine validated their feelings and experiences of their own bodies.[35] Patients also followed certain protocols before, during, and after treatment for best results. Diets received particular attention as Hahnemann believed that certain foods could adversely affect the medicine's power. "It may be readily conceived that everything which exercises a medicinal influence on the patient should be removed from his regimen and mode of life," counseled Hahnemann, "in order that the effects of such minute doses may not be destroyed, overpowered, or disturbed by any foreign stimulant."[36] Acute diseases had very specific rules, while those suffering from chronic illnesses followed more general guidelines largely aimed at the elimination of foods that kindled disease. Forbidden foods included smoked meat and fish, duck, turtle, sausages, pastries of any kind, sugar, cinnamon, and alcohol. And if anyone needed a reminder to not eat rotten food, rancid cheese and butter were also prohibited.[37]

Hahnemann had a particular problem with coffee. He drew clear distinctions between "food" and "medicine." "Medicinal things are substances that do not nourish, but alter the healthy condition of the body," wrote Hahnemann. Medicine taken unnecessarily by healthy people "deranges the harmonious concordance of our organs, undermines health and shortens life." For Hahnemann, coffee fell squarely into this category of medicinal food. Worse, many people drank coffee daily and certainly in amounts far larger than a safe infinitesimal dose. Hahnemann came to blame the beverage for nearly all chronic suffering and general ill health.[38]

Two decades later, in 1828, Hahnemann changed his mind. He realized that perhaps he'd been too hasty in his condemnation of coffee, as his observations revealed the inadequacy of homeopathy in treating chronic sufferers, even among the coffee abstainers. Rather than discounting what he witnessed or rationalizing his data to fit his theory, Hahnemann altered his hypothesis to account for his observations: a very scientific approach to the problem. While he wasn't ready to fully embrace coffee, he would allow that maybe it wasn't the principle cause of suffering. Chronic diseases, Hahnemann now explained, stemmed from deep disturbances of the body's vital forces known as "miasms." Contagious and hereditary, these miasms surfaced when people lived in unhealthy states for extended periods of time, and their presence pointed to a more fundamental problem in the body than the current illness. Hahnemann's miasms bore much in common with the ancient idea of contagion from miasma, or bad air, filled with malodorous and poisonous particles much discussed by Hippocrates. Hahnemann divided his miasms into three primal types: syphilis, sycosis, and psora. Syphilis caused many diseases of the nervous system and sycosis many sexual diseases and joint infections. Hahnemann labeled psora the "oldest, most universal and most pernicious," having existed for thousands of years and causing seven-eighths of all chronic illnesses. Characterized by skin eruptions that reflected the inner diseased state, Hahnemann blamed psora for hysteria, epilepsy, gout, cancer, impotence, mania, and countless other afflictions. Because of the deep-seated nature of these miasms, treatment could take weeks longer than acute cases and required patients to take short whiffs of diluted remedies so as to not overwhelm their severely debilitated systems.[39]

Hahnemann's new theory of miasms did not sit well with many of his followers. Encouraged to think critically by homeopathic theory and Hahnemann himself, homeopaths demanded that Hahnemann further clarify its principles before they would incorporate it into their treatment regimen. Hahnemann refused. "He who does not walk on exactly the same line with me is an apostate and a traitor, and with him I will have nothing to say," declared Hahnemann in a pompous tone not unlike that of Thomson before him. These hostile remarks led some homeopaths to split with him, declaring their old leader, now in his seventies, past his prime. But they did not abandon homeopathy. Followers pledged to stick with their original convictions and to ignore what they saw as Hahnemann's more irrational claims.[40]

These internal divisions did nothing to slow homeopathy's rapid colonization of Europe. Regular doctors from across the continent, many of them young and just starting out in the field, flocked to Hahnemann to receive personal tutorials in homeopathic therapy. They returned home and set up clinics of their own and taught homeopathy to colleagues. Homeopathy also caught on with the European aristocracy, who hungered for the newest and most scientific innovations. Members of the German and British royal families patronized several homeopaths, including Hahnemann himself.[41]

Though it was created to wipe out sickness, it was, ironically, epidemic disease that enhanced homeopathy's reputation and contributed to its explosion in popularity. During an outbreak of cholera in Europe in 1831, Hahnemann advised sufferers to take homeopathic doses of camphor (from the camphor tree), cuprum (copper), and veratrum (a plant commonly known as false hellebores). He also prescribed fresh air and frequent baths for the healthy, and advised the quarantine of those who had already contracted the disease. Since the primary treatment for cholera is rehydration, Hahnemann's wa-

tered-down cures likely helped to replace some lost fluids while isolation and his hygiene recommendation prevented its spread. These
relatively benign remedies contrasted sharply with treatments by
regular doctors, whose harsh and largely ineffective heroic response
with purging and bleeding likely only hastened dehydration and did
little to heal or win the confidence of people seeking relief. Although
Hahnemann knew no more about the cause and proper treatment of
cholera than regulars, the relative success of his method and higher
survival rate of his patients played a major role in winning homeopathy additional friends and supporters on both sides of the Atlantic in
the 1830s and 1840s.[42]

Late in his life, Hahnemann surprised his followers by marrying
French artist Marie Melanie d'Hervilly and moving from his German
home in Kothen to Paris in 1835. Hahnemann established a lucrative
practice in an elegant mansion and taught homeopathy to his new
wife, who soon began practicing by his side. Controversial until the
end, even with his aristocratic clientele, Hahnemann found himself
defending his theory and his method until his death in 1843.[43]

Homeopathy arrived in the United States with Hans Burch Gram
in 1825. Born in Boston but trained in Europe, Gram first learned of
homeopathy while studying medicine at the Royal Medical and Surgical Institute in Copenhagen. Returning to the United States, Gram
established a successful homeopathic practice in New York City and
created an apprenticeship program to train the first generation of
American homeopaths. But Gram's New York City enterprise was
soon eclipsed by activity in Philadelphia, which emerged as the first
true center of American homeopathy thanks largely to the efforts of
several German immigrants.[44]

By far the most influential of these immigrants was Constantine
Hering, who became known as the father of homeopathy in America. Hering first learned of homeopathy as a medical student at the
University of Leipzig in the 1820s, where he received a commission
to write a book refuting Hahnemann and his theories. Rather than
disagree with Hahnemann, though, Hering found himself impressed
with Hahnemann's work and homeopathy's potential. His convictions
strengthened after he contracted a severe infection in his finger after
an autopsy. The wound became so bad that amputation seemed all
but necessary until a friend persuaded Hering to try a homeopathic

dose of arsenic as a last resort. His infection resolved and led Hering, grateful for his ten fingers, to declare, "The last veil that blinded my eyes to the light of the rising sun was rent and I saw the light of the new healing art dawn upon me in all its fullness. I owed to it far more than the preservation of a finger. To Hahnemann, who saved my finger, I gave my whole hand and to the promulgation of his teachings not only my hand, but the entire man, body and soul."[45] He soon abandoned regular medicine for homeopathy and joined a zoological expedition to South America, where he carried out provings on a variety of plants and animals on the side, including a particularly risky trial with snake venom.[46]

Hering first heard stories about the bushmaster, the largest poisonous snake in the New World, while encamped in the Amazon Basin in Suriname in 1828. A zealous convert to his new system, Hering reasoned that the snake's lethal venom might be beneficial in infinitesimal doses, so he paid locals to capture a snake so he could collect its deadly saliva for observation. The venom was so toxic that even the process of preparing and diluting the poison for homeopathic dosing made him delirious. Hering mixed the venom with lactose and conducted a proving on himself while his poor wife recorded the results. He woke up the next morning lucky to be alive. Fever, delirium, and a "frantic struggle for breath" were just a few of the symptoms she listed. The venom Hering collected became the first snake poison ever researched for medical purposes. Even today, doctors and researchers continue to study the usefulness of snake venom and poisonous animals in medicine.[47]

Hering and his alcohol-preserved bushmaster arrived in Philadelphia in 1833. Finding a handful of like-minded immigrant homeopaths in his new city, he quickly organized the Hahnemann Society, the nation's first homeopathic medical organization. Two years later, he became president of the world's first homeopathic medical school, the North American Academy of the Homeopathic Healing Art, in Allentown, Pennsylvania. Instruction, conducted entirely in German, included lectures on medical botany, dietetics, surgery, obstetrics, anatomy, physiology, and the history of medicine. Financial difficulties forced the school to close in 1842, but not before sending out a host of evangelistic graduates eager to carry the homeopathic faith to the rest of the country.[48]

Hering went on to found several other homeopathic schools, including the Homeopathic Medical College of Pennsylvania in 1848, which became the national leader in homeopathic education. Twenty years later, in 1869, the school merged with another homeopathic school to become the Hahnemann Medical College of Philadelphia with Hering as dean and chair of materia medica. Homeopathic instruction continued at the school into the 1950s, a lasting vestige of the school's origins and a reflection of the strength of homeopathy as a medical practice into the twentieth century. Besides his educational endeavors, Hering continued to experiment with remarkably risky provings. In 1849, he experimented with the newly discovered explosive nitroglycerine, curious about its possible therapeutic value for headaches after learning of Italian scientist Ascanio Sobrero's observations that it produced throbbing, violent head pain when placed on the tongue. He confirmed the effect in his volunteers with dilutions of less than one three hundredth of a drop. Hering also reported changes to the pulse, observing that nitroglycerin caused "contraction" and "oppression" of the chest. Decades later, regular doctors adopted nitroglycerine as a treatment for the chest pains associated with heart disease, for which it is still widely used today. Hering also wrote more than forty books on homeopathy, the most important of which was the popular home-health manual *The Homeopathic Domestic Physician*. The book found a wide audience among regular doctors interested in learning about homeopathy as well.[49]

The number of homeopaths in the United States expanded rapidly. By 1860, the nation had more than two thousand practitioners. They formed local and state organizations and in 1844 established the first national medical organization, the American Institute of Homeopathy (AIH), to improve the quality of the field. Constantine Hering became its first president. It surely wounded many regular doctors' pride to see one of their supposedly unscientific rivals forming an organization to implement standards and improve medical practice before they had organized to do the same.[50] Three years later, in 1847, regular doctors established their own national organization, the American Medical Association.

While the AMA may not have explicitly formed to fight homeopathy, it's not hard to imagine that motivation behind the organization's actions. One of the AMA's first orders of business was to effectively ban homeopaths from ever becoming members by rejecting a homeopathic education as unscientific and inadequate to the task of training doctors. This despite the fact that the content of homeopathy's two-year training program was nearly identical to that of regular medicine. Homeopaths' understandings of bodily function and how to find and study disease did not differ from those of their regular peers. Even more, before 1860, the majority of homeopaths were regulars who had converted or those who offered a mixed practice of heroic and homeo-pathic therapies.[51]

Education was a serious matter for homeopaths, who organized the American Institute of Homeopathy in part to improve training and standards. They particularly wanted to reign in "physicians from pretending to be competent to practice homeopathy who have not studied it in a careful and skillful manner."[52] Homeopathic schools opened all over the country, more than twenty by the end of the nine-teenth century. The majority also admitted women, unlike regular medical schools, though some homeopaths did share the conviction of regulars that women were better served by female medical colleges. Only a year after its founding, the AIH resolved to admit only mem-bers who had completed a "regular course of medical studies," homeo-pathic or regular, and who had passed an examination, far stricter criteria than existed for membership in the AMA.[53]

Soon after forming, the AMA passed a code of ethics barring members from even consulting or associating with homeopaths at the risk of expulsion from the organization. It was no idle threat. "No one can be considered as a regular practitioner, or a fit associate in consultation, whose practice is based upon an exclusive dogma, to the rejection of the accumulated experience of the profession," read the code.[54] One Connecticut doctor was ousted from his local medical society after talking over a case with his wife, who was studying to become a homeopath. One observer wryly noted that his error might have been overlooked "had he consulted with another man's wife upon topics not purely medical." Another was expelled for purchasing milk sugar, a standard dilution ingredient, from his local apothecary.[55] Anyone calling him- or herself a homeopath was deemed "unfit" for consultation on patient care, even if it came at the patient's request. At the same time, no regular doctor could serve a patient under the care of a homeopath until the homeopath was dismissed, no mat-ter how desperate the situation and need for assistance. Local and state medical societies held meetings to determine if regular doctors who had converted to homeopathy should be allowed to retain their membership; most voted no. The Medical Society of the County of New York, which had gone so far as to give Hahnemann an honorary membership in the organization, rescinded the honor a few years later as homeopathy's ideological and financial threat to regular medicine grew more apparent.[56] From the 1850s onward, medical societies used the consultation clause to successfully keep homeopaths from practicing in publicly funded medical institutions, medical schools, and the medical departments of the military.[57]

The AIH took a far more restrained and tolerant approach to regular medicine. That's not say that some members did not want to extinguish regulars, but the AIH never became a vehicle for launching attacks. Most of the first AIH members graduated from regular medical schools and considered themselves equal to their regular peers. They tended to view homeopathy as a specialty requiring additional training on top of the basic medical education in anatomy and body function rather than a wholly separate form of medicine. Homeopaths also avoided confrontation with regulars to set themselves apart from other irregular healers who routinely derided regular medicine as a matter of course. Continually denigrating regular medicine, determined the leaders of the AIH, would not further homeopathy's mission. To maintain the dignity of homeopathy, the AIH passed resolutions urging respect in speeches and writing and discouraging actions and words unbecoming to members of a professional scientific field. Dr. Jabez P. Dake reminded members at an 1858 AIH meeting in New York that "we can never expect charitable and kindly treatment from others unless we exhibit it ourselves."[58]

Most Americans, however, did not know or did not care that there was any difference between the two types of doctors. They cared only who made them feel better, and if they could do so without the painful side effects, all the better. Homeopaths advertised better cure rates for all diseases than regular medicine. Whether or not their cures actually worked, homeopathy likely did far less to inhibit recovery than regular doctors with their courses of bleeding, purging, and blistering. Homeopathic remedies also tasted better and cost less despite the labor involved in mixing and diluting, so more people could afford to try them. The mildness of Hahnemann's remedies made them especially useful for treating young children. Constantine Hering observed that children would no longer need to be bribed with money or cookies to "drink the nasty dose."[59]

Homeopathy's style proved as attractive as its pleasant flavors. Patients loved the personal attention they received from homeopaths in appointments that often lasted an hour or more and frequently covered everything from medical symptoms to sleep patterns, clothing preferences, exercise regimens, and eating habits. Hahnemann encouraged homeopaths to develop interview techniques to construct vivid pictures of their patients and to learn the peculiarities of each medicine by experimenting on themselves. "The key to the individuality of each patient is not found in the symptoms he has in common with others, but in those which distinguish him from others," wrote Hahnemann.[60] Doctors listened attentively to every patient complaint so they could prescribe remedies tailored to every symptom down to its finest subtlety. A gnawing hunger called for a different remedy than a gnawing in the stomach; a shooting pain in the left arm differed from a twitching of the same arm. Thorough examinations set the homeopath apart from the regular doctor, who, according to Hahnemann, did not "deign to investigate the case of disease thoroughly, but generalizes it in an off-hand way to suit his own convenience, labels it with one of his systematic names, and invests a treatment to correspond."[61] Homeopaths faulted regular doctors for cramming as many appointments into a single day as they could to maximize profits, which led to hasty, one-size-fits-all prescribing rather than the individualized medicine that made homeopathy so attractive and, they claimed, so effective.

Perhaps even more than the personal attention, though, Americans loved that homeopaths gave them the power to treat themselves. Taking a page from Samuel Thomson's botanic book, homeopaths offered home health tools to lay practitioners in the form of instructional manuals and medical kits. Home health guides and kits produced by both regular and irregular healers became fairly common by the middle of the nineteenth century. Most contained laborious instructions for preparing and consuming medicines made from roots, herbs, or common household products. The homeopathy kit was different: it came with bottles of ready-to-use remedies. Unlike Thomsonism, which approached nearly every sickness with the same six-step regimen, homeopathy provided a specific remedy for specific complaints. The accompanying guide helped users identify symptoms and corresponding remedies. The kits cost between two and ten dollars and ranged in size from a small pocket case for individual use to large chests for treating the whole family. Having prepared medicines right at hand, like today's over-the-counter remedies, allowed anyone to diagnose and treat quickly. These kits were not intended to replace doctors, however. Unlike the Thomsonians who disdained formal medical training and wanted to put doctors out of business, or even the hydropaths, who drew no distinction between formal and self-taught practitioners, homeopaths intended their kits for use on uncomplicated illnesses or in the absence or unavailability of trained homeopaths.[62]

Thousands of homeopathy kits were sold, most from local pharmacies. Typical of his prominence in American homeopathy, Constantine Hering produced the first and most popular homeopathic text and kit in the 1830s. Hering's kit cost five dollars and came with a copy of his book *The Homeopathic Domestic Physician* and a small box of forty-six numbered remedies keyed to the book. He instructed users suffering from multiple complaints to look up every symptom before deciding on a remedy. He then offered directions for administering doses and the health regimen to follow, including regular baths and exercise, to ensure best results. Homeopaths embraced hygiene and dietary reform as both complements to healing and good preventative medicine. Most of these practices came from outside homeopathy, but the additions made homeopathy much more appealing and relevant to patients, many of whom were already practicing vegetarianism, temperance, hydropathy, and other lifestyle reforms. In all, Americans had their choice of more than thirty homeopathic manuals and kits, reflecting the immense interest in and popularity of homeopathy among the public.[63]

Homeopathic kits served as advance agents and popularizers of homeopathic principles. The authors and creators of domestic texts and kits became household names and their services were highly sought after by patients. This was particularly helpful for winning converts among women, who had long served as the caretakers of family health. The kits seemed to work. In 1869, the American Institute of Homeopathy estimated that nearly two-thirds of homeopathy's adult patients were women. The benefits were not completely one-sided in favor of the homeopaths, though. Armed with a homeopathic kit, women found an empowering public role beyond their immediate homes as health providers for their communities, as Elizabeth Cady Stanton discovered in her own life.[64]

Not every homeopath supported the sale and use of home medical kits, however. Even as they recognized the importance of the kits in attracting followers, some homeopaths worried that the kits made them look like quacks rather than medical professionals. Some wondered if the use of vials of premixed remedies to popularize domestic homeopathy had degraded their true mission to personalize medical science. They also recognized that too much self-reliance on the part of their patients had a detrimental effect on their pocketbooks. By the mid-nineteenth century, some homeopaths encouraged the publication of guides for use by professional homeopaths only.[65]

Meanwhile, homeopaths attended to and won converts among some of the most prominent members of American society. Businessman John D. Rockefeller; President Grant's vice president, Schuyler Colfax; Lincoln's secretary of state, William Seward; and President James Garfield all used homeopathy. Many were drawn to the scientific foundation of homeopathy, even if they could not explain how or why it worked. All that really mattered was their positive experience with homeopathic remedies. New England transcendentalists such as educator Bronson Alcott, abolitionist William Lloyd Garrison, educator Elizabeth Peabody, and poet Henry Wadsworth Longfellow became some of homeopathy's earliest supporters. They liked its metaphysical emphasis on sense perception as well as physical pain in the process of discovering and determining patient care. Transcendentalists as a group tended to oppose institutions that fostered inequalities in education and status and to support those that encouraged self-direction and self-knowledge, which made them, in many ways, natural allies of irregular medicine. Hahnemann's attention to the mental and physical symptoms of disease and the spiritual essence of his healing substances, as well as homeopathy's domestic use, seemed to mesh perfectly with the transcendental worldview. Homeopathy's connections and relationships with these well-known Americans made for lucrative practices and proved marketing gold for well-connected practitioners.[66]

Among the many writers to seek help from homeopathy was

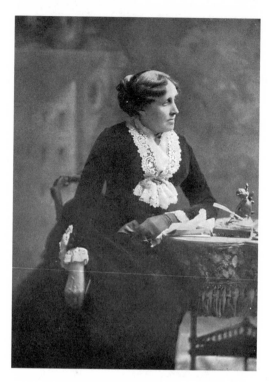

Writer Louisa May Alcott found relief for her chronic ill health in homeopathy. (Wikimedia Commons)

Louisa May Alcott, who relied heavily on Boston homeopath Conrad Wesselhoeft (the son of Brattleboro hydropath Robert Wesselhoeft) for her chronic pain. Given mercury for typhoid fever in the early 1860s, Alcott believed, not unreasonably, that it had ruined her health and caused her near continuous pain. Alcott experimented with a variety of forms of pain relief, including mesmerism and botanicals, but found the most consistent and lasting relief in homeopathy. Alcott kept careful track of symptoms throughout her life, and more recent studies of her illness have suggested that she may have actually had systemic lupus erythematosus, the most common form of the disease. The relief she found in homeopathy was likely a placebo effect as the disease has no cure, though the remedies may have helped lessen inflammatory flare-ups if she did have lupus. So enamored was she with homeopathy's powers, Alcott even wrote it into her stories. When Beth falls ill with scarlet fever in *Little Women*, her older sister Jo prescribes homeopathic Belladonna, one of the earliest homeopathic remedies, as treatment. Regular doctors usually treated scarlet fever with bleeding in an attempt to relieve the flush of the patient's skin that gave the disease its name. Alcott also dedicated her final novel, *Jo's Boys*, to Wesselhoeft. In the book, Jo's student Nan treats a dog bite with a homeopathic remedy. A bright and "scientifically minded" girl, Nan later decides to use her skills to pursue a career as a homeopathic physician.[67]

That's just the kind of message author Elizabeth Stuart Phelps hoped to send to other women as well. In 1867, the twenty-three-year-old Phelps decried the misery of the American woman burdened with unrewarding housework or leisured idleness. Her writings posed the arguments of *The Feminine Mystique* nearly a century before Betty Friedan. "Next to ill-health, the principal cause of women's unhappiness—for women are not happy—is the want of something to do," she wrote. "Whether for self-support, or for pure employment's sake, the search for work—for successful work, for congenial work—is at the bottom of half the feminine miseries of the world."[68] Phelps's essay proposed some potential career paths for women to consider—a few less than thrilling options like filling out insurance policies and trimming bonnets among them—but she saved her greatest praise and encouragement for women in medicine: "Be a doctor? And be sure that you could be few things more womanly or more noble."[69] Phelps returned to the topic of women in medicine again and again in essays, columns, letters, and short stories; few were as vocal in their call to increase the number of women in medicine. Homeopathy's receptiveness to aspiring women practitioners drew Phelps's enthusiastic praise and personal devotion to its tenets. Her 1882 novel *Dr. Zay* featured a strong and capable woman who dedicates her life to homeopathic medicine and social reform. So great was Phelps's love of homeopathy that she even named her dog after Hahnemann.[70]

But while many women practiced homeopathy, membership in the American Institute of Homeopathy remained closed to them for several decades. That had not stopped women from applying for admittance to local and state societies, where membership validated their professional skills and more generally granted them full participation in their professions. American homeopaths tended to see women as useful allies in their fight against regular medicine, so many male homeopaths encouraged, or at the very least tolerated, the greater activism and involvement of women in homeopathy, while regular doctors remained largely unwelcoming to female practitioners. Even so, many male homeopaths worried that admitting women into the AIH would discourage men from joining the field and harm its reputation among the general public. Finally, in 1869, George W. Swazey, president of the Massachusetts Homeopathic Medical Society, put the "woman question" up to a vote at the annual meeting of the AIH. Only two years earlier, members had denied a woman's application for membership by a close vote. Rather than let the issue continue to hang over them, Swazey pushed for an official decision. Swazey chose not to frame the issue as a matter of equality but rather as an official recognition of the prominent place women already had attained in the field. "The question is whether, after having encouraged women to enter the profession, educated them, taken their money, permitted them to practice, and fraternized with them, we shall now debar them from the privilege of our larger institutions," declared Swazey.[71] A majority agreed with him and cast their votes in favor of women's admission the following year.[72] The American Medical Association, in contrast, would not admit its first female members until 1915, almost fifty years later.[73]

Once the doors to the AIH opened to them in 1871, women became active participants in the organization, presenting papers, chairing committees, and enlarging the materia medica with drugs specifically tested on women. American homeopaths had begun calling for more comprehensive testing on women in the 1830s and 1840s to improve and upgrade the provings. Homeopaths believed that sexual differences made men and women react differently to the same medications, so to treat women effectively, women had to be enlisted in the essential work of testing. It was an unprecedented step at a time when women's health was rarely discussed, much less seriously considered and extensively researched. The provings gave women a specific framework in which they could make important contributions to the science of the profession. The inclusion of women in testing homeopathic drugs from its early days made homeopathy particularly appealing to twentieth-century feminists, who were often critical of women's exclusion from drug trials in the United States. Not until 1993 did the National Institutes of Health mandate the inclusion of women in clinical trials, more than a century after homeopathy.[74]

Among the first women to join the AIH was Philadelphia homeopath Harriet Judd Sartain. Born in Waterbury, Connecticut, in 1830, Sartain enrolled at the American Hydropathic Institute in New York City at the urging of her aunt and uncle. There, she fell under the instruction and counsel of Mary Gove Nichols, who likely encouraged her pursuit of a medical career. After her term at the Hydropathic Institute, Sartain went on to Cincinnati's Eclectic Medical Institute. One of the country's best-known and largest medical schools outside of New York and Philadelphia, the school was also one of the few places where women could earn a medical degree in the 1850s. It was here that Sartain likely learned about homeopathy, the field in which she would ultimately take a leading role. If anyone doubted Sartain's commitment to her career, it was certainly not her eventual husband, Samuel, whom she rebuffed after his initial offer of marriage in July of 1854. "Now my plans for the future. First to outlive the objections against me here [in Waterbury] as a Physician and to establish myself in my profession," she declared. "I must be an independent woman, able to stand alone."[75]

Although she eventually gave in to Samuel's proposal, Sartain did not relinquish her professional ambitions. She soon had a thriving homeopathic practice in Philadelphia, the largest of any female medical practitioner in the city and one of the most successful operations in the city, male or female, regular or irregular. She became one of the founding members of her county homeopathic medical society and, one year later, the first woman elected to the Pennsylvania State Homeopathic Society. Even with her successful practice and membership in these organizations, Sartain, and women like her, continued to face some discrimination from her homeopathic peers. In 1883, Sartain founded the Women's Homeopathic Medical Club of Philadelphia, largely in protest of the all-male Hahnemann Medical College of Philadelphia, which remained closed to women until 1941 despite repeated appeals from female homeopaths. School administrators recognized the importance of women in the profession but feared that coeducation would discourage male applicants and cause a decline in the financial support they depended on for survival. Separate organizations for female homeopaths were the exception, though, and by the 1880s, nine of the nation's eleven homeopathic colleges admitted women. Most women preferred direct involvement in coeducational homeopathic institutions and found acceptance, albeit begrudgingly in some cases, in their profession's formerly all-male medical organizations.[76]

The battles within homeopathy paled beside the growing war against it in regular medicine, though. Besides barring homeopaths from membership in their medical organizations, regular doctors attempted to cripple homeopathy with words, so much so that the anti-homeopathy screed became virtually its own literary genre. One of the earliest and most famous attacks came in 1842 from irregular medicine's most eloquent and ardent foe, the irrepressible Oliver Wendell Holmes. Over the course of two lectures on the subject of "Homeopathy and Its Kindred Delusions" delivered before the Boston Society for the Diffusion of Useful Knowledge, Holmes dealt a devastating blow to homeopathy as he picked apart Hahnemann's theories and found them lacking, to say the least. "When one man claims to have established three independent truths [like cures like, high dilutions, and the psora] which are about as remote from each other as the discovery of the law of gravitation, the invention of printing, and that of the mariner's compass, unless the facts are overwhelming and unanimous," he proclaimed, "the question naturally arises, Is not this man deceiving himself, or trying to deceive others?" Hahnemann's claim that smaller doses exerted larger effects was to Holmes like saying that a "pebble may produce a mountain." Homeopathic doses were so dilute, he argued, as to be the equivalent of doing nothing at all. Fortunately for homeopaths, Holmes noted that the vast majority of patients under any form of treatment will eventually recover. So advocates of every system, homeopathy included, asserted Holmes, could thus claim to cure a large number of patients regardless of scientific proof of efficacy.

Holmes also investigated the validity of Hahnemann's use of ancient authors and texts to support and give lineage to his doctrines. A cursory examination led Holmes to conclude that Hahnemann had cherry-picked and exaggerated the evidence. Worse, he cited texts inappropriate for medical use to prove his points. Taking Hahnemann's assertion that the smell of a rose can both cause and cure fainting as an example, Holmes noted, with obvious disbelief, that Hahnemann quoted that fact "from one of the last sources one would have looked to for medical information, the Byzantine Historians." Hahnemann's reference to how Princess Eudosia restored a person who had fainted with rosewater struck Holmes as "pedantic folly" if Hahnemann saw "confirmation of his doctrine in such a recovery as this." To Holmes, homeopathy was a "pretended science" comprised of little more than a "mingled mass of perverse ingenuity, of tinsel erudition, of imbecile credulity, and of artful misrepresentation."[77]

Much of the ink and anger aimed at homeopaths came from the growing threat that the field posed to regular medicine. Homeopathy's popularity among middle- and upper-class Americans decreased the earnings and influence of regular doctors among the very people they most wanted as patients. It also incensed regulars that educated Americans with common sense and money to spend would chose homeopathy over them. Homeopaths themselves were not the poorly educated—and thus easily dismissed—frontiersmen who practiced Thomsonism. While regulars lambasted homeopathic theory as absurd, they were not blind to the popular appeal of its painless approach to healing. Even Holmes, troubled by the slow progress of medical science, could acknowledge the deficiencies of his own brand of medicine. "I firmly believe that if the materia medica, as now used, could be sunk to the bottom of the sea, it would be better for mankind, and all the worse for the fishes," he wrote in the 1870s. While he still believed homeopathy ridiculous, Holmes did offer backhanded praise. Homeopathy's dilute "no remedy" remedy served as a "lesson of the healing faculty of Nature," an important and much-needed reminder to regular doctors.[78] Moreover, homeopathy took an approach to investigation and research that had a better claim to science than the mostly trial-and-error assessments of bloodletting and calomel. Until regular medicine offered more effective treatments, homeopathy only continued to gain adherents and power.[79]

By the 1880s, some regular doctors had begun to ignore the AMA's ban on consulting with homeopaths. A few even suggested the ban should be lifted. Some homeopathic remedies also made it onto the prescription pads of regulars in the second half of the nineteenth century. Popular remedies in both regular and homeopathic fields included arnica for pain relief; rhus for rheumatism and skin disorders; nux vomica for digestive disorders, heart disease, and nerve conditions; and pulsatilla for menstrual cramps, testicular swelling, insomnia, and tension headaches. Regulars routinely gave rhubarb and ipecac for dysentery, aconite for fever, and nitric and muriatic acid for chronic stomach inflammation, treatments common in homeopathy, though usually in diluted form.[80] At the same time, though, several scientific discoveries began to change the medical playing field. The germ theory of disease, the introduction of sterile surgery, advances in lab science more generally, and the discovery of a bacterial cause for diseases such as anthrax, conjunctivitis, and tuberculosis seemed to prove that illness did not spring spontaneously from bad air or from spiritual disruptions.[81] Many regulars hoped that these new discoveries would finally separate the legitimate doctors—themselves—from what they considered the obvious quackery of homeopathy in the public eye.

Against these new scientific discoveries homeopathy began to question itself and its practices. Was the psora the same as germs? How did the vital force relate to the germ theory? What role did lab tests play in diagnoses? Some homeopaths did not think any revisions or reconsiderations of homeopathic theory were necessary. If the remedies worked, and they felt they obviously did, why should homeopathy change? Communication between the doctor and patient structured the examination and determined the therapy. Nothing else was necessary or important, pure homeopaths argued. More practically, though, these medical advances did pose challenges to certain structural elements of the field. Lab science seemed to threaten the very methods and therapies that made homeopathy distinct (and so attractive to patients) by turning attention away from the individual and toward impersonal and reductionist test results. They also put rural homeopaths at a disadvantage. Rural practitioners seldom had the technology and facilities available at urban clinics and hospitals, not to mention the fact that one of homeopathy's selling points had been the simple and affordable equipment necessary to get started. These medical developments had the potential of lessening the overall number of homeopaths and patients.[82]

Many more homeopaths, perhaps because of their background in regular medicine, embraced scientific advances in medicine. These "mixers" saw themselves as part of a progressive field that would evolve with new medical knowledge and technology. They pushed for the incorporation of new discoveries to improve healing but also to maintain their professional status and to counter the belittlement of regular doctors who declared homeopathy so weak and ineffective that it had no place in academic institutions and was best left to home practice. In truth, most homeopaths had long employed a combination of homeopathic and regular therapies, sometimes mixing in some hydropathy, mesmerism, or other irregular methods as well. They honored and respected Hahnemann's work but did not accept all of his ideas. While nearly all subscribed to the law of similars, the doctrine of infinitesimals had never garnered uniform support among American homeopaths, and more abandoned the idea as the century went on.[83] Louisiana homeopath William Holcombe argued that dosage, "from the crude natural substance up to the highest infinitesimals, should be open to the choice and the practice of every candid and sensible man."[84]

By the 1870s, some homeopaths joined regulars in seeking specialized medical training in Europe, and homeopathic medical schools began to incorporate bacteriology, microscopic pathology, and other laboratory sciences into the curriculum. Similar efforts were under way in regular medical schools. In the last decades of the nineteenth century, both homeopathic and regular medical schools raised standards for graduation, lengthened training sessions, and increased tuition. Medical students now had to have completed at least two years of high school for admittance and then nine months of medical school classes spread over four years. At some homeopathic medical schools, students demanded the same education as their rivals so that by the 1890s, the curriculum at homeopathic schools in urban areas nearly matched those of regulars. The founder himself also got a makeover to fit the newly scientific times. The new Hahnemann was painted as a cool clinical scientist who searched for truth based on empirical research in a lab.[85]

The AIH took an open-door approach to the divide over pure and mixed homeopathy. In an 1870 speech before its members, AIH president Carroll Dunham, a professor and dean at the New York Homeopathic Medical College, asserted that mixing remedies, alternating and rotating them, and even giving massive doses did not indicate a disregard for homeopathic principles. A traditional homeopath himself, Dunham nonetheless argued against placing restrictions on medical practice and vigorously supported accepting anyone who sincerely applied for membership in the AIH. He reminded his colleagues of the struggles they had all faced against restrictive laws imposed by regulars that had interfered with their own investigation and experimentation, shutting out all new thoughts and insights that might have been gained from such work simply because of competition and a differing viewpoint. Four years later, the AIH voted to remove the word "homeopathy" from its membership requirements.[86]

By 1891, the United States had approximately fourteen thousand practicing homeopaths. Most major US cities had homeopathic medical colleges. The University of Michigan taught both regulars and homeopaths under one roof, with regulars teaching those intending to practice regular medicine and homeopaths teaching the remedies of the materia medica to future homeopaths. In 1890, Mark Twain wrote in the pages of *Harper's Magazine* that Americans should be "grateful that homeopathy survived the attempts of allopathists to destroy it." Homeopathy, Twain declared, had "forced the old school doctor to stir around and learn something of a rational nature about his business."[87]

Stir around they had. Homeopathy's assault on heroic drugging and bleeding, not to mention its popularity among middle-class Northeastern intellectuals, had pushed many regular doctors toward milder treatments by the 1860s. Some regular doctors lessened their use of heroic doses and began using fewer interventions, depending more on nature's healing power. These regulars didn't necessarily admit that they had been wrong. Some argued, instead, that the nature of disease had changed as society changed and so now required milder treatments.[88] New York doctor Dan King observed that "perhaps Hahnemann did not live wholly in vain. Although not actually a messenger from Heaven ... he seems nevertheless to have had an important mission indirectly to accomplish. Through the use of his empty and inert means, we have been enabled to see what the innate powers of the animal organization can accomplish without medical interference. We have been taught to rely more upon these, and less upon art, and have seen the wonderful influence which the mind has over the bodily functions." King predicted that a doctor would now "lay a gentler hand upon his patient" thanks to homeopathy.[89] To be sure, the decline in heroic treatment resulted from several developments, not the least of them being the discovery of new drugs, but regulars willingly and gleefully gave homeopathy credit for showing that patients "would very generally get well without any drugging at all."[90]

Homeopathy continued to grow and change. By 1900, homeopaths were increasingly stressing their similarities with regular medicine and had refashioned their profession as a supplemental therapeutic field. Rather than seeing this as a capitulation to regular medicine, many homeopaths instead saw themselves as keeping up with the latest advances in science. Some homeopaths argued that the germ theory and laboratory evidence revealed the power of small organisms to affect the human body, which validated Hahnemann's belief in infinitesimals even if many homeopaths had abandoned the practice of small doses. But as homeopathic medical schools added new courses, laboratories, and clinical opportunities for students, the actual study of homeopathy moved into the background. The reduced attention to homeopathy and the concomitant emphasis on the same subjects taught in regular medical schools provided applicants with few compelling reasons to choose homeopathy over regular medicine. At the same time, regular medicine's continued refusal to acknowledge homeopathy as a partner or even a factor in the emergence of scientific medicine caused the number of practitioners taking up the cause to decline. By 1923, all but two homeopathic medical schools had closed or converted into regular medical schools. Homeopathy, at least on the professional and academic level, had converged with regular medicine to the point of disappearing within it by the early decades of the twentieth century.[91]

Professionalization and scientific advances had a hugely negative impact on female homeopaths. The shift to lab and hospital work and away from the home, small practices, and homeopathic institutions moved homeopathy into a world largely dominated by paid male administrators and physicians. Increased educational requirements for admittance to medical school also made it hard for women, who continued to struggle to attend school in a culture that did not value professional women. Women lost their voice and active role in this new order of medicine. They didn't stop practicing homeopathy, however. Women continued to diagnose and treat patients, and worked particularly hard to preserve homeopathy as a distinct medical alternative even as it faded from institutional settings.[92]

By the 1920s, a small group of Hahnemannian traditionalists remained dedicated to their founder's ideas. They strictly adhered to the law of similars, the minimum dose, and the single remedy, and they saw homeopathy's fall from institutional power not as a victory for science, as regulars hailed it, but one of politics. The growing power of regular medicine, argued homeopath and birth-control advocate Mary Ware Dennett, infringed on people's freedom to make personal choices regarding their health. In 1924, Hahnemannians Julia Minerva Green and Julia M. Loos founded the American Foundation for Homeopathy to support pure homeopathy and to establish a national network of local leagues to train lay practitioners and build demand for "real" homeopathy. Women took a particularly active role in the AFH and its affiliated leagues, producing publications, teaching classes, and providing support to fellow homeopaths. In the 1960s and 1970s, as a new generation discovered homeopathy, the AFH and its leagues became primary sources of information, providing the critical link between the traditional homeopathy of the nineteenth century and the revitalized homeopathy of today. To these new followers, many of them feminists, homeopathy represented personal freedom, self-reliance, and a democratic alternative to the elitism of regular medicine, much the same values that drew women's rights leader Elizabeth Cady Stanton more than a century earlier.[93]

Julia Green never lost faith that homeopathy would rise again, insisting that homeopathy would thrive "when this materialistic age has passed and a better, more spiritual one arrives."[94] While few would consider the 1980s a less materialistic time, by that time homeopathy had made a comeback. Homeopathy remains one of the nation's most popular alternative therapies, even as it's unlikely to ever regain its nineteenth-century prominence and power. Today, an estimated 3.9 million adults use homeopathy, some through purchases of over-the-counter products labeled homeopathic and others through visits to a practitioner.[95]

Although regulars mercilessly ridiculed them for their mysticism, homeopathy was not alone in its attention to the healing power of things unseen in the nineteenth century. Mesmerists shared the homeopathic belief in invisible forces that could be activated or turned to the task of restoring a natural state of health. Hahnemann himself praised mesmerism's benign treatment, "[of] whose efficacy none but madmen can entertain a doubt."[96] He believed, like the mesmerists did, that a healer transferred his mental power to the medicine. In homeopathy, this happened in the dynamization process of diluting remedies, where mesmerism used touch. Hundreds of thousands of people on both sides of the Atlantic fell quite literally under the spell of Franz Anton Mesmer and the invisible healing solution he called animal magnetism.

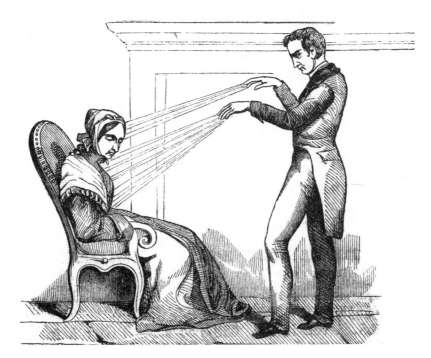

Franz Anton Mesmer and his followers held patients literally entranced as they directed the flow of an invisible force they called animal magnetism through the bodies of their patients. (Wellcome Library, London)

CHAPTER FIVE

Hypnotized
Mesmer and His Mental Magic

In 1862, Mary Patterson entered the Portland, Maine, office of mental healer Phineas Quimby in tatters. Pale, weak, and emaciated, the forty-two-year-old Patterson, her wavy brown hair pulled back from her face, could barely carry herself up the stairs into the waiting room. She had been sick her entire life, missing much of school as a child and writing despairing poems from her bed about death and the meaninglessness of life as a young adult. Low in energy, emotionally unstable, and subject to spells of pain, Patterson tried regular care, homeopathy, hydropathy, and a Grahamite vegetarian diet, but nothing worked. Most of her life had been consumed by a constant search for someone who could provide her with lasting relief. She desperately hoped that someone might be Quimby.

Phineas Parkhurst Quimby, or "Park" to his friends, had experimented with mesmerism and magnetic healing since 1838. Concluding that a patient's trust and rapport with the healer led to cures, Quimby attempted to connect with his patients mentally and physically. He talked over their disease, massaged their hands and arms, tried to adopt and feel their symptoms himself, and encouraged them to think differently about life and health. His success with this method made him a national figure.

After only a week in Quimby's care, Patterson's health improved dramatically. The woman so enfeebled she could not step out of her carriage alone was, only days into her treatment, climbing the 182 steps to the dome on top of Portland's city hall unassisted. No one

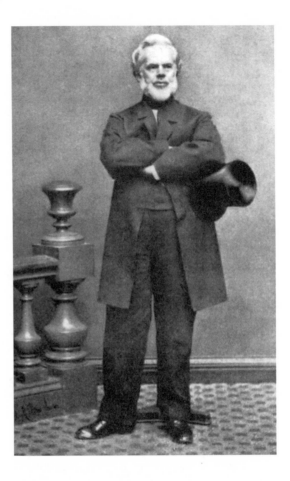

Phineas Parkhurst
Quimby taught his
patients that good
health came from
positive thinking.
(Wikimedia Commons)

was more astonished than Patterson herself, who before long was de-
voting her days to the practice and further study of Quimby's method.
Only a few years later, Patterson, soon to be known through another
marriage as Mary Baker Eddy, would introduce her own new medical system. She called it Christian Science, and it quickly became the
largest homegrown healing faith in American history, following in the
long and potent path of mental cures and magnetic fluids that had
begun more than a century earlier in Europe as mesmerism.[1]

Like phrenology, mesmerism began in late-eighteenth-century Vienna with the experimentation of an established regular physician. In
the 1770s, Franz Anton Mesmer began to test an idea he'd first had
in medical school about the body's vital force. Just as gravity affected

the behavior of the sun, moon, and planets, Mesmer proposed that the "nervous fluids" that coursed through the body made humans as susceptible as the tides to the universe's invisible gravitational forces. He based his theory on those of the sixteenth-century alchemist Paracelsus, who had suggested that the human body could attract corresponding planetary effects. The idea of bodies influenced by unseen and unexplainable powers was nothing new in medicine, nor even unusual in an eighteenth-century world that seemed alive with powerful unseen forces. Isaac Newton's gravity, Benjamin Franklin's electricity, even the miraculous hot-air balloons of Jacques Charles and the Montgolfier brothers that lifted humans into the air were just a few of the powerful new forces turning heads and firing scientific thought in Europe.

The idea of nervous fluids had an even longer lineage. Roman physician Galen had speculated in the second century CE that bodily movement and sensation resulted from animal spirits that formed in the brain and flowed outward through hollow ducts in the nerves. This idea dominated thinking about the function of the nervous system for centuries even as the composition of those spirits and the mechanics of actual nerve function adapted to the latest scientific trends and discoveries. Gradually, the idea of animal spirits came to be replaced with "nerve fluid," though the general concept of a substance moving through the nerves remained much the same. Like vitalism's core concept of a life force that animated all living beings, it was widely believed that disruptions in the free flow of this nervous fluid caused disease.[2]

Unlike his predecessors, though, Mesmer suggested that a physician could learn to control the flow of these invisible forces from outside the body. It was a startling idea. Not only that, he believed he could also restore the internal harmony that signaled health. He theorized that illness might be cured with magnets. Since they, like celestial bodies, could influence other physical entities without actual contact, he wondered if magnets could also redirect the body's nervous fluid. In 1774, Mesmer tested his theory on twenty-nine-year-old Franziska Oesterlin, a "hysteric" who experienced convulsions with vomiting and fainting. Mesmer treated and observed Oesterlin for two years. During an attack, Mesmer placed one magnet on her stomach and another on each of her legs. Almost immediately, Oesterlin reported feeling "painful currents of a subtle material" moving within her that eventually traveled downward to her extremities. Her spells soon subsided and did not return for hours. Mesmer repeated the treatment many times over the following weeks with the same success. He finally declared her entirely cured.[3]

Mesmer was unique among irregular healers for starting with a theory rather than a treatment. He assumed that some force did act on the body, and modified his therapy based on the results of his empirical tests. At first, Mesmer thought the magnets cured. But he soon found that he could provoke the same reaction in other patients that he had with Oesterlin using wooden objects and other nonmagnetic materials—even the simple stroke of his finger. Magnets could cure, but so, it seemed, could a lot of other things. Mesmer determined that the effects he witnessed must not be the ordinary magnetism known since ancient times but something else entirely: a separate imperceptible natural force that he called "animal magnetism." Modern slang associates animal magnetism with sexual attraction, but Mesmer conceived of his force as the compelling power behind all kinds of interactions and attractions. Animal magnetism transmitted influence from and between all physical objects, from metal rods to water, food, and even the hat on a patient's head. Once magnetized through touch or simply the wave of a hand, the object became indistinguishable from a real magnet, which Mesmer became convinced was merely a conductor of animal magnetism.[4]

Based on his new discovery and his experiences treating Oesterlin, Mesmer revised his theory to center on this "magnetic substance." Sticking to vitalism, he claimed that human health depended on the unimpeded flow of animal magnetism, which he believed to be a real physical albeit invisible substance, through the body. Interruptions or imbalances in the stream caused organs to falter, deprived of sufficient amounts of this vital force to operate properly. Disease was the inevitable result.[5] Removing the obstacle became the key to healing.[6] His theory had a beautiful simplicity. Tracing disease back to a disturbance in the body's supply of magnetism meant that all disease had one cause and thus one treatment, a universal method of healing like Thomson's goal of restoring bodily heat. Mesmer's theory reduced medical science to a straightforward set of procedures aimed at supercharging the nervous system with the life-giving energy that would keep people healthy, no drugs required.[7] Armed with his new theory, Mesmer resolved to "dedicate my remaining life" to saving his fellow man from disease.[8]

Excited about his discovery and a bit prone to excess, Mesmer decided that if some animal magnetism was good, then more must be even better. He infused magnetism into every aspect of the patient experience. Patients napped between magnetized sheets, bathed in magnetized water, ate from magnetized plates and silverware, and strolled the grounds of his estate in magnetized clothing. Mesmer also played a magnetized glass armonica, a musical instrument that essentially mechanized the experience of rubbing the rim of a crystal glass with a wet finger. Mesmer was a virtuoso on the instrument, which was invented by Benjamin Franklin, who would, ironically, later lead an investigation that condemned Mesmer's scientific claims. Franklin's armonica consisted of a series of glass bowls in graduated sizes that turned on a foot-powered spindle. Players touched the rotating rims with moistened fingers to produce high and haunting pitches with a slight vibrato. Thousands of glass armonicas were built and sold. For Mesmer, music was not just ornament or background accompaniment: rather, the music communicated, propagated, and reinforced the flow of animal magnetism.[9]

Word of Mesmer's healing success spread rapidly throughout Vienna, but scandal erupted when Mesmer claimed to have restored the sight of the talented pianist Maria Theresia Paradis. Eighteen-year-old Paradis had been blind since age three. Her parents had tried everything to cure her, summoning the best medical talent in the city, who applied leeches and plasters, prescribed purgatives and diuretics, and shocked her eyes with Leyden jars. Nothing worked. As a diversion from her malady, Paradis began music lessons and so impressed Austrian empress Maria Theresa with her musical skills as an eleven-year-old that she earned a government stipend for her musical education. Mesmer had known Paradis's family for several years when he boldly proposed to her parents in 1777 that his animal magnetism might restore the young pianist's vision. They agreed with his assurance that he was up for the challenge. After a series of treatments, Mesmer declared her sight restored. But vision turned out to be troubling and confusing to Paradis, and her piano skills dramatically declined. Some said she also might have fallen in love with Mesmer and maybe he with her, rumors that outraged and scandalized Viennese society. Her angry parents snatched Paradis away from Mesmer, worried about losing her pension and perhaps also the loss of her marketing cachet as the blind pianist. Once she was away from Mesmer, her blindness quickly returned. The incident sparked responses both vitriolic and gleeful from critics who jumped at the chance to ridicule Mesmer and his method. Discredited in the eyes of the medical profession, Mesmer abandoned Austria for Paris in 1778.[10]

One year later, Mesmer reflected on the Paradis incident in his *Memoir on the Discovery of Animal Magnetism*. "I was being taxed with eccentricity," he wrote, "my tendency to quit the normal path of Medicine was being construed as a crime."[11] Despite his troubles in Vienna, Mesmer's reputation and fame as an extraordinary healer preceded him to Paris. His worldly manners, intellect, sturdy good looks, and unabashed confidence gave Mesmer quick access to Parisian social circles even with his strong German accent and scandal-tinged character (though this being Paris, it may have intrigued more than it repelled). Soon, more patients than Mesmer could possibly treat individually besieged his office.[12]

Never one to miss a potential business opportunity, Mesmer introduced a magnetized instrument known as a baquet to meet the demand for his services. He had discovered a few years earlier that he could magnify his powers by standing with one foot submerged in a bucket of water. The baquet was simply a larger wooden bucket with a cover. Flexible iron rods that concentrated the flow of energy passed through the lid for patients to apply to specific body parts. Most important for Mesmer's business, though, the baquet allowed as many as twenty patients to gather around and receive treatment at the same time. Mesmer kept four in his treatment rooms in Paris. One baquet was reserved for the poor who received treatment at no cost, while the other three had to be reserved far in advance and cost roughly the same price as a ticket to the Paris Opera.[13] Patients gathered around the tub and joined hands to form a complete "magnetic" circuit. Once they were settled, the treatment—and show—could begin.

A flashy and theatrical entertainer, Mesmer entered the darkened room wearing gold slippers and flowing lilac robes. He circled the room, sometimes stopping to play the glass armonica to prepare the patients for the flow of magnetism. Large mirrors on the walls reflected any errant fluid back toward the assembled patients. Mesmer then passed slowly from patient to patient and gazed deeply into their eyes. His intense and enthralling stare immobilized and entranced clients, literally mesmerizing them and giving birth to a new term in connection with Mesmer himself. Passing his hands and magnetized wand over each patient, Mesmer provoked screams, sweating, fits of hysterical laughter, dramatic convulsions, and fainting. Mesmer, like hydropathy's Priessnitz, called these extreme effects the "crisis," and he considered them the goal of the treatment. Nerve fluid must be pushed to its maximum velocity and intensity to dissolve and expel the obstruction from the body while simultaneously reactivating the life force of the patient. The frenzied responses passed like a chain reaction around the baquet and sent everyone into fits, an effect that emphasized Mesmer's control over the room and his subjects.[14]

To help him with his growing practice, Mesmer took on associate Charles-Nicolas Deslon, a medical professor at the University of Paris and the private physician to the Count d'Artois, brother to King Louis XVI. Deslon's credentials brought prestige and visibility to Mesmer's practice, but more important, it brought him into contact with the French aristocracy, who would prove to be some of his most ardent and faithful supporters in Europe.[15] More than one hundred patients a day, women, men, and children, aristocratic to working class, passed through his doors and under his hypnotic gaze. By 1784, only six years after settling in Paris, Mesmer estimated that he had treated more than eight thousand people.[16]

Patient accounts of what it felt like to be mesmerized are scarce since most patients claim that it's difficult, if not impossible, to credibly witness an altered state in one's self. To do so, an individual would have to be astute and alert at the exact moment the intended phenomenon, insensibility through crisis, took effect. Most patients awoke from the experience remembering nothing.[17] Even so, in the mid-nineteenth century, a Lady Rosse described her experience under the care of British clergyman and mesmerist William Scoresby. Anxious at first, "the moment I was settled on the sofa, with my hands in his— all apprehension vanished," she claimed, as "a calmness, a delightful resignation to his will came over me. My eyes were irresistibly drawn to his and in vain did I combat the superior power of my Mesmerist. A pleasant thrill ran from my fingers throughout my body towards my feet—my heard pounded with joy." Seconds later, "the faces and figures of those around me dissolved, one melting into another until the last vision of them seemed to vanish in Dr. Scoresby's eyes. He was no longer Dr. Scoresby to me, but my all, part of myself; what he wished, I wished. In fact the attraction astonished me. The cares, the interest in this life ceased. I felt no longer a common mortal but infinitely superior and yet felt my Mesmeriser far superior to myself."[18] English writer Harriet Martineau recorded similar sensations in the 1840s at the hands of mesmerist Spencer Hall. Twenty minutes into her session, she "became sensible of an extraordinary appearance" that "seemed to diffuse itself through the atmosphere,—not like smoke, nor steam, nor haze,—but most like a clear twilight, closing in from the windows and down from the ceiling, and in which one object after another melted away." The experience left her feeling hot, sick, and suffering from a "disordered stomach" for several hours after her session. But those sensations were gone by evening. Martineau soon found herself feeling a "lightness and relief" from the sickness that had kept her bedridden for several years.[19]

Some people found themselves so taken with Mesmer's powers that they wanted to become practitioners of animal magnetism themselves. Mesmer was at first reluctant to share his system with anyone, convinced that he alone truly understood animal magnetism. He eventually agreed to share some parts of his system—but not without a monetary and psychological price to those who wished to learn. Mesmer's more affluent disciples paid an enormous amount of money for the honor of membership in the Society of Universal Harmony, a semisecret organization founded in 1783 that mixed business, mesmeric education, and fraternalism. Like Thomson, Mesmer demanded absolute devotion from his disciples, but he felt no need to show any gratitude of his own in return. No one was allowed to add, modify, or subtract anything without his permission. Anyone who suggested alternative or contrary ideas was thrown out. Despite these strict conditions, chapters of the society soon existed in most major French cities. Men from some of France's most illustrious and aristocratic families joined, including the French hero of the American Revolution, the Marquis de Lafayette. Benjamin Franklin's grandson William Temple Franklin also joined, though he would later tell his grandfather that he was merely curious.[20] The society made Mesmer rich. It also transformed what had begun as one's man closely guarded secret into the common knowledge and shared enthusiasm of an influential group of men.

But despite his success and incredible wealth, Mesmer remained dissatisfied. He was desperate for official recognition of his discovery from a scientific institution that would validate its importance to current understandings about life.[21] "I dare to flatter myself that the discoveries I have made will push back the boundaries of our knowledge of physics as did the invention of microscopes and telescopes for the age preceding our own," boasted Mesmer in his memoir.[22] Members of the Academy of Sciences of Berlin did not agree with Mesmer, however, and they rejected his theory as nonscientific and "unworthy of the smallest attention" after witnessing his cures.[23] The Royal Society of Medicine ignored his requests to present his ideas to its members, as did the Faculté de Médecine at the University of Paris.[24] Even outside these institutions, regular doctors remained largely unimpressed with Mesmer and his magical force. Although some regulars acknowledged that he likely did succeed in curing some patients, they argued that these patients suffered from psychological rather than real, physical ailments so any attention would likely produce positive results. Not to mention the fact that his drugless system and single healing method made the medical profession largely superfluous, never an easy path to medical legitimacy. One English doctor scoffed that mesmerism bore as much relation to medicine "as astrology does to astronomy."[25]

Mesmer's biggest challenge came in 1784 when King Louis XVI set up a royal commission to investigate his claims. Far less enamored of Mesmer than his wife Marie Antoinette and eager to determine the veracity of a theory inflaming both widespread acclaim and condemnation in Paris, the king appointed five members of the Academy of Sciences and four prominent physicians from the Faculté de Médecine to the case. Chaired by the witty and worldly Benjamin Franklin, the only foreign member of the team, the commission comprised most of France's leading scientists of the time, including the chemist Antoine-Laurent Lavoisier, the astronomer Jean-Sylvain Bailly, and physician Joseph-Ignace Guillotin, who was to achieve greater fame for an invention that would later cost his fellow commissioners Lavoisier and Bailly their heads. The subject of their investigation would not be Mesmer himself, who refused to cooperate, perhaps feeling the investigation biased from the start, but Mesmer's disciple Charles Deslon, who gave them full access to his practice.[26]

The commissioners first spent one day a week in Deslon's clinic receiving treatment. They each sat around the baquet while Deslon tried to magnetize them. Nothing much happened over three months of weekly visits. "Not one of the commissioners felt any sensation, or at least none which ought to be ascribed to the action of the magnetism," read the report.[27] Observing Deslon's work with other patients, the commission recognized that a number of patients showed what appeared to be the crises Mesmer described. The effects impressed even the jaded commissioners: "nothing can be more astonishing than the sight of these convulsions."[28] But the commission's charge was not to determine whether Mesmer's treatment had any beneficial effects but whether animal magnetism—a new force of nature—actually existed.

Franklin's gout and other illnesses made travel difficult, so Deslon agreed to perform experiments at Franklin's home in Passy outside Paris. In one experiment, a blindfolded woman was told that Deslon was in the room magnetizing her. Almost immediately, she began shuddering and crying out in pain, lapsing into crisis within minutes. The only trouble was that Deslon was nowhere near her—he was not even in the same room. Another experiment had Deslon supposedly magnetizing a woman from behind a door. Even when he was not present, the patient showed visible changes. When the reverse experiment was conducted on the same woman with Deslon trying to magnetize her but without her knowledge, nothing happened.[29]

On another day, Deslon magnetized an apricot tree in Franklin's backyard with his special magnetized cane. He then blindfolded his subject, a twelve-year-old boy suffering from an unspecified illness. Once blindfolded, the boy stumbled clumsily around the yard toward the trees. "They made him embrace several trees for two minutes," wrote Franklin's fourteen-year-old grandson, Benjamin Franklin Bache, observing the proceedings. "At the first three trees . . . he said that he felt a numbness which redoubled at each tree."[30] Besides numbness, at the first tree, nearly thirty feet from the magnetized tree, the boy began to sweat, cough up phlegm, and complain of severe head pain. At the second tree, still further from the magnetized tree, his head pain increased. He appeared dazed and bewildered. Moving on, the boy claimed that the magnetic force felt even stronger. He complained of a tingling sensation like a light electric shock that increased with each tree, even as he walked farther and farther away from the magnetized tree. The experiment ended suddenly when the boy fainted.[31]

These experiments suggested to the commissioners that those people who felt the effects of the treatment had high expectations and vivid imaginations. "If the symptoms are more considerable and the crisis more violent at the public exhibition, it is because various causes are combined with the imagination, to operate, to multiply and to enlarge its effects," wrote the commissioners. They concluded, "This agent, this fluid has no existence."[32]

Released in August of 1784, the *Rapport des Commissaires* became an immediate sensation. More than twenty thousand copies sold, and summaries of the commission's findings appeared in publications ranging from *Gentleman's Magazine* to the *London Medical Journal*. The report itself was notable for being one of the first, if not the first, instance of blinding of subjects in a medical trial, a practice now essential to modern medicine. Mesmer, unsurprisingly, refused to accept the commission's report. He argued that it was unfair and politically motivated since the commission's scientists had the most to lose from the veracity of his claims. He was particularly infuriated that the commissioners had based their results on treatments administered by Deslon, though Mesmer himself had refused the commission's invitation to participate. Many of Mesmer's followers also protested the commissioners' conclusions. They claimed vivid memories of the animal magnetism entering and leaving their bodies, if little else of the actual experience, and asserted their belief in the mystical power of the baquet. Mesmer soon left Paris and traveled through Europe before spending his final years near his birthplace in Germany, where he died in 1815.[33]

Mesmerism itself was far from dead, however—it was just getting started. The same year that the commission's report appeared to discredit magnetism, Amand-Marie-Jacques de Chastenet, the Marquis de Puységur, made a spectacular discovery that breathed new life into the movement. The eldest of three brothers in a respected aristocratic family, Puységur began experimenting with magnetism on the peasants who worked his estate in Buzancy in northern France in 1784. They proved willing subjects for his new healing art. Among the first to come to him was a young shepherd named Victor Race who had spent several days in bed with what appeared to be pneumonia. Puységur magnetized Race, but rather than experiencing the crisis that Puységur expected, he instead found that the young man fell into a strange peaceful sleep. This wasn't like any sleep Puységur had seen before. Although he appeared to be sleeping, Race soon began to talk about his problems. Puységur worried that these unhappy thoughts might aggravate Race's illness, so he tried to change the subject to happier topics. He suggested that Race might imagine himself dancing at a party and taking part in a shooting contest. Puységur's suggestions set Race into motion. He stood up and began walking. He pantomimed dancing. He shot a gun. Race not only appeared to be awake and aware of his surroundings, he also seemed more intelligent and well spoken than normal. After an hour experimenting with this new kind of magnetic crisis, Puységur calmed Race down and brought him back to consciousness. Race recalled nothing that had happened.[34]

Intrigued, Puységur magnetized Race again some days later to similar effect. Puységur soon found that many of his workers fell into these unusual, sleeplike states of consciousness. Lacking a baquet of his own, Puységur mesmerized a group of peasants tied around a magnetized tree and observed the results. Like Race, these entranced patients appeared brighter and more receptive to their surroundings and to other people. They recalled long-forgotten memories in minute detail and answered questions with an intelligence unexpected in those with a peasant's education and background. Even better, when Puységur asked them about their illnesses, many could offer a complete case history and diagnosis that usually held up under further investigation. These patients claimed they could see their own insides like human X-rays. Some even prescribed remedies and could predict the day the illness would finally pass. A select few achieved what Puységur called "extraordinary lucidity" and could perform feats of telepathy and clairvoyance. Once, Puységur claimed he used magnetism to bring a supposedly dead dog back to life. Puységur named these unusual effects "mesmeric somnambulism" or "magnetic sleep."[35]

Quite inadvertently, Puységur discovered the human unconscious, a strange new world just below the threshold of ordinary consciousness. Mesmer, perhaps feeling spurned by the attention lavished on Puységur, claimed that he had actually discovered somnambulism many years before, but it seems unlikely. Although Mesmer's name is the one remembered, Puységur's discovery dramatically shifted the debate over mesmerism and the substance of animal magnetism. The remarkable effects produced by mesmerism now seemed to have not a physical cause, as Mesmer had claimed, but a psychological origin, the mechanisms of which would consume many scientists, philosophers, and doctors in the nineteenth century.[36]

The relationship between patient and healer, always important but secondary to the actual fluid itself under Mesmer, became the primary component of Puységur's brand of magnetism. Mesmer himself had paid little attention to psychological factors. He did not concern himself with questions about the patient's attitude or belief going into treatment, or the effect the magnetizer might have on the patient.[37] Puységur rejected Mesmer's claim that the redistribution of the physical fluid of animal magnetism induced the healing crisis. He instead explained his therapeutic success as a mental effect produced by the mesmerist's will over the vital power. The crucial variable in the mesmerizing process, according to Puységur, was the magnetist's ability to gain some control over the patient that then allowed the patient to slip into the somnambulistic state.[38] "I believe in the existence within myself of a power. From this belief derives my will to exert it," explained Puységur in a 1785 address to the Strasbourg Masonic society. "The entire doctrine of Animal Magnetism is contained in the two words: *Believe* and *want*. I *believe* that I have the power to set into action the vital principle of my fellow-men; I *want* to make use of it; this is all my science and all my means."[39] Patients had internal capabilities that he as the magnetizer could activate and manipulate through the magnetizing process. And that control changed the role and responsibilities of the patient. Where before, Mesmer had treated a seated and mostly passive patient, Puységur's method demanded the active involvement of the patient in the healing process. Mesmerized patients needed to move, talk, and, most important, discern illness in themselves and others, becoming both performer and diagnostic tool.

Intrigued by Puységur's discovery, some regular doctors experimented with using somnambulistic trance in their own practice. Alexandre Bertrand, Ambroise Liebault, and Hippolyte Bernheim were among the scientists who further examined Puységur's theory and claimed to have proved the existence of an unconscious mental state.[40] Alleviating the pain of surgery seemed like the most promising application of somnambulism. The need was great as anesthetics did not exist until the introduction of ether in 1846; most surgical patients endured the terrible pain of surgery with little more than a strong drink and a broom handle held between clenched teeth. Parisian mesmerist Pierre Jean Chapelain participated in one of the first mesmeric surgeries in April 1829. He entranced a sixty-four-year-old woman known as Madame Plantin while surgeon Jules Cloquet successfully removed her cancerous breast. Cloquet recounted his accomplishment before the Section on Surgery of the French Royal Academy of Medicine a few days later. Several members of the Academy questioned Cloquet's story, even though a later account of the surgery by a Scottish authority on somnambulism, John C. Colquhoun, reported that the woman "continued to converse quietly with the operator [magnetizer], and did not exhibit the slightest sign of sensibility" during the procedure. When she awoke, she "did not appear to have any idea, any feeling of what had passed in the interval." The success of the surgery spurred further investigations of mesmerism in medical treatment.[41] In 1837, somnambulistic surgery came to England at the suggestion of John Elliotson, a well-respected regular doctor at London's University College Hospital. Mesmerism, he insisted, had a huge future in modern medicine. It was not Elliotson's first maverick act—he had also been the first doctor in England to use a stethoscope. Drawn to the new and exciting, Elliotson argued that medical progress required experimentation and risk. He amazed observers with his surgical demonstrations on deeply mesmerized patients. After witnessing one of his mesmeric displays, writer Charles Dickens became an Elliotson disciple and used his magnetic skills on his family and friends. He also wrote mesmerism into his unfinished novel, *The Mystery of Edwin Drood*. Unfortunately, Elliotson's colleagues were less unimpressed with mesmerism than Dickens. In 1838, the University College Hospital passed a resolution banning the use of mesmerism within its doors, a move that essentially booted Elliotson out of his job. He left and eventually started a journal devoted to the study and promotion of mesmerism and phrenology. He also established the London Mesmeric Infirmary, a hospital devoted to mesmerism, in 1850.[42]

These medical experiments also gave mesmerism a new name. In 1841, Scottish physician James Braid began dangling bright objects before the eyes of his subjects to induce trance. Braid had first witnessed the phenomenon in a demonstration by Parisian showman and magnetist Charles Lafontaine. At first he wondered if the patients faked their trances, but he soon came to believe that the effects Lafontaine caused were genuine. The real question then concerned the nature of the effects and the agent that produced them. Braid's observations and experiments led him to reject animal magnetism outright, concluding instead that somnambulism had a purely psychological and subjective source, most likely rooted in suggestion. Though most mesmerists disagreed with his theory, many began using the name he coined for the practice in 1842 as a way to dissociate his findings from mesmerism and the antics of traveling showmen: hypnosis. His method of inducing trance also inspired the popular image of the hypnotist waving an object before his patient.[43]

Mesmeric mania finally hit American shores in the 1830s, only a few years after phrenology had first suggested the wondrous possibilities of the mind. Although some educated Americans knew of it already from its introduction in the 1770s, mesmerism only gained widespread popularity in the United States with the arrival of Frenchman Charles Poyen de Saint Saveur. A twenty-year-old medical student and self-styled "Professor of Animal Magnetism," Poyen came to Boston in 1836 to spread his magnetic faith. But much to his surprise and dismay, he found himself talking about a subject that few Americans knew anything about. It wasn't the first time a Frenchman had tried to introduce mesmerism to America. In 1784, General Marquis de Lafayette, an enthusiastic member of Mesmer's Society of Universal Harmony, wrote to his friend and mentor George Washington promising to reveal to him "Mesmer's secret, which, you can count on it, is a great philosophical discovery." Though sincere in his enthusiasm, Lafayette had overstepped his bounds. Not only did he not have Mesmer's permission to make such an offer, even worse, when King Louis XVI heard of his letter, he scornfully asked Lafayette, "What will Washington think when he learns that you have become Mesmer's chief journeyman apothecary?" Washington chose not to get involved, perhaps heeding the advice of Thomas Jefferson, who, appalled by the irrational popularity of mesmerism in France, handed out copies of the negative conclusions reached by Franklin's royal commission that very year.[44]

Poyen had discovered mesmerism during his medical studies in Paris. Suffering from a nervous ailment that defied standard medical treatment, Poyen eventually sought the services of a mesmerist and was impressed with the effects. He then traveled to Martinique and

Guadeloupe in the West Indies and met French planters using magnetism to heal their slaves in cases Poyen found "altogether remarkable." Poyen stayed and studied magnetism and somnambulism for a
year before deciding to move to New England for its cooler climate
and healthful maritime air. His mesmeric study had also imbued him
with a messianic message for the American people: the hidden secret
to human happiness and well-being.[45]

Poyen embarked on a lecture tour of New England soon after he
landed. He did little to transform the theory he had first learned in
Europe. Poyen believed that Puységur's discovery of the somnambulistic state was the most important scientific discovery of animal magnetism, and perhaps the most important in all of science. Larding his
lectures with medical magic tricks, Poyen demonstrated the magnetic
state of consciousness to awestruck audiences. He hired a clairvoyant who could supposedly read the thoughts of audience members
as well as the contents of sealed envelopes while under a mesmeric
trance. Colonel William Stone, editor of the *New York Commercial
Advertiser*, admitted to his "times of laughing at animal magnetism,"
but after seeing Poyen, Stone changed his mind. Mesmerism had to
be seen to be believed. "Nothing hitherto published upon that subject,
is so wonderful by far, as the facts of which we were witness," declared Stone. After witnessing a blind girl under trance read a sealed
letter at a demonstration in Providence, Rhode Island, Stone hailed
mesmerism as "not only marvellous [sic] in our eyes, but absolutely
astounding."[46]

During his lectures, Poyen picked volunteers from the audience
to undergo trances. They sat onstage while Poyen waved his arms
over and around them to heighten the activity of their internal animal magnetism. Poyen usually succeeded in hypnotizing about half
of his volunteers. Loud hand clapping and jars of ammonia passed
under their noses failed to evoke even the slightest response or nose
twitch. To the audience, these volunteers appeared to have with-
drawn completely from the physical world. Crowds thronged to see
family and friends transformed before their eyes.[47] "The gossip of the
city is of Animal Magnetism," wrote Ralph Waldo Emerson to his
brother William on January 13, 1837. "Three weeks ago I went to see
the magnetic sleep & saw the wonder."[48] The trance subjects themselves, like Poyen's own medium Cynthia Gleason, became featured

players in the performances. Poyen's exhibitions proved to be great theater, mimicking the drama that had so captivated and entertained Parisians in Mesmer's time. It also had the unfortunate side effect of disenfranchising mesmerism from the serious consideration of the American scientific community, which highly disapproved of pairing frivolity with science.[49]

While people certainly came for the entertainment, many others sought Poyen's medical care. Like Mesmer, he attempted to direct the flow of animal magnetism to the diseased part of the body with his hands. These patients generally remembered nothing of their mesmeric trance but still declared themselves cured when they awoke. Poyen boasted the successful treatment of everything from rheumatism and back pain to liver disease and nervousness. Newspaper articles and letters to the editor from patients following his appearances tended to support his healing assertions.[50]

Word of Poyen's healing methods spread rapidly throughout New England and the rest of the country. Poyen was an able and evocative speaker bursting with egotism, and his message played on growing public confidence in the promise of science to bring about a better world. He prophesied that mesmerism, when fully accepted by "intelligent and fast progressing" people, would make America "the most perfect nation on earth."[51] For an American public with a boundless sense of destiny, Poyen's message found eager ears.[52]

But while many Americans enthusiastically embraced mesmerism without question, others were not so sure. The idea of a force with the power to influence human behavior led some to worry about what horrors could result if it were left uncontrolled or put in the hands of the untrained or immoral. Many ministers thought that mesmerism might undermine religious faith with its similarities to the healings performed in the New Testament. They worried that some followers might conclude that the miracles described in the Bible were simply mesmerism and that Christ raised the dead through animal magnetism rather than anything divine. Some mesmerists did, in fact, make that claim, perhaps hoping to capitalize on religious skepticism or to link magnetism to a long and ancient history.[53] These religious concerns tended to fade as mesmerism claimed more and more converts. Many evangelicals came to embrace mesmerism's potential to demonstrate the hidden powers of the mind. Mesmerists put patients through an intense physical and mental experience that "restored the body to harmony," but also happened to look an awful lot like a religious conversion experience. The visible changes seen in patients under trance seemed to testify to the utter transformation possible when people came under spiritual guidance. Both revivalists and mesmerists argued that confusion and self-doubt would continue until people gave themselves over to a higher power, which for mesmerists was animal magnetism and for the religious, God. In America, the two became increasingly entwined.[54]

The sexual overtones of the mesmerizing process, however, worried far more Americans, and these worries were not as easily dispatched as religious concerns. It was, after all, an act where a passive patient, often female, willingly yielded all mental resistance to comply with the physical gestures of a powerful and usually male mesmerist. Individual treatment often relied on close proximity between doctor and patient. Sitting face-to-face, the doctor usually enclosed the patient's knees between his own. He then began touching and stroking the patient's body, often paying particular attention to the abdomen. Many could not help but suspect improper passions at work, an accusation that dogged mesmerism from the very beginning, particularly as most reports of mesmeric malfeasance involved female patients. In fact, members of the original French commission had secretly submitted a second report to Louis XVI warning of the indecencies to which Mesmer's science and method were inherently prone. The king had a personal stake in this as his wife, Marie Antoinette, had been among Mesmer's greatest fans.[55] Eighteenth-century comics, writers, and musicians seized on mesmerism's erotic implications, satirizing the treatment in cartoons and bawdy verses that congratulated Mesmer for conquering so many women. Mesmer repeatedly denied that he took liberties with his female patients, but the gossip continued unabated.[56]

These concerns crossed the Atlantic with Poyen. The publication of the anonymous but American-written *Confessions of a Magnetizer*, in which the author boasted of taking advantage of his more attractive patients after placing them in a trance, certainly did nothing to quell suspicions and fears.[57] Soon, a whole genre of scare literature featuring evil mesmerists who seduced innocents appeared on the publishing scene. Timothy Shay's *Agnes; or, The Possessed, A Revelation of Mesmerism* (1848) told the story of a young woman who leaves her fiancé after falling under the spell of mesmerist Monsieur Florien during a tooth extraction. Her exceptional magnetic conductivity leads Florien to abduct Agnes for further experiments. She's eventually rescued by her fiancé, who tracks her from Boston to New York City. Fortunately, he finds that the young Agnes has not been compromised. Florien's wife assures the fiancé that Agnes has remained pure under her watchful eye. In case the message was not clear enough, Shay warns of the dangers of mesmerism and its "disorderly, and therefore, evil origin" in both the preface and afterward of his tale. In a more enduring book, *The Bostonians*, Henry James compares mesmerists to vampires feeding on the animal magnetism of their unknowing patients.[58]

Mesmerism both fascinated and repelled Nathaniel Hawthorne, who used its power dynamics as a theme and cautionary tale. In *The House of the Seven Gables*, the hardworking carpenter Matthew Maule entrances the snooty beauty Alice Pyncheon and uses his powers in selfish revenge after she spurns his affections. The acts he subjects her to eventually result in her death. Mesmerism appears again in *The Blithedale Romance* in which the passive and receptive Priscilla is exploited as a stage performer. But despite these dark portrayals of mesmerism, Hawthorne also found similarities between himself as an artist and the mesmerist: both create characters, the author in his stories and the mesmerist of his patients under trance and often of himself as well; explore intimate lives; and hold others spellbound. The negative view prevailed in his own life, though, as Hawthorne was unwilling to entertain his wife Sophia's interest in mesmerism. He told her to "take no part" in "magnetic miracles" to prevent the possible violation of her soul by the mesmerist.[59]

The patient-mesmerist relationship did not have to be this way, though, counseled Joseph Francois Deleuze. The French mesmerist devoted an entire section of his mesmerism manual *Practical Instruction in Animal Magnetism*, first translated into English in 1837, to choosing the right magnetizer. He counseled women to seek the services of other women since patients commonly developed a deep affection for the magnetizer. Female modesty was also at stake since magnetism tended to produce "spasmodic movements" in women that were "not proper for a man to . . . witness."[60]

Concern for women could turn quickly to scorn, however, if a woman voluntarily participated in mesmerist shows as a volunteer or, worse, as a clairvoyant. Immoral, greedy, and attention seeking were just some of the insults hurled by critics at these women. But mesmerism offered poor women an opportunity for economic and social advancement far from the dangers of the factory floor in a culture that afforded them few choices. Poyen's own clairvoyant, Cynthia Gleason, had worked in a textile mill in Rhode Island when she sought his care for chronic stomach pain. Her skills while under mesmeric trance "of discerning the symptoms of disease, and prescribing appropriate remedies for them" impressed Poyen, who hired her on as his traveling assistant. By the time she died in 1847, Gleason had amassed a small fortune for her work as a clairvoyant somnambulistic healer, first for Poyen and then on her own. With hundreds if not thousands of people attending some demonstrations, it wasn't hard to understand why some factory girls preferred this more lucrative and potentially star-making job. Mesmerists also preferred female assistants because of the widespread belief that women more easily succumbed to trance than men.[61]

Women participated in mesmerism as far more than passive subjects, though. They also used its healing power for their own gain and benefit. Women loved mesmerism's potential to reduce the pain of childbirth. Just as the mesmeric trance could be used as an anesthetic in surgery, it found a welcome home in the home health-care regimen of some midwives. Once there, it never really left, as hypnobirthing is still in use today with more than one thousand practitioners in the United States, online courses, and classes offered at some major hospitals.[62]

Other women became mesmerists themselves. As in other irregular fields, female mesmerists treated women almost exclusively. Most appear to have received little public notice, as the uproar over potential liberties taken by male mesmerizers over supposedly helpless female patients dominated popular conversation. A female mesmerist named Elizabeth angrily denounced accusations of immorality from regular doctors in the pages of the mesmerist journal the *Zoist*. "But *why*, and on *what account* and *proof*, are mesmerists to be thus stigmatized?" she asked. "Are then mesmerists, as a class, 'notoriously' worse than other people? There must be some distinguishing character belonging to them." She asserted that mesmerists "proudly boast among their number, refined and educated females, possessing highly intellectual attainments."[63]

The United States soon crawled with itinerant mesmerists. In

Boston alone, more than two hundred magnetizers sold their services by 1843. Dozens of books with do-it-yourself instructions appeared on store shelves to train and tempt would-be home mesmerizers with the promise of health and self-improvement. Methods of inducing trance varied from practitioner to practitioner. Nearly all passed their hands over the body, but where some made actual contact, others simply moved their hands over and around the body. Some imitated Mesmer and used a metal wand to conduct the flow of animal magnetism. Still others dragged phrenology into the mix and tried to direct their magnetic powers toward particular parts of the brain associated with one or more phrenological traits.[64] All mesmerists could agree on one thing, though: one person had the power to gain control over another.[65]

As mesmerism's disciples became more numerous and enthusiastic in the United States, the movement fell ever further away from respectability in the eyes of regular medicine. In 1844, the *Boston Medical and Surgical Journal* expressed the frustrated bewilderment felt by many in the medical establishment. "In after times, the history of the mesmeric infatuation in New England will be read with surprise, and produce a train of feeling much like that developed by reading an account of the witchcraft mania in the ancient town of Salem."[66] A writer in the *New-Hampshire Gazette* wondered, "Can it be possible, that among enlightened men, in this age of light, the pretended wonderful art or science of 'animal magnetism' can gain a moment's credence!"[67] The apparent ease of inducing mesmeric trance did inevitably draw enterprising showmen who drew large crowds with what amounted to carnival sideshow hypnotism. For these practitioners, mesmerism was nothing more than entertainment and profit. And as with other irregular healing movements, these showmen degraded all of mesmerism in the eyes of regular doctors eager to find fault with their competitors.[68]

Other regulars questioned mesmerism's healing claims. They charged magnetizers with overstatement and deception for making extravagant claims about unseen and unknown forces to dupe the witless. They accused patients of faking trances to gain access to free medical care or of actually being hired actors. The patient's "grimaces, manipulations, and jargon of words is all a farce to deceive the ignorant . . . hoaxed out of much small change, at the expense of their wit."[69]

To combat these accusations and make the case for the seriousness of their science, American mesmerists offered detailed neurophysiological observations and made hypotheses based on contemporary medical knowledge. Mesmerist John Bovee Dods suggested that the body breathed in animal magnetism from the air and transformed it into vital fluid for human use. Several mesmerists proposed that animal magnetism took the form of electrical impulses when it entered the nervous system. Others suggested that the brain exuded animal magnetism. All were convinced that science would eventually account for this new and wholly unexplored autonomous psychological realm. Aware of the power of suggestion and expectation in determining behavior, mesmerists became the first Americans to directly study the psychodynamics of interpersonal relationships. Most mesmerists accepted that suggestion and prior expectation affected the patient's susceptibility to trance, but they, like Puységur before them, did not believe that this could account for all of their data. Subjects in the highest mesmeric state reported feeling a distinct, and in some cases, tangible force emanating from their nervous systems. Afterward, most could not remember the details of the trance experience, but many clearly recalled feeling something inside them moving around. For mesmerists, the physical existence of animal magnetism seemed undeniable based on their data. Many believed it also gave their theory greater significance because it proposed both a new psychological realm as well as a new natural force in the universe. Mesmerists promoting even the most psychological versions of their method never abandoned the idea of an invisible fluid. This commitment to animal magnetism distinguished mesmerism from opposing theories and other mental cures. As a result, American mesmerists were not as interested in pursuing the notion of suggestion as some European scientists, such as neurologist Jean-Martin Charcot and his student Sigmund Freud, would be later in the nineteenth century. Charcot found aspects of mesmeric trance useful in treating certain psychiatric patients, while Freud used hypnosis in his career to recover repressed memories. But until then, mesmerist articles and charts in the 1840s and 1850s represented some of the most significant attempts of the period to explore the nature of consciousness and the mind-body connection.[70]

Almost as abruptly as he arrived, Poyen left the United States and returned to France in 1839. But by then, the movement he spawned had developed a life of its own. Both P. T. Barnum's American Museum and Ruben Peale's New York Museum of Natural History and Science drew crowds at twice-daily demonstrations of mesmerism and clairvoyant somnambulism that combined, like the museums themselves, sensational and over-the-top entertainment with education. Competition grew so fierce between the two museums that each actively poached popular magnetizers from the other with the timeworn lure of higher pay and greater prestige.[71] Outside of cities, small-town and rural Americans relied on traveling mesmerists to provide them with medical instruction and entertainment. These itinerants tried to make a career out of demonstrating their mesmeric skills to fellow Americans.

These public displays injected mesmerism into the lives of the American lower and middle classes. Mesmerism, not unlike its fellow irregular healing systems, provided one answer to a growing popular demand for new and more satisfying worldviews outside of religion. Exploring the unconscious mind and the mind-brain connection through trance states allowed Americans to learn about themselves and their true nature outside the walls of the churchyard.[72] Followers believed, or certainly hoped, that mesmerism was not a hoax, but a healing tool with real scientific and therapeutic benefit.

One of these Americans was Phineas Parkhurst Quimby, who expanded mesmerist philosophy into a total philosophy of life. A clockmaker by trade, Quimby sat spellbound in the audience as Poyen demonstrated the astonishing powers of animal magnetism on a stop in Belfast, Maine, in 1838. After the lecture, Quimby nearly assaulted Poyen with questions about this mysterious mental fluid. Poyen told Quimby that he, too, could develop his own mental powers if he devoted himself to its study. It was all Quimby needed to hear. He set aside his clocks and followed Poyen from town to town until he mastered the practice of mesmerism. His dedication prompted Poyen to compliment his "exceptional magnetic powers and great power of concentration."[73] Before long, Quimby had a magnetic practice of his own back in Belfast.

Quimby soon joined forces with Lucius Burkmar, a young man particularly adept at mind reading and clairvoyance while under a mesmeric trance. Once magnetized, Quimby directed Burkmar to

use his clairvoyant powers to diagnose illnesses in patients and prescribe medicinal remedies. At other times, Quimby dispensed with
Burkmar and instead transmitted the magnetic energy from his own
brain into his patient's body. The two took to the road in 1843, providing demonstrations and enacting miraculous cures. Newspapers took
note, and soon the former clockmaker from Maine was being touted
as the world's leading mesmerist.[74]

As time passed, though, Quimby began to doubt that animal magnetism alone could explain his healing successes. The startling accu-
racy of the diagnoses that Burkmar produced so amazed patients that
they tended to put their full trust in the curative power of Quimby
and Burkmar. But Quimby wondered if the remedies worked more
on what the patient believed about her disorder than on what actually ailed her. Was Burkmar simply using his telepathic skills to read
the patient's mind rather than to diagnose the actual physical illness?
Was he perceiving what the patient already supposed about the illness and simply providing confirmation of that thought? Most of the
remedies Quimby prescribed were innocuous enough substances to
prove equally effective (or ineffective) on any number of diseases, so
it was hard to know what actually did the healing.[75] Quimby's speculations about Burkmar led him to a radical conclusion: rather than
suppose that what a person believed contributed to healing, Quimby
determined that the patients' beliefs were actually the cause of all
their symptoms. This idea bears much in common with what are now
known as somatoform (or psychosomatic) disorders, where physical
symptoms result from psychological causes. Quimby, however, felt
that this was the origin of most, if not all, disease.[76]

Starting from the assumption that the human mind comprised
all beliefs, Quimby rationalized that if a person is "deceived into a belief that he has, or is liable to have a disease, the belief is catching
and the effects follow from it."[77] Quimby wasn't the first mesmerist to
suggest a psychological origin for disease, but unlike his predecessors
who pointed to a magnetic fluid imbalance as the primary problem,
Quimby specifically identified faulty ideas as the main cause of disease. "All sickness is in the mind of belief," proclaimed Quimby. "To
cure the disease is to correct the error, destroy the cause, and the effect
will cease."[78] His theories moved mesmerism one step closer to clinical psychology.

Before Quimby, neither regular doctors nor mesmerists were really prepared to deal with problems that did not have an obvious physical cause. Doctors were uncomfortable with diseases that lacked a discrete, material, and easily explained origin. Without an understanding of their basis or the presumption that they even existed, the pain and discomfort of mental health issues and symptoms of psychological origin rarely received the social recognition that would grant these illnesses legitimacy. Mental and emotional disorders tended to be classified as ephemeral or hypochondriacal, so most Americans could find little consideration or relief for mental health issues. Quimby, on the other hand, based on his new theory of disease, expanded the scope of the mesmeric cure to provide the support patients needed to constructively manage life's difficulties. He still believed strongly in animal magnetism, which he thought flowed to the nervous system and conscious mind from some deeper, unconscious part of the mind that he believed existed as an actual physical place, but he now assigned human beliefs to a new interventionist role as control valves or power switches regulating the flow of magnetism from the conscious to the unconscious mind. Wrong beliefs could block this flow and disrupt the body's internal harmony by placing it solely at the mercy of outside conditions. Deprived of these essential energies, patients eventually lapsed into disease. The healer's job was to engage with clients on a one-on-one basis to overcome their negative and self-defeating attitudes, a proto–talk therapy. This discussion allowed the healer to identify the wrong beliefs that were causing the outward symptoms and to then heal the patient with new, more positive thoughts. Armed with his new mentalistic theory of disease, Quimby no longer needed Burkmar or any clairvoyant, and the two parted ways in 1847.[79]

Quimby instructed patients to "come with me [mentally] to where the trouble is, and you will find . . . it is kept hot and disturbed by your mind being misrepresented."[80] His treatment consisted of a combination of straightforward mesmerist technique and a self-induced altered state of consciousness. In this state, Quimby claimed he could see a kind of vapor cloud enveloping his patient's body, similar to an aura, that contained all of her "ideas, right and wrong. This vapor or fluid contains the identity of the person."[81] He could see events long forgotten and, presaging Freud, suppressed opinions and feelings contained in this mental fog. While in this superior mental state, Quimby engaged with the cloud to transmit his mesmerically acquired healing forces telepathically from his own person to the patient. He used this force to instill faith in the patient that she was healthy and that any negative thoughts were wrong.[82]

Quimby described his treatment process when he visited a Mr. Robinson who had been confined to his bed for four years. He explained how he'd take up Robinson's feelings "one by one, like a lawyer examining witnesses, analyzing them and showing him that he put false constructions on all his feelings." Robinson was skeptical of Quimby at first but allowed him to proceed, his arguments being "so plain that it was impossible not to understand." By the end of the session, Robinson "felt like a man who had been confined in a prison for life" who had just been given "a pardon" and "set at liberty." The next day, he felt better than he had in years and "had no desire to take to [his] bed" again.[83] Quimby's skill and method proved so powerful that he even treated people through the mail. In this "absent treatment," Quimby professed to be present for the patient in spirit through the written word.[84]

Quimby's mind cure had an appealing simplicity about it, even as the explanations he offered for his healing powers often defied reason and skirted the edges of the fantastic. Describing his mesmeric state, Quimby claimed to travel into the "land of darkness with the light of liberty, [to] search out the dungeons where the lives of the sick are bound, enter them and set the prisoners free."[85] He couldn't explain his powers; he knew only that they worked. When offered one thousand dollars for his secret, he was forced to confess, "I don't understand it myself."[86] His willingness to admit that he did not know everything was a far cry from other irregular healers, who tended to lash out at those who asked too many questions or required clarification. Right beliefs led to health and happiness. Human misery resulted from listening only to the outward world and losing touch with the body's inner mind and spiritual self. The key element, Quimby counseled, was to identify internal rather than external reference points of self-esteem and worth, a message so modern and familiar as to not seem out of place in any women's magazine or self-help book today. "Disease is something made by belief or forced upon us by our parents or public opinion," wrote Quimby. "Now if you can face the error and argue it down you can cure the sick."[87] Listen to your inner voice. Don't let other people distract you from the life you were meant to live. Quimby was the Oprah of the nineteenth century.

In case anyone questioned the religious implications of his theory as they had of mesmerism, Quimby made sure to spell it out. His "Science of Health" reunited the wrong-thinking mind with the divine internal spirit of Christ. Quimby asserted that he established inner rapport with the Christ-like spirit contained inside every person when he healed. Quimby's mesmerist psychology seemed to verify a common belief that humans possessed both a lower animal nature and higher spiritual nature. Phrenologists also made this distinction by locating the traits associated with animals in the lower part of the brain and the more religious and moral faculties in the lobes. By turning the mind inward toward its own psychic depths and God's emanative powers, people could grasp the true purpose of their lives in the physical world; under Quimby, mesmerism now offered a way to conceptualize a theological viewpoint in psychological terms. The mind-cure approach to well-being decreed that everyone had power over their own psychological realm, even if modern life had seemingly stripped away every other aspect of control. Quimby's cure presented both a Christian and scientific approach to life that many nineteenth-century Americans wanted and that he occasionally referred to as "Christian Science."[88]

By 1865, nearly twelve thousand patients had come to Quimby's Portland, Maine, office for treatment. Most came out of sheer desperation after regular doctors had given up hope of a cure. Patients came for relief of everything from consumption and smallpox to cancer, diphtheria, and nervous ailments. Quimby was skilled at putting people at ease. His interest and compassion astonished his patients, who were unused to doctors listening so intently and seriously, especially to emotional complaints.[89]

One of the patients to appear on Quimby's doorstep was Mary Patterson, soon to be Mary Baker Eddy, in 1862. Quimby with his patient ear and healing mind worked wonders on Eddy. She was so inspired by his healing process that once well, she resolved to take up a career in Quimby-style mental healing. A few months later, Eddy gave her first public lecture on "P. P. Quimby's Spiritual Science Healing Disease as Opposed to Deism or Rochester-Rapping Spiritualism," the last a reference to the mysterious and ghostly knockings that

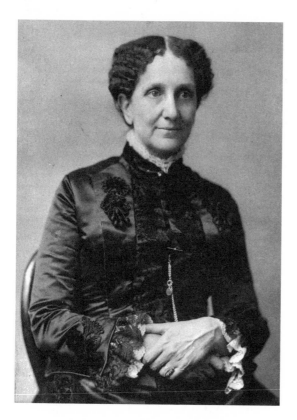

Mary Baker Eddy introduced her own new medical system, "Christian Science." (Library of Congress)

inaugurated the spiritualist movement in Rochester, New York. With this talk, she anointed herself Quimby's first spokesperson. Unfortunately for Eddy, her mentor died the next year, on January 16, 1866, temporarily robbing her of her inspiration and role model.[90]

Two weeks after Quimby's death, though, Eddy discovered the path to her future. After a fall on an icy street left her largely confined to bed, Eddy found sudden relief from her painful injuries while reading passages from the Bible on Christ's healing ministry. The "presence and power of God seemed to flood her whole being" and she stood up "healed."[91] She could not explain what happened, but she knew beyond a doubt that her recovery resulted from her reading of the Gospel. From this experience, she developed a theory based on the premise that disease resulted from one's alienation from God. Like

Quimby, she believed that illness existed in the mind; her reading of the Bible told her that it was not inherent in God's creation. Since "God is good" and "God is all," Eddy reasoned that evil, a category under which disease naturally fell, therefore could not possibly exist. "Evil is but an illusion," Eddy counseled, a misbelief that needed to be changed. It was an idea that largely conformed to Quimby's practice. She then took the extreme step of negating the existence of the physical body itself. Eddy argued that God lived in the spirit that existed in the mind, and since God was everything, what people thought of as their physical body was in reality only another misguided belief. In theory, she wrote, "a man could live just as well after his lungs had been removed as before, if he but thought he could." She named her new approach to healing "Christian Science," ignoring or perhaps not caring that Quimby had sometimes used that name for his system. She also disavowed any debt to her mentor and claimed only divine revelation, even though her theory appeared to be little more than Quimbyism embellished with biblical references.[92]

Eddy published her findings in *Science and Health with Key to the Scriptures* in 1875 and four years later, in 1879, founded the Church of Christ (Scientist). The church soon became one of the fastest-growing denominations in the country, counting more than 200,000 members by 1925. Local churches and instructional institutes opened around the country, and several thousand Christian Science healers, more than 80 percent of them women, began practicing.[93] Eddy also opened a school, a first for any of the mesmerist and magnetist mind cures in the United States, in 1881. The Massachusetts Metaphysical College graduated hundreds of doctors of Christian Science, who helped spread her message and technique from coast to coast. She'd begun teaching students more than a decade before, in 1868, promising lessons in a method "with a success far beyond any of the present modes."[94]

Christian Science boasted an impressive record of cures. Healing "testimonies" appeared as a monthly feature in the *Christian Science Journal*, which launched in 1883. In its pages, people claimed to have been cured of cancer, blindness, and gunshot wounds to the chest. When a stage curtain descended on the head of an operatic prima donna, it delivered a "staggering blow" to her "delicate little nose." But after a visit with a practitioner of Christian Science, her swollen nose and badly bruised eyes had healed completely.[95] Not all believers went to visit a Christian Science doctor. Some attempted to cure themselves by reading *Science and Health*. One Seattle woman reported that thirty years of constipation cleared up after she read Eddy's book. Another woman in Salt Lake City declared the broken arm she suffered in a bicycle accident healed after ten minutes of reading. Eddy expected patients to try to heal themselves first. This is partly why she put so much work into editing and refining *Science and Health* throughout her life, undertaking eight major revisions and issuing more than four hundred printings.[96]

Few irregular theories struck regular doctors as more ridiculous than Christian Science, particularly Eddy's denial of the very existence of physical bodies. After Eddy reported saving the life of a pregnant woman and her twelve-pound infant, Chicago physician Edmund Andrews sarcastically remarked that, for having no body, "this bouncing offspring" had produced "a very satisfactory result" for the mother.[97] Another case found a Christian Science healer called to attend to a sick cow. Once recovered, the cow chased the doctor around the barnyard until a hired man scared him off with a pitchfork. The story prompted one regular doctor to wonder if the line of "non-existence of matter has to be drawn at enraged animals."[98] American journalist Ambrose Bierce got in on the fun, too, writing in his *Devil's Dictionary* that Christian Science was superior to regular medicine because it "will cure imaginary diseases, and they cannot."[99] Eddy's claim that the death of her husband in 1882 was caused by a mental poison delivered by an enemy mesmerist earned the scorn of the *Cincinnati Daily Gazette*, which claimed that, in fact, he had suffered from arsenic poisoning. "Mrs. Eddy's theory reminds one of the old stories of witchcraft, in which the tormenter made an image of the person he wished to afflict, and by sticking pins into it and otherwise misusing it, caused the live victim to feel pain as if he had been directly attacked," stated the *Gazette*. "This is the nineteenth century, but the traditions of the seventeenth still survive."[100] An autopsy conducted by Dr. Rufus Noyes concluded that Eddy's husband had died from heart disease, but Eddy refused to believe him, even after Noyes went to the extraordinary length of bringing her his heart on a tray and showing her the diseased parts.[101]

Harvard physician Richard Cabot was more generous, writing that "most" of the cures claimed by Christian Science were probably true if gauged by the power of suggestion and placebo. Tabulating cures proclaimed in Christian Science journals, Cabot proposed that at least three-quarters were of psychological rather than physical ailments.[102] Many regulars agreed that Christian Science probably worked for hysterics, worriers, and sufferers from "imaginary maladies," but for serious cases like smallpox and heart disease, they called Christian Science a danger to public health. Some Christian Scientists were accused of murder, but most were acquitted on the grounds that patients were free to express their religious beliefs. To avoid further legal trouble, though, Eddy advised her followers to decline patients seeking help for infectious or contagious diseases as well as seriously ill children.[103]

Eddy herself also provoked the heated cries of her critics in the religious and medical circles she sought to displace with her own medical-religious system. Clergymen portrayed her as a boa constrictor who had "coiled herself around the Christian system, breaking all the doctrinal bones of Christianity," while she covered them in slime so they would "go down easy." Others saw her as a spider attempting to "beguile simple souls into her web" and "devour them."[104] In human form, she was an "enchantress," cruelly enticing the innocent with "the sweet cup of her sorcery," before revealing to the ensnared masses that she was "not a beautiful maiden, but an old hag" leading "the sons of men downward to darkness and woe."[105] Clearly, Eddy's gender and not just her theory played a large part in the attacks. Developed and led by a woman, rather than just allowing women to take part, Christian Science posed a unique threat to both regular medicine and traditional religion. Prevailing views held that women who promulgated unorthodox views or who did not fulfill their female duties were insane, unpleasant "mental harridans." Some declared Christian Science to be little more than the delusions of a hysterical woman. Ralph Wallace Reed asserted that practitioners of "psychological medicine" would "have no difficulty in diagnosing her case" of major hysteria. Widespread stereotypes of women's intellectual inferiority made others declare Eddy simply incapable of reason and scientific inquiry and thus pronounce her system impossible to take seriously, dismissing it as a movement of women, even as it grew into an international phenomenon.[106]

Despite Eddy's critics, Christian Science only continued to grow and spread among women and men. The large number of men who helped to expand the church and spoke out in its favor belied the image of Christian Science as an organization of hysterical women. Letters in the *Christian Science Journal* found followers coming to Christian Science primarily for healing but also for a more satisfying understanding of God. Both men and women confessed themselves unable to reconcile themselves to the idea of a God who caused or even allowed so much suffering in traditional religion. Eddy's insistence that God did not cause evil in any form and her advice to have a hopeful state of mind comforted those theologically and medically disillusioned.[107] As more people converted, Christian Science Reading Rooms for the study and purchase of books opened around the country and continue to operate to this day. The *Christian Science Monitor* continues to publish national and international news with a daily religious feature. Church members can be found in more than 130 countries.[108]

Christian Science was not the only mental healing group to emerge after Quimby's death. Two other Quimby patients, Warren Felt Evans and Julius Dresser, along with Dresser's wife, Anetta, interpreted the growing public interest in mental health as a calling, and they set up mental healing practices in Boston. Unlike Eddy, they fully acknowledged their debt to Quimby. With no prior training other than what they had observed from Quimby, Evans and the Dressers continued to clarify and refine their intellectual understanding of mental healing, picking up pieces of nearly every metaphysical idea they happened across, be it Christian, spiritualist, Transcendentalist, Buddhist, Swedenborgian, mystic, or otherwise. Their enthusiasm proved contagious and helped to spread their increasingly popular brands of healing around the country. These and other like-minded thinkers contributed to what became known as the New Thought movement, a loosely organized group that shared a conviction—if little else—that the mind can solve all human problems. "Minds are forces," they argued, and could be harnessed with proper instruction.[109]

Publishing a stream of articles and books, New Thought authors attempted to systematically apply the principles of mesmerism and other metaphysical ideas to everyday life. They advised readers to adopt mental habits that duplicated the thinking associated with the mesmeric state of consciousness, in effect taking the "right beliefs" that Quimby sought to place in people's minds and turning them into complete descriptions of how people ought to think and act.[110]

In practice, this resulted in a flood of surefire mind-cure solutions to problems in marriage, work, or home life. Books with titles like *Thought Is Power*, *How to Get What You Want*, and *Making Money* transformed belief in the power of the mind to cure illness into a whole life philosophy largely centered around positive thinking.[111] "Within yourself lies the cause of whatever enters your life," advised Ralph Waldo Trine's 1897 *In Tune With the Infinite*, which sold more than two million copies. "To come into the full realization of your awakened interior powers, is to be able to condition your life in exact accord with what you would have it."[112] Frank Channing Haddock offered practical, hygienic advice for "acquiring magnetism" and what he called "success-magnetism" in his *Master of Self for Wealth, Power, and Success*, recommending "scrupulous cleanliness of the body, without and within," "sweet, sound and early sleep," and a balance of "work and recreation."[113] These books, many of them best sellers, dramatically increased the number of people who came into contact with American mesmerist ideas of the mind's extraordinary powers to shape one's external circumstances. It also obscured mesmerism's history and original applications.

While mental healing systems that grew out of mesmerism proliferated, by 1900 mesmerism itself had quietly disappeared as a subject of popular interest. American mesmerists, while successful, had never established mesmerism as a professional medical science. No official schools of mesmerism were established. No professional organizations formed. Many magnetic healers abandoned their mental healing practices after a few years in favor of more metaphysically inclined psychological theories, a trend that only increased after Quimby's death. Some mesmerists became spiritualists, concentrating their mental powers on speaking to the dead in the spiritual realm that they believed the mesmeric state activated. The actual practice of mesmerism languished in the 1870s and mostly expired in the 1880s with the emergence of psychology as a professional scholarly field. These new psychologists sought to demonstrate the superiority of their psychology to its philosophical predecessors by writing articles denouncing mesmerism and mind cures as speculative, irrational, and unscientific.[114]

Although mesmerism itself never achieved scientific acceptance, it spawned many legitimate scientific fields and stimulated new strains of inquiry. Mesmerism, like phrenology, was one of the first in a long line of American popular psychologies that promised to impart the secret to personal renewal. Mesmerism differed from phrenology, though, in that it had nothing specifically to do with the brain as an organ but rather envisioned the mind and thought itself as a physical force. Where phrenology put a detailed map and vocabulary for self-development into the hands of Americans, mesmerism provided them access to their innermost mental domains. While other scientists, physicians, and healers alluded to the potential of the mind to cure, Mesmer was the first to elevate the mind to primacy in the healing process, inspiring waves of cures and healing movements based on mental powers.

In many ways, though, Puységur's name is the one we should know. His discovery of the unconscious mind through somnambulism led to the first truly psychological treatment, and his method and emphasis on the psychological, rather than Mesmer's focus on an imperceptible physical fluid, became the standard form of mesmerism (despite the name) practiced in the nineteenth century. He observed and recorded all of the core elements of modern hypnosis: the idea of a therapeutic connection between the magnetizer and subject, an altered state of consciousness with noticeable lucidity in some patients, and the near total amnesia of the trance experience that followed. Experimentation with somnambulism led to the development of dynamic clinical psychology as scientists, including Sigmund Freud, used data provided by entranced patients to formulate the rudiments of psychoanalysis. By the late nineteenth century, the act of bringing someone into a trance state, now known as hypnosis, had finally won the scientific and medical backing that Mesmer had so desperately craved in his own life.[115] Mesmerism's ideas and healing successes stimulated public interest in the inner workings of the mind and laid the groundwork for psychology, psychiatry, and the modern use of therapeutic hypnosis as a healing tool.

But if mesmerist practice mostly disappeared in its original form, the pop-cultural image of a flamboyant doctor turned mystical scientist and the idea of altered states certainly did not. Virtual travel through altered states like that induced by mesmeric trance has become a staple of books and movies. Think of the *Matrix* movies, where heroes act in a virtual space while their physical bodies sit immobilized. A similar idea underlies the plots of the movies *Avatar* and

Inception. Books like *The Secret* and those of Eckhart Tolle promoting the power of thought to change lives continue to sell briskly.

As with phrenology, mesmerism spoke to a deep-seated desire to unlock the potential of the mind for human use. To know and understand ourselves and others, to be better people, to cure what ails us—these are goals humans are still striving to achieve. The idea that the answers might lie within continues to mesmerize.

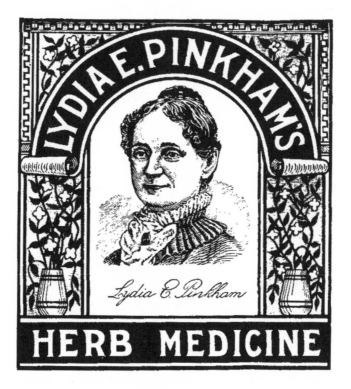

Lydia Pinkham marketed a patent medicine that bore her name and, unusually for the time, her face. She was one of few woman entrepreneurs in a crowded and predominantly male patent-medicine marketplace.
(Wikimedia Commons)

CHAPTER SIX

Selling Snake Oil
Patent Medicine

Despite the common belief, most patent medicines did not contain snake oil. Snake oil did exist, however. Clark Stanley, better known as "The Rattlesnake King," likely inspired the association with his "Snake Oil Liniment," which cured everything from rheumatism and sciatica to lumbago, frostbite, and sore throat. Stanley claimed to have learned of snake oil's healing powers from his years as a cowboy out west with the Hopi Indians in the 1870s and 1880s. He shared his discovery with the public at the 1893 World's Columbian Exposition in Chicago, where he pulled live snakes out of a sack, slit them open, and plunged their bodies into boiling water. As the fat from the snakes rose to the top, Stanley skimmed it off, mixed it with his previously prepared oils, and sold his liniment freshly made to the crowd that gathered to watch the spectacle. A few years later, in 1897, he published *The Life and Adventures of the American Cowboy: True Life in the Far West by Clark Stanley, Better Known as the Rattlesnake King*, which explained cowboy life, contained lyrics to cowboy songs, and, of course, promoted the healing wonders of his snake-oil liniment. Stanley's liniment became so successful that a reporter who visited his office in Beverly, Massachusetts, found it filled with snakes, some more than seven feet long, slithering around the room and up his arms. He claimed to have killed three thousand snakes in 1901 alone to meet demand for his product. Stanley's was not the only snake-oil remedy on the market. Consumers could also find Tex Bailey's Rattle Snake Oil, Tex Allen's Rattlesnake Essential Oil Compound, and Monster

Brand Snake Oil, among others, which capitalized on American fascination with cowboys, the Wild West, and Native Americans. Snake oil itself had an even longer history in Chinese medicine, in which people had rubbed the fat of the Erabu sea snake, not rattlesnakes, on aching joints for centuries.[1]

Snake-oil salesmen like Stanley exemplify the image most people have of "quack medicine": the charlatans making outlandish claims to make a buck off the gullible. These quacks, as popularly conceived, marketed bottles of alcohol blended with a few herbs and spices as cure-alls for dread diseases both real and imaginary. They hawked medicine on street corners and onstage, turning medicine into magic and beguiling audiences with the idea that anything was possible.[2] Medicine was serious, not a game, cried regulars, and it was certainly not entertainment. Regular doctors tended to paint those who sold patent medicines and medical devices with the broad brushstroke of quackery, but the lines of legitimacy remained far from clear in the nineteenth century.

Nicholas Boone of Boston placed what is believed to be the first American patent-medicine ad, in the *Boston News-Letter* in 1708: "Daffy's Elixir Salutis, very good, at four shillings and sixpence *per* pint Bottle."[3] The remedy was not Boone's own invention but an English remedy from the late seventeenth century said to cure innumerable ailments from rheumatism, gout, and scurvy to the King's Evil, a lymph infection popularly believed only curable by the royal touch, a commodity even harder to find in colonial America than a trained doctor.[4] Colonial Americans imported English patent remedies that they learned about from newspaper ads. These ads tended to be mostly lists and not the drawings and screaming headlines yet to come. Although many colonists concocted their own home remedies from herbs and other botanicals, British patent medicines remained the premade remedy of choice for those that could afford them until the American Revolution disrupted trade. American pharmacists, who before the war had sometimes counterfeited medicines by refilling and reselling old British bottles with their own remedies, found a robust market for their wares in an independent United States eager to break ties with all things British. Struck with a new nationalist fervor, Americans began to demand made-in-America medicines.[5] These homegrown remedies rarely contained any new or special ingredients. Most consisted of herbs and drugs found in the standard drug formularies and home medical guides of the day.[6]

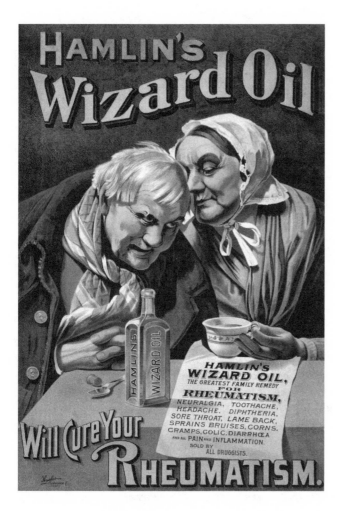

An advertisement for one of many patent-medicine "cures." (Library of Congress, from a print by Hughes Lithographers, Chicago, via Wikimedia Commons)

The nineteenth century revolutionized the patent-medicine trade. The commercial and printing advances of the new century changed the relationship between seller and consumer from one that was face-to-face to one at a distance—and one of trust gained through the printed word. The greater numbers of newspapers, books, and magazines in circulation gave Americans more and new ways to learn about and engage with science. It also exposed them to ads for patent medicines. Consumers eager to exercise their purchasing power found an ever-increasing array of medical devices, pills, and health regimens to try, the megavitamins, glucosamine, and green coffee beans of their day. The flood of products made for a fiercely competitive marketplace among sellers. To make their products stand out, medicine makers developed name brands with distinctive packaging and bottle designs, proclaimed testimonial success, and made extravagant healing claims.[7]

Thomas W. Dyott became the first American patent-medicine baron. A pharmacist in Philadelphia, Dyott marketed his Robertson's Infallible Worm Destroying Lozenges nationally. He claimed the pills were named for his Scottish physician grandfather, but the line was likely a lie. Agents sold his lozenges in cities and towns across the country. Together with his newspaper advertisements, Dyott became nationally known for his cure in the 1810s. By the 1820s, Dyott had generated a quarter-million-dollar fortune off the sale of his remedy. He purchased a glass factory to bottle his own medicines and constructed a model company town, Dyottville, for his employees. The town included a hospital, athletic fields, a church, schools, and farms. He also opened a bank that printed its own money. Dyott's face graced every bill. The 1837 national economic panic did Dyott in, though, and he lost much of his fortune.[8]

Despite the use of the name, most of these remedies were never patented. The name "patent" likely came from the British practice of granting a "patent of royal favor" on eighteenth-century remedies, which then allowed medicines to feature the crest of the king on the label. To actually file for a patent in the United States would have required sellers to reveal the ingredients, which most were loath to do. The mystery added to a remedy's selling power and mystique. It also provoked some of the biggest complaints about patent medicines from regular doctors and represented a sharp break from other forms of irregular health care that made a virtue of their transparency. Makers did, however, trademark their product names and label design. Ads and product labels tended to boast that the remedies were painless, nice tasting, and nonmineral, direct shots at the practices of regular doctors and right in line with their irregular compatriots. In fact, many patent-medicine makers were motivated by the same factors that contributed to the rise of Thomsonism, homeopathy, hydropathy, and the other irregular health systems: the arrogance of regular doctors and the dangers of heroic medicine.[9]

Impatient with doctors who "physic us to death," Lydia Estes Pinkham devised her own remedy that she promised would make her the "Saviour of her Sex" in the 1870s.[10] Born in Lynn, Massachusetts, in 1819, Pinkham grew up in a reforming household in a town well known for its passion for agitation and social improvement. Pinkham's parents left the local Quaker church after members refused to endorse the abolition of slavery in the 1830s. In its place, Pinkham's mother Rebecca introduced the family to the science-based theology of Emanuel Swedenborg and later to spiritualism. The Pinkhams' devotion to the antislavery cause made their home a popular meeting place for abolitionist leaders, including journalist William Lloyd Garrison, writers and activists David and Lydia Maria Child, and the Quaker poet John Greenleaf Whittier. The family counted Frederick Douglass, Lynn's most famous resident, as a close friend. Just down the street lived the Hutchinsons, a family of singers who would later become famous for their social reform ballads, including the satiric song "Go Call the Doctor, & Be Quick, or Anti-Calomel" with its dozens of verses highlighting the greed, ignorance, and indiscriminate dosing of regular doctors. Raised in this environment, it's hardly surprising that the adult Pinkham supported abolition, spiritualism, women's rights, temperance, and eventually, irregular medicine.[11]

Lydia married Isaac Pinkham in 1843, raised four children, and took on the traditional role of domestic healer for her family. She used old family remedies and cures from home medical guides, particularly John King's *American Dispensatory*, which combined traditional European botanic remedies with plants from the New World. She carefully noted all her favorites in a notebook labeled "Medical Directions for Ailments." Her healing acumen brought neighbors to her door seeking advice and the homemade medicines she brewed on her stove and generally gave away for free to those in need. One of her most popular was a remedy designed especially for the health of women. But Pinkham wasn't selling—at least not yet.[12]

The Pinkhams were hit hard by the economic depression that followed the fiscal panic of 1873, and they struggled to remain financially afloat in the 1870s. In 1875, several women from Salem ventured to the Pinkhams' home seeking to purchase six bottles of her female remedy. Although Pinkham usually refused payment, with her family's money troubles, she reluctantly accepted five dollars.[13] Her son Daniel immediately saw the marketing potential. "Mother, if those ladies will come all the way from Salem to get that medicine, why can it not be sold to other people," he reportedly exclaimed. "Why can't we go into the business of making and selling it, same as any other medicine?"[14]

He was right. Advertisements for Radway's Relief, Holmen's Liver Pad, Dr. Williams' Pink Pills for Pale People, and Hale's Honey of Horehound and Tar filled newspapers, netting many of their makers a healthy income. She would not even be the only woman selling in the Boston area, as Elizabeth Mott already offered an herbal remedy and hydropathic regimen to women based on her Medicated Shampoo. Pinkham had her doubts, but Daniel and his brother Will's enthusiasm and her family's declining circumstances finally convinced her to go forward. By the spring of 1875, "Lydia E. Pinkham's Vegetable Compound" for "female weakness" entered the crowded patent-medicine marketplace.[15]

Pinkham registered her label and trademark with the United States Patent Office in 1876. Like most patent medicines, Pinkham's Vegetable Compound was actually a proprietary remedy. Only the name and label were trademarked and enjoyed government protection. The recipe remained a closely guarded secret.[16]

Both the name of Pinkham's remedy and the ingredients she chose owed much to Samuel Thomson and other botanic healers. Pinkham's notes for her original formula called for unicorn root, life root, black cohosh, pleurisy root, and fenugreek seed, botanical elements used for generations. Many irregulars still recommend both black cohosh and fenugreek seed to women suffering symptoms of menopause today. The ingredients and perhaps even the basis of the recipe itself came from Pinkham's favorite *American Dispensatory*, which contained descriptions, properties, and uses for every known medical botanical remedy. Even the author of *American Dispensatory*, John King, owed much to Thomson, as he was a practitioner of Eclecticism, a medical movement that came out of the splintering of Thomsonism earlier in the century. Thomsonism had also spawned strains of imitator patent-medicine makers who cashed in on public enthusiasm for botanicals and their distaste for mineral drugs to market plant preparations throughout the nineteenth century. Despite a general unwillingness to reveal their active ingredients, patent medicines happily screamed what they did not contain: namely calomel. While other irregular systems, too, influenced patent medicines making related theoretical claims, Thomson's influence in this field was far wider and longer lasting, with Lydia Pinkham a clear successor of his botanical enthusiasm.[17]

The public disgust with heroic therapies that helped to make botanicals as well as homeopathy and hydropathy so popular began to make inroads into the practices of regular medicine by the middle of the nineteenth century. In 1835, prominent regular physician Jacob Bigelow argued that some diseases would naturally cure themselves in a critique of heroic therapy presented before the Massachusetts Medical Society. Bigelow understood that it was difficult for doctors to stand by and do nothing but warned that their attempts to intervene too often left them unsure "whether the patient is really indebted to us for good or evil." He counseled caution and, sounding every bit like an irregular healer, suggested that the role of the doctor was to remove obstacles in nature's healing path.[18] Easier said than done for many practicing doctors, who wondered why anyone would call for a doctor if all they could do was stand aside and wait. Those that did try to implement more conservative use of bleeding and calomel faced resistance from some patients conditioned to expect a big effect from medical care. It was a problem that both regular and irregular medicine wrestled with throughout the nineteenth century.[19]

Even so, by the Civil War, heroic medicine was in retreat. Regular doctors could no longer ignore the criticism of Thomsonians, mesmerists, and hydropaths or the economic threat posed by homeopathy. Reflecting evolving attitudes and the shifting medical landscape, Surgeon General William Hammond banned the prescription and use of calomel and tartar emetic from the healing arsenal of the Union army in 1863. Hammond's decision created a furor in medical journals.[20] Hammond was compared to the "irregular charlatans" who "habitually seek popular favor by denouncing well-known remedies employed by the regular profession."[21] The criticism was not enough to overturn Hammond's order, however, and the use of calomel and bleeding decreased after the war. Some regular doctors continued to use heroic medicine exclusively into the 1880s, but most began replacing bloodletting and calomel with new pharmacological remedies containing primarily alcohol, opium, and quinine.[22]

Despite these changes, these new drugs were not a far departure from heroic medicine's emphasis on demonstrable relief from illness, as well as its often horrific consequences. Large doses of opium and alcohol produced side effects just as bad if not greater than those of calomel. Regular medicine's increasing reliance on drugs also produced an economic and cultural climate particularly well suited to a boom in patent medicine. Alcoholic proprietary tonics, bitters, and opiate-laced elixirs found a ready market among Americans habituated to their increasing use by regular doctors. During the Civil War, soldiers eagerly consumed medicines laced with alcohol. The US Army had abolished the alcohol ration in 1832, replacing it with coffee and sugar, so patent medicines provided an affordable way for soldiers to imbibe without running afoul of military rules. Patent medicines soared in popularity during and immediately following the Civil War, with total sales of $75 million by 1900. Improved transportation, wider circulation of newspapers, and cheaper manufacturing costs also enabled patent-medicine makers to expand distribution in the late nineteenth century. At the same time, professional mudslinging over the use of patent medicines became a favorite pastime of regular doctors, who seemed to have no problem overlooking their own misuse of alcohol, morphine, and quinine, liberally prescribed. Regulars were likely just as responsible as the patent medicines they viciously attacked for poisoning people and contributing to the rise of medically induced alcoholism.[23]

Pinkham's Vegetable Compound, too, contained alcohol. Brewing her early batches on a stove in her cellar, Pinkham first macerated the herbs and then suspended them in 19 percent alcohol for preservative purposes. The end product came in at forty proof. Pinkham was herself a temperance advocate. But she had no problem with using alcohol as medicine.[24]

Alcohol was a medical mainstay of the late nineteenth century for its low cost and wide availability. Though it was first prescribed for its stimulant effects, the discovery of germs turned alcohol into an internal cleanser, able to kill germs in the body's hard-to-reach places. Alcohol was prescribed for a variety of ailments, from anemia and heart disease to typhoid and tuberculosis. In 1878, Pinkham prescribed herself a teaspoon of whiskey mixed in two tablespoons of milk before meals for pneumonia. This was a small dose, however. Many regular doctors recommended doses the equivalent of five shots a day. Alcohol was not just for adults. Medicinal doses for children ranged from half a teaspoon to two teaspoons given every three hours, certainly enough to inebriate a small body. Pinkham's own alcohol-based remedy advised three spoonfuls a day, hardly enough to cause serious drunkenness and certainly no threat, Pinkham believed, to everyday temperance.[25]

Pinkham's business operated as a family venture. Her sons spread

the word through handbills and pamphlets while Pinkham worked
on production and ad copy. Although hesitant at first to get in the
medicine-selling game, she had clearly done her homework on the
type of marketing language likely to appeal to customers. The bright
blue label proclaimed "LYDIA E. PINKHAM'S VEGETABLE COMPOUND:
A Sure Cure for PROLAPSUS UTERI or falling of the Womb, and all
FEMALE WEAKNESSES. . . . Pleasant to the taste, efficacious and immediate in its effect, It is great help in pregnancy, and relieves pain during
labor. For All Weaknesses of the generative organs of either Sex, it is
second to no remedy that has ever been before the public, and for all
diseases of the Kidneys it is the Greatest Remedy in the World."[26]

Although the label claimed to offer relief to both women and men,
Pinkham aimed her remedy squarely at women. Like Lydia Fowler,
Mary Gove Nichols, and many other irregulars, Pinkham believed
that women suffered needlessly and ignorantly at the hands of regular doctors. She offered her Vegetable Compound as a way to help
women, and she used her gender as a selling point. "Only a woman
understands a woman's ills" became her ad slogan.[27] Purchasers could
trust that she was in fact who she said she was, too, after her grandmotherly image became the public face of the remedy.

Pinkham's son Daniel had hit on the idea of putting a woman's
face on the label in 1879. On an earlier trip to Brooklyn, he'd noticed
that "folks seem to be all tore up on home made goods" and he wondered how he could use that to his family's advantage. Several years
later, he looked at his mother and realized that he had found the perfect model for made-at-home goods. At sixty years old, Pinkham had
a maternal air and a warm and caring face. She truly had made her
remedy on her home stove, and had used it effectively for years before making it commercially available. No advertising man could have
made up someone better. Pinkham's grandmotherly face conveyed
sympathy and compassion in a single image. Her gray braid pulled
back in a bun and her respectable black silk dress and white collar instilled trust in her authority and the safety of her remedy. Who could
believe that this kindly woman would intentionally hurt anyone? The
label also convinced skeptics that there was a real person behind the
product. The same could certainly not be said for all patent remedies
bearing someone's name.[28]

The Vegetable Compound was not the first patent remedy to
feature a portrait, but it was the first to use a woman. Pinkham's

photograph made her a national figure. It appeared in newspapers and on druggists' counters. Newspapers found other uses for her image as well. Because editors had so few pictures of women, Pinkham's face stood in for other news-making women, including the much younger actress Lily Langtry and even Queen Victoria.[29] Pinkham's face made advertising history.

Patent-medicine sellers pioneered American advertising techniques and strategy. In part, they had no choice. With thousands of remedies available for sale and dozens of new medical systems, patent-medicine makers had to keep their product names on the tips of people's tongues with near continuous ad campaigns. Demand tended to drop precipitously when the ads stopped. In the 1830s, the emergence of the penny press, which generally sold sensational tabloid news at just one cent per issue, caused circulation to soar and bolstered the advertising of patent medicines.[30]

Critics condemned the penny press for running patent-medicine ads. The papers defended themselves by appealing to the common sense of their readers to judge the truth of the advertising claims. "Some of our readers complain of the great number of patent medicines advertised in this paper," declared the *Boston Daily Times*. "To this complaint we can only reply that it is our interest to insert such advertisements ... without any inquiry whether the articles advertised are what they purport to be. That is an inquiry for the reader who feels interested in the matter, and not for us, to make." It was the same pitch made by irregulars to the common sense and judgment of ordinary Americans, and to their ability to make their own decisions. Patent medicines proved a perfect match for the penny papers since the incredible claims of the sellers nearly matched the sensational stories appearing inside.[31]

Advertisements for patent medicines exploited nearly every human need and emotion. They also appealed to the common man and woman using the same simple and direct language shared by all irregular healers. Fear played a significant role. Death, disease, suffering, and evil became familiar and grim advertising themes. Labels, too, came filled with skulls and tombstones. Pinkham's own early advertisements ran in single columns with blaring headlines that resembled news stories to trick readers into thinking they were news so they would keep reading. "LIFE'S WOES," began one headline. "THOUSANDS DYING ANNUALLY, From Causes to the World Unknown, While

Other Thousands Are Being Restored to Health, Hope and Happiness by the Use of LYDIA E. PINKHAM'S VEGETABLE COMPOUND, The Positive Cure for Female Complaints." Another ad capitalized on a recent murder case to suggest the horrors that could result from untreated female weakness. "A FEARFUL TRAGEDY—A Clergyman of Stratford, Conn., KILLED BY HIS OWN WIFE. Insanity Brought on by 16 years of Suffering With Female Complaints the Cause. LYDIA E. PINKHAM'S VEGETABLE COMPOUND, The Sure Cure for These Complaints, Would Have Prevented the Direful Deed."[32]

Sex sold. Many patent medicines promised to restore sexual vitality. The Reinhardt brothers of Milwaukee declared themselves specialists in "private and secret diseases particular to men," which was the polite way of saying they treated erectile dysfunction and STDs. Sexual weakness and other sexual diseases, both real and imaginary, ran rampant throughout the nation in the late nineteenth and early twentieth centuries—or at least that's what the Reinhardts led their patients to believe. Roping in patients with printed literature and advertisements making hard-to-resist promises, Willis Reinhardt and his brothers handed out diagnoses of sexual dysfunction and took in thousands of dollars in return.[33]

A repetitive emphasis on suffering in many ads forged what came to be known as the "pain and agony" pitch still used in medical advertising today, though with a slight reduction in the melodrama.[34] "Grim death has taken darling little Jerry, The son of Joseph and Seveva Vowels; Seven months he suffered with the dysentery, And then he perished with his little bowels," read one ad for Castoria.[35] Others emphasized feelings of "constant pain," "dull, heavy pains," and "severe burning and sharp pains." Critics charged that the extensive detail gulled the healthy into believing themselves sick. Ad men countered that detailed lists of symptoms instilled confidence in users that the manufacturer knew what he was doing, and that "most ailing people get a morbid satisfaction in reading vivid descriptions of their sickness."[36]

Mythical and historic figures sold remedies for all kinds of complaints. Before moving to Milwaukee in 1901, the Reinhardts operated a fraudulent medical institute in Minneapolis known as the Heidelberg Institute, as famous for its cures as its fantastical waxworks window displays. Among the most dramatic was "The Dying Custer," which featured Custer flat on his back while a machine pumped his chest up and down as though he were taking his last breaths.[37] The Roman goddess of medicine, Minerva, sold a pill for venereal disease while Ben-Hur offered cures for kidney ailments. Patriotism was frequently called into service as were ads that capitalized on the foreign and mysterious, such as Mexican Mustang Liniment and Dr. Drake's Canton Chinese Hair Cream. American Indian remedies also proved sufficiently exotic and ancient as to have been a major selling point, reflecting a belief that Indians possessed secret healing wisdom unknown to whites.[38]

Patent-medicine manufacturers did not rely solely on newspaper and magazines, however. They promoted their products in every way imaginable. They distributed pamphlets, books, calendars, joke books, and cookbooks. January, the *New York Times* sarcastically noted in 1860, has become the month of the "medicated almanac," a "tremendous engine for the dissemination of its author's views—approaching the unsuspecting victim, as it does, in the delusive guise of a calendar, and seducing him into the purchase of three bottles before the first eclipse."[39] The W. H. Comstock Company, better known as the home of Dr. Morse's Indian Root Pills, sent out millions of almanacs annually, including editions in Spanish and German, beginning in the 1850s and continuing several decades into the twentieth century.[40] Pinkham initially distributed a four-page "Guide for Women" that discussed health issues particular to women and explained how her remedy could provide much-needed relief. The Pinkhams also printed posters and illustrated cards.[41] The Reinhardt brothers seized on the long tradition of home medical manuals and produced their own, known as *The Home Private Medical Advisor*, which they sent free of charge to people around the country. Written in "plain language for the young people, the unmarried, and the married," the Reinhardts' guide was part instructional text and part advertisement, supposedly written by an unnamed doctor known as "The Master Specialist." Since they claimed to treat sexual diseases, a home guide was also a good way for patients to avoid the embarrassment of making a trip to their offices.[42]

Other sellers took their messages outdoors. They splashed advertisements on the sides of buildings and on fence rails. Promoters offered to repaint entire barns for those farmers willing to give one side over to an advertisement. Anywhere a train, ship, or wagon passed was prime territory. Rocks, trees, and even the faces of cliffs were called into service for medical sales.[43]

Still others hit the road to win customers. Scientific shows emerged in the United States in the 1830s on the heels of the explosion in printed materials that made science more accessible to the general public. Public demonstrations of science and technology found enthusiastic audiences eager to see and decide for themselves what they had only had the opportunity to read about in books and newspapers. It's what made Johann Spurzheim's phrenological tour of New England the hit of the 1832 season, and what drew hundreds to the mesmeric displays of Charles Poyen in 1836. The nineteenth-century science lecture and entertainment circuit did not just include people on the margins of science and medicine, though. Without the state support and patronage system that existed for science in Europe, American scholars had to cultivate audiences to win popular backing for their research and projects.[44] "He must exhibit his disinterestedness, enthusiasm, and learning before large audiences; he must be constantly before the public in newspapers, periodicals and popular books," lamented one writer in an 1867 article in the *Nation*.[45] Eminent Yale chemist and geologist Benjamin Silliman gave frequent public lectures in the 1830s and 1840s. Perhaps to distinguish himself from the theatrics of other itinerant lecturers, Silliman asserted that he "had been successful in making the subjects on which I had spoken intelligible and attractive, without diminishing the dignity of science."[46] Even so, Silliman was known as a talented showman who loved dazzling demonstrations. In the 1840s, he grew particularly fond of the oxyhydrogen blowpipe, an early kind of blowtorch that he used to create pyrotechnic displays. His assistant claimed these displays provided "no lull or intermission" and were a "constant appeal to the delighted senses."[47] Popular science came in a variety of forms with no clear separation—except perhaps in the minds of the performers and their critics—between good and bad science, regular and irregular, or high and low culture.[48] And with intense competition for audiences among itinerants and scholars, lectures and presentations became more lively and creative out of necessity.[49]

Medical shows and lectures thrived by mixing science with wonder and surprise to educate, heal, and hopefully, sell. The shows established a healer's authority and authenticity because audiences could literally see with their own eyes the miraculous cures that were possible. Patent-medicine sellers followed in this tradition, often putting on elaborate productions that had little overtly to do with healing but provided tremendous entertainment. Some dressed as wizards or shamans and told dramatic tales of how they discovered their remedy, a practice common among irregulars of all types. Self-improvement and American progress also figured into the displays, as sellers made sure to demonstrate how their remedies would lead to a better, more perfect world. Patent medicine shows tended to perform a night or two and then move on quickly, hitting the road before customers had a chance to discover that their much touted and hoped for remedy might be no remedy at all.[50]

While it's tempting to label the tactics and theatrics of itinerant medicine sellers as quackery, many took their lecturing and doctoring seriously. Charles Came was a self-taught scientist and medicine man who toured upstate New York in the 1840s and 1850s selling patent medicines and offering electrical healing demonstrations. Posters announcing his arrival in town included a long list of diseases he could cure, including liver disease, paralysis, bronchitis, ulcers, and rheumatism. His lectures were accompanied by music from mechanical organs, magic lantern projections, and slides for presentations on everything from astronomy and phrenology to the Bible, architecture, and fungi. He also had a telegraph that audience members could use to send messages to each other. Vases on both sides of the stage shot flames into the air. Such promotions and theatrics make Came appear easily categorized as an out-and-out charlatan: that is, until he opened his mouth to speak. During his lectures, Came spoke about the promise of electricity to heal, but he also demonstrated Galileo's insights on the speed of falling bodies using a pneumatic device containing a feather and a coin inside a vacuum. He carried an orrery, a device showing the relative positions and motions of bodies in the solar system that he used to teach about astronomy. Came's appearances were like a tour through a science museum. He also stayed in towns longer.[51]

Unlike the itinerant healers who offered quick fixes before leaving town, Came carefully tended to his patients, often hanging around for several days to treat certain cases as required. In 1850, he traveled to Michigan to care for his sister after several local doctors had tried and failed to heal her mysterious illness. His success in treating her, likely with a combination of patent medicines and electricity, won him more patients. After treating several others, he reported that the townspeople would "not hear about my going home," though he did eventually break free. Came also used his remedy on himself and his family, a sign that he believed in and took his own medications seriously. He wrote home often advising on remedies for his children. He also sent home money. And with the few cents he charged men—even less for women and children—to attend his lectures and demonstrations, his was not the lucrative scam that regular doctors would accuse itinerants like Came of running.[52]

Life on the road was hard. Like Samuel Thomson in his early years, Came spent months away from his family, traveling constantly to eke out a living. Competition for audiences and buyers was fierce. Women sellers often had an easier time because they faced little competition: there were few women doctors and even fewer treatments for female-specific ailments. Even so, nothing about performing on the road was easy for men or women: itinerancy made for a life of endless uncertainty and exhaustion. Many healers simply preferred a fixed address and the comforts of home that a regular medical practice often afforded.[53]

Although patent-medicine advertisements and shows encouraged self-diagnoses, many also cultivated direct relationships with their clients. Pinkham's ads urged women readers to write to her for advice. She promised to personally answer each one at no cost to the writer. Her kind and sympathetic face provided a personal touch that made readers feel comfortable seeking her advice and trusting in her response. Appealing to Victorian modesty, Pinkham promised that only women would ever read or even touch the letters. Encouraging women to write her also pulled potential customers away from regular doctors. One ad asked, "Do you want a strange man to hear all about your particular diseases?" Soon, dozens of letters arrived each week. By 1909, Pinkham's ads claimed that the company files contained "over one million one hundred thousand letters from women seeking health."[54]

True to her word, Pinkham answered each one, though she was forced to hire a correspondence department to take her dictation as the letters increased in frequency. Many sought her advice on problems that had plagued them for years with no answer in sight. "Dear Mrs. Pinkham, I have been afflicted with a malady that my physician frankly tells me he has never met with before and I write to ask you the cause and what the cure [is]," wrote one woman. She went on to describe a mouth infection that had turned her gums and cheeks white and left her face and throat swollen and painful. Her lower back was in "constant pain," her urethra enlarged and painful, and her general condition utterly fatigued. Pinkham knew just the problem. "You have taken virulent poisons in the form of medicine that has caused disease of the mucous membranes," she wrote. From the symptoms, Pinkham declared that the woman suffered from mercury poisoning that resulted from overdosing with calomel. Heavy doses of calomel had resulted in similar cases of mercury poisoning throughout the nineteenth century. That this woman's doctor could not identify her symptoms underscores the difficulties women faced in getting proper medical care; many doctors did not recognize or know how to treat women's complaints, and some doctors also shied away from full examinations for fear of offending female modesty. Pinkham advised the woman to bathe with hot water, eat fibrous foods, drink warm broths, take walks, and to get plenty of fresh air. Of course she also recommended a course of her Vegetable Compound but instructed her to take it in dry form as the alcoholic version would aggravate her symptoms.[55] It was straightforward advice that made sense to her patients as well as promoting the health hygiene common to hydropaths. It probably even helped her.

The Reinhardts also offered advice to patients through the mail from their Milwaukee offices, though perhaps of a more dubious quality. Readers of their *Home Private Medical Advisor* were urged to write for advice on all aspects of love and sexuality to save themselves from the tremendous pain that might result from mistakes. Sexual diseases offered a particularly ripe platform for healers like the Reinhardts to ply their services. While some sexual dysfunction was real, most of the cures offered by people like the Reinhardts embodied the specific anxieties of the Victorian age about the body and pleasure. Sexuality was seen as both a benevolent power and a source of misfortune and danger for nineteenth-century men and women. Many believed that sensual desires could easily become insatiable and lead to moral degradation and suffering, a belief callously played up by both quacks and moral reformers at public expense. Sexuality, so the story went, had to be controlled and directed to achieve its benevolent effects. Into this arena marched the Reinhardts, eager to "treat" and bill those they diagnosed as being on the perilous path to sexual excess and downfall.[56]

Diagnostic forms included in their home manual asked about

common, nonspecific symptoms such as headaches and dizziness as well as subjective questions about the "strength of manly power," and a man's bashfulness around women. These forms also asked about previous experience wearing an electric belt, providing the suggestion for a treatment that figured prominently in the Reinhardts' arsenal. With this information, the Reinhardts offered a free diagnosis and suggested a course of treatment that was not free, of course, but was, so they claimed, guaranteed to work.[57]

Regular medicine found much to hate in healers like Lydia Pinkham, Charles Came, and Willis and Wallis Reinhardt. Financially, patent-medicine sellers presented a formidable challenge to regular medicine. Although they called 1906 a lean year, the Reinhardt brothers pulled in $34,357.40 in business from 485 patients, at an average price of $71 per person (more than $1,500 in today's dollars).[58] The money that patent-medicine sellers spent on advertising assured them a wide audience and the potential for profit far in excess of a regular doctor confined to one town or city. Patent sellers also had vocal and powerful supporters. Newspaper publishers actively defended patent-medicine sellers because their livelihood depended, in large measure, on their ads, which made regular doctors' efforts to stop patent medicines more challenging. In Wisconsin, the Reinhardts paid the Wisconsin Newspaper Association to lobby against state efforts to pass medical licensing laws. They also urged newspaper editors to oppose any bills that attempted to restrict medical advertising on the grounds that these laws violated the freedom of the press.[59]

To regulars, advertising by any means smacked squarely of quackery. The American Medical Association's 1847 code of ethics specifically prohibited advertising and condemned propriety patents. "It is derogatory to the dignity of the profession to resort to public advertisements, or private cards, or handbills, inviting the attention of individuals affected with particular diseases," read the statute. "To boast of cures and remedies, to adduce certificates of skill and success, or to perform any other similar acts. These are the ordinary practices of empirics, and are highly reprehensible in a regular physician."[60] The only legitimate way for regulars to publicize themselves in the eyes of the AMA was through presentations of scientific papers at local medical societies, teaching in medical schools, or working in clinics. Of course, many regular doctors used other means, including making public presentations, to win patients. In his commencement address before the 1867 graduating class of the Medical College of Georgia, Dr. Henry H. Tucker reminded students that "the man who goes about seeking patients proves, by that very fact, that patients do not seek him, and that is the very best evidence that he is not worth seeking."[61] The AMA also drew a sharp distinction between ethical remedies made of known ingredients advertised only to doctors and unethical patent remedies that bypassed doctors in a cloak of secrecy to go directly to the consumer. The distinction was impossible for the AMA to enforce with its limited resources, and many regular doctors prescribed patent remedies despite ignorance of their contents. By 1902, patent medicines and machine-made tablets accounted for 20 to 25 percent of all prescriptions at apothecaries in New York, a number likely similar in states across the country.[62]

But to druggist R. V. Pierce of Buffalo, New York, the "holy horror" that regulars expressed toward the "advertising doctor," "liberally bestowing upon him the epithet of quack" was ridiculous. He, instead, suggested that the difference between regulars and patent-medicine sellers was more a matter of style than substance. The doctor "announces *himself* a graduate, talks learnedly and gives notice to the public in *some* way that he is ready to serve them," wrote Pierce. "He may make a great display in style, manner, dress, pretensions, writing for the newspapers, exhibiting literary pedantry, referring to the superior facilities afforded by some particular school or society to which he belongs." All of these, declared Pierce, "are but *modes of advertising* professional wares; in short, are artful, though not refined tricks, resorted to for private announcement."[63] Pierce's sarcastic appraisal of medical advertising may have had a personal motive, as regular doctors routinely attacked pharmacies that carried propriety remedies. Many druggists claimed they could not live on the sale of prescriptions alone and that they had little control over the products that consumers came asking for by name. They also pointed out that many of those patent medicines, including Radway's Ready Relief and Holman's Liver Pad, came with the endorsement of regular doctors right on the label.[64] Others, like Dr. James's Fever Powders and Dr. Hooper's Female Pills, were the branded remedies of regular doctors.[65]

Pinkham also sought the endorsement of regular doctors even as she ridiculed them for the inefficacy of their therapies for women's troubles. While many patent medicines used patient testimonials as promotion, many of Pinkham's female customers were reluctant to appear in advertisements for embarrassing female problems. Druggists, on the other hand, did so willingly, happy for the free advertising. A few regular doctors did as well, including Dr. John S. Carter of Erie, Pennsylvania, who declared that he "shall continue to prescribe your Vegetable Compound." The endorsement of a doctor, or even someone pretending to be one, gave patent medicines an air of authenticity and efficacy. Customers may have lost patience with regular therapies, but they still gravitated toward products with a professional seal of approval.[66]

Some regulars not only affixed their name to some labels but accepted money from patent-medicine sellers themselves. Even as the American Medical Association condemned advertising as unethical and immoral (and those who placed such ads as far worse), the organization's periodical, the *Journal of the American Medical Association*, featured pages of ads for patent medicines, which it, like the penny press, depended on for revenue.[67] The hypocrisy of such an act was not lost on all regular doctors. A paper presented before the Pennsylvania State Medical Society in 1894 charged the AMA with promoting quackery by allowing patent-medicine ads to appear under its imprimatur. It certainly was not the only regular medical journal to run such advertisements. The *American Lancet*, another medical journal, responded to the accusations by essentially pointing a finger at the other journals and crying "but they do it too!" "It is hardly to be expected that the ASSOCIATION will advise that the JOURNAL be deprived of an income of $8000 yearly, by refusing advertisements which its rival weeklies accept," declared the *American Lancet*. The paper went on to assert that reputable doctors, "by long and severe training," have learned to "distinguish between the true and false in all medical matters" and asked what all that training was good for if it did not "enable him to detect the falsehood?"[68]

Even worse, many regulars ran their own advertisements in newspapers and magazines. In 1866, the *Boston Medical and Surgical Journal* lamented that many doctors had gone far beyond the bounds of professional decorum that allowed for a simple announcement of a change of address or notice of the resumption of practice. "Now we find the newspapers of this city every day containing the advertisements of members of our body which can in no way be distinguished from those of some professional quacks," the *Journal* moaned. "Not satisfied, moreover, with seeking notoriety by special and extra puffs in the columns of the daily journals, disgraceful exhibitions of machinery and written promises to cure are conspicuously presented to the gaze of the passerby in office windows, pamphlets containing accounts of wonderfully successful cases are published for public distribution, and self-laudatory circulars are issued for the medical reader."[69] In a crowded medical field, in a profession that did not always pay well, regulars had to do something to stand out from the crowd. But how to do it while maintaining the dignified image demanded of them by medical societies and by the fledgling profession itself posed a seemingly irresolvable conundrum.

Regulars also condemned patent-medicine sellers for their inferior or nonexistent medical education. "In almost every instance they are prepared by men who "know little of medicines beyond their names," and nothing of the physiology or diseases of the system," proclaimed Dr. Hunter in the *New York Daily Times*. "How few [patients], indeed, look beyond the advertisement by which they are induced to purchase the nostrum, to inquire into the professional character of its assumed discoverer! Did they do so, they would be somewhat startled to find that, in almost every instance, his medical education is scarcely superior to their own."[70] While it was likely true that nearly all patent-medicine sellers had no formal medical training, the same could also be said of many regular doctors, who were self-taught or learned through an apprenticeship. In the absence of licensing laws, medicine was a field open to nearly everyone. Lydia Pinkham came from a long line of female healers who practiced medicine on family, friends, and neighbors. Her success in applying herbal remedies earned her respect and standing as a healer long before she even considered turning her home practice into a business. To those who considered them ignorant of medical practice, most patent sellers took the same line as other irregular healers, arguing that experience trumped education and book learning every time.[71]

Dr. Hunter's attack suggested, too, as many other regulars would also claim, that patients were partly to blame for blindly accepting the claims of patent medicines. But Americans had long tended to their own health with only the occasional intervention of a doctor. Self-dosing was both a habit of choice and necessity. Patent medicines easily meshed with American notions of self-reliance, common sense, and self-confidence in dealing with most health problems. This culture would begin to change a bit by the end of the nineteenth century. Americans became more urban and thus closer to trained medical care, and they grew more accustomed to relying on the specialized skills and knowledge of experts, but even so, the affordability of many patent medicines and the high value placed on the cure allowed patent medicines to thrive into the twentieth century.[72]

Patent medicines easily swallowed and exploited new scientific ideas without the agony and divisiveness that plagued other irregular systems. The germ theory of disease proved no deterrent to patent sellers, who began marketing germ whackers like William Radam's Microbe Killer. Another seller marketed the Pillow Inhaler, a pillow filled with medicines said to destroy germs while the patient slept. Each new scientific discovery or therapeutic advancement seemed to find a place in patent medicine. Without an underlying theory or a national network of practitioners, patent-medicine makers could adapt far more seamlessly to the changing medical landscape and latest health fads than other irregular healing systems. Patent medicines took advantage of medicine's theoretical prospects and thrived on its persistent weaknesses in daily therapeutic care.[73]

All of this is to say that despite the excoriating rhetoric of regular medicine, patent-medicine makers were not all charlatans preying on the innocent and gullible. Nor did their business tactics by necessity mark them as unethical and dangerous. Regular doctors had a complicated relationship with advertising, alcohol as medicine, and self-promotion. For centuries, regular doctors had gathered ingredients and mixed and prepared most of their own remedies, so ready-made and easily purchased patent medicines represented direct competition and a formidable financial challenge to regulars. Everyone advertised in some way, but patent-medicine sellers tended to take better advantage of these new avenues for reaching their audience than regular medicine. Prosperity took many different paths and forms in nineteenth-century medicine. Some healers opted for the individualism of an independent business while others found a home in the collective security of an established trade in a culture that sanctioned a wide range of medical practices. Healers like the Reinhardts surely did operate a quackish and exploitative business, but the case seems far less clear for Charles Came and Lydia Pinkham.[74]

The commercial climate of the nineteenth century encouraged people to believe that health, like nearly everything else, was a tangible good that money could buy. In some ways, regulars helped to foster the market for patent medicines by encouraging patients to trust in their pills and tonics that, just like patent medicines, often contained opiates and alcohol as primary ingredients. At an average cost of a penny a pill, patent medicines seemed like a good value for the money and cost far less than a visit to the doctor. These remedies also suggested speed and convenience, factors as appealing today as they ever were in the past. Impatient about illness, Americans still treat themselves more than they seek professional medical care, and usually without consulting or even informing their doctor. For the sick, whether a remedy was bought at the pharmacy on a doctor's prescription or from a traveling medicine man likely made little difference in the nineteenth century's hit-or-miss climate of relief and cure. In the absence of therapies with proven effectiveness, patent medicines made sense.[75]

Consumer confidence determined, in large measure, the success of the remedy. Many customers swore by the effectiveness of particular medicines and took them regularly. Patent-medicine makers used advertising to develop direct relationships with their users. They identified problems and provided the solution. Repeat sales were critical, and some remedies served satisfied customers for decades. Wistar's Balsam of Wild Cherry for coughs and consumption, for instance, "which has effected some of the most astonishing cures ever recorded in the history of Medicine," was on the market for more than one hundred years. Some products still around today began life as patent medicines. Angostura bitters, Coca-Cola, Dr. Pepper, tonic water, and Hires Root Beer were all once patent medicines. They also appealed to temperance advocates, a growing market in the late nineteenth century. Early recipes for root beer, for instance, often called for sassafras, a root with a potent flavor noted since at least the early nineteenth century for its medicinal use as a cleansing tonic, laxative, and blood purifier. Hires marketed its root beer as a cure-all, claiming that it was "soothing to the nerves, vitalizing to the blood, refreshing to the brain." Dr. Pepper was also sold as a remedy for a variety of health problems, including impotence, as it was said to restore "vim, vigor, and vitality." A treatment for headaches and depression, Coca-Cola got its name from two of its medicinal ingredients, kola nuts and coca leaves, the raw source of cocaine. Just how much cocaine was in the original 1885 formula is unknown, but by 1902, the drink contained as little as one four hundredth of a grain per ounce of syrup. Coca-Cola was hardly alone among patent medicines for its use of cocaine, as the drug's harmful effects were not generally known; the drink became cocaine-free in 1929. Many other products that date from the heyday of patent medicines are still used for medical purposes but have altered ingredients and toned down the spectacular health claims in the ensuing decades. These include Geritol, Doan's, Phillips' Milk of Magnesia, and Luden Brothers Cough Drops.[76]

Manufacturers of patent medicines reversed the standard production process of the era. Rather than collect and fill orders, patent-medicine makers made a product and created demand through psychological lures and vivid advertising; it was a new way of doing business that pioneered the modern systems of manufacturing, advertising, and distribution.[77]

The host of contemporary publications condemning patent-medicine sellers as ignorant and inept contributed to the rise of the modern conception of consumer protection. Sensational exposés in the nation's newspapers and magazines along with the cries of regular doctors whipped up government and public concern about the contents and practices of patent medicines. The American Medical Association lobbied for legislation affirming its belief that drug decisions should be left to regular doctors alone. In 1905, the AMA began requiring drug companies that advertised in its journals to prove that the drug worked as it was claimed to do. Progressive Era legislators, however, while expressing faith in science to reveal the truth, also strongly believed that people must be given information in order to make their own decisions. The same idea motivated the muckraking journalism of Upton Sinclair against the meatpacking industry and Samuel Hopkins Adams's "The Great American Fraud," a multipart exposé of patent medicines: the right of the public to know. While Adams's work, along with the two-volume *Nostrums and Quackery*, a compilation of articles from the *Journal of the American Medical Association*, named names of patent sellers and assigned blame fearlessly and bluntly, neither succeeded in shutting down patent medicine. The first federal drug regulation, the 1906 Pure Food and Drug Act, prohibited false or misleading drug labels and required sellers to list the presence and amount of dangerous ingredients, including alcohol and cocaine, but not every ingredient. The act did not prohibit false therapeutic claims, and though subsequent legislation attempted to do so, proving an intent to defraud or harm on the part of the manufacturer turned out to be virtually impossible. In short, the law allowed patent-medicine makers to determine what their labels said for the most part but demanded that whatever they said about the ingredients at least be true. It was up to the public to read the label and assume responsibility for its choices: in other words, buyer beware.[78]

The Reinhardts' business ended with their expulsion from the medical field in Wisconsin. Although they boasted hundreds of happy patients, not every case turned out well. Once patients ran out of money, the Reinhardts proclaimed them cured and turned them away if they tried to come back. If a patient got an attorney to enforce his claim, the Reinhardts nearly always settled out of court and returned some of the money. One man, after paying more than five hundred dollars for treatment of his "sexual weakness," told the Reinhardts that he "had paid them sufficient money to be cured" as they were treating him "for all diseases that human flesh is heir to." The Reinhardts locked the door and told the man he could not leave until he paid them an additional hundred dollars for treatment. He gave them everything he had, eighty dollars, so they would release him and stop all further treatment.[79] This and other cases led the state to restrain the Reinhardts on civil and criminal charges. The charges did not stick, but in 1908, the Milwaukee County district attorney reached a settlement with the brothers that forbade them from running or participating in any medical business in Wisconsin ever again.[80] It was a decision hailed in the pages of the *Journal of the American Medical Association*, which commended the Wisconsin Board of Medical Examiners for its persistence in finally securing the closure of the Wisconsin Medical Institute.[81]

Lydia Pinkham's Vegetable Compound, on the other hand, is still on the market. Though Pinkham herself died in 1883, her company carried on. The remedy that saved her family from financial ruin in the 1870s created a fortune that her descendants, unfortunately, fought bitterly over for decades into the twentieth century. But the product, if not the original formula, survived, and Pinkham's face still graces packages of her eponymous remedies, still giving comfort, if not care, to those in pain. Other patent medicines are still available in the twenty-first century. Proprietary remedies touting proven formulas for weight loss, energy, stamina, and immune health abound in health food and vitamin stores and in the pages of popular magazines.

The Pure Food and Drug Act of 1906 and subsequent regulations helped to constrain some makers and curbed the use of narcotics, cocaine, and alcohol, but it also pushed some toward medical devices, which were more lightly regulated. Electrical belts, brushes, and vests proved particularly popular in the early twentieth century. Williams' Electric Batteries, an electric box with different applicators attached, claimed to help rheumatism, neuralgia, and nervousness while also affording "constant amusement in the home circle."[82] The government also placed restrictions on drug advertising to consumers through most of the twentieth century, but in 1997, the Food and Drug Administration issued new guidelines that allowed for direct-to-consumer advertising as long as the drug maker provided information about risks and benefits—the long list of side effects that zip by in small print and speed reading on television and radio. Drug makers once again have a direct and independent relationship with consumers just as they did in Lydia Pinkham's day. Federal laws now regulate the extravagant claims and harmful ingredients of the past, but the Reinhardts' "sexual weakness," rebranded erectile dysfunction, and other ailments are now treatable in pill form (in this case, Viagra and Levitra) by regulars. Though many of these remedies still require a prescription, patients ask for remedies by name, and doctors often have trouble denying their requests, particularly with a payment structure based on patient satisfaction.[83]

Patent medicines made many promises to their users, the most potent of which may have been their claim to treat seemingly intractable problems. Holes in medical knowledge provided opportunities to medical entrepreneurs and reformers alike in the late nineteenth century, and into one of these gaping holes stepped the osteopaths and chiropractors.

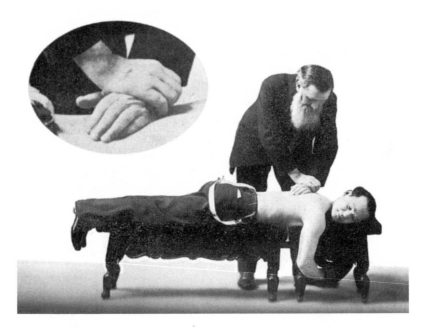

Daniel David Palmer demonstrates his chiropractic method of spinal adjustments, designed to alleviate pressure on the nerves that he believed caused disease.

CHAPTER SEVEN

Manual Medicine
Osteopathy and Chiropractic

Time began on September 18, 1895. Or at least it seemed that way to magnetic healer Daniel David Palmer, who restored Harvey Lillard's hearing with a touch. An African American janitor at Palmer's Davenport, Iowa, office building, Lillard had lost his hearing seventeen years earlier while working in a cramped and stooped position. He told Palmer he suddenly felt something "give way in his back." Suddenly, the world went mute, so much so that he "could not hear the racket of a wagon or the ticking of a watch." Learning of Palmer's healing skills, he came seeking help.

Palmer listened to Lillard's story with interest. He'd been investigating the cause of disease and exploring drugless approaches to healing for several years. "One question was uppermost in my mind in my search for the cause of disease," wrote Palmer. "I desired to know why one person was ailing, and his associate, eating at the same table, working in the same shop, at the same bench, was not. Why?" Examining Lillard, Palmer found a vertebra out of alignment—the possible source of that feeling of movement Lillard felt in his back. Intrigued by the possible connection, Palmer persuaded Lillard to let him try to knock the vertebra back into place. Palmer "racked it into position" with two adjustments, freeing the nerves that had "been paralyzed by the pressure." Soon, Lillard could hear as well as before.[1]

That September day soon assumed legendary proportions in chiropractic lore. The "First Adjustment" became year zero, the point in time from which all else could be measured, according to the masthead of the chiropractic periodical *Fountain Head News*. From that moment on, each passing year gained one "A.C.," the number of years "After Chiropractic."[2]

Palmer was not alone in the late-nineteenth-century medical marketplace for manual manipulation. Osteopathy had emerged in the 1870s and offered patients another form of drugless therapy based on bodily adjustment. The similarity did not end there. Both systems began in the Midwest and found their most enthusiastic followers and practitioners in predominantly rural areas. Both pushed for legitimacy, not by fighting against laws and standards as the Thomsonians had before them, but by fighting *for* licensing laws and implementing guidelines to improve the quality of their schools and practitioners nearly from the start. Both were riven by internal disputes between those who remained true to their founders' vision and those who saw the benefit of dabbling in many forms of healing. And perhaps most strangely of all, both systems were founded by haphazardly educated frontiersmen born in log cabins, who, as adults, were known for their scraggly beards and dynamic personalities, and who at one time practiced magnetic healing and claimed divine inspiration for their theories.

Osteopaths and chiropractors were not the first to notice the potential health benefits of the physical manipulation of the human body. In ancient Greece, Hippocrates described how to correct dislocated joints through pressure and adjustments, techniques that guided practitioners for centuries. The methods described in "On the Articulations" and "Instruments of Reduction" were not for the weak of stomach.[3] For dislocated shoulders, Hippocrates first advised pulling the forearm back to the spine while simultaneously bending the arm upward at the elbow to snap it back into place. For particularly stubborn or chronic dislocations, he advised cauterizing the shoulder by passing red-hot irons through the skin of the armpit until it "burnt to the opposite side" while pushing them "forward with the hand." The high heat was essential so the irons could pass through "as quickly as possible."[4] Hippocrates also described methods for reducing vertebra displacement on a treatment table fitted with various straps, wheels, and axles that bore a passing resemblance to the modern chiropractic adjustment table. Chiropractors clearly thought so, too, as many still claim Hippocrates as the true founder of the chiropractic technique. In the second century CE, Roman physician Galen won wide acclaim for reversing the paralysis in the right hand of the scholar Eudemus by adjusting the vertebrae in his neck. Galen's writings include frequent mentions of Hippocrates' manipulative techniques as well as his own recommendations for standing and walking on dysfunctional areas of the spine.[5]

This ancient and respected origin made manual manipulation an important treatment option for subsequent generations of European doctors. Tenth-century Persian polymath Avicenna included the Hippocratic manipulative methods in his influential five-volume *al-Qanun fi al-Tibb*, or *The Canon of Medicine*, published in numerous editions in Europe and used as a textbook in many medieval European medical schools. In the sixteenth century, French military surgeon Ambroise Paré practiced spinal manipulation and repeated many of Hippocrates' techniques in his writings on the vertebrae. German surgeon Johannes Scultetus carried the tradition into the seventeenth century with the publication of *The Surgeons Store-House*.[6]

But despite this long lineage, by the eighteenth century regular medicine had largely abandoned the technique. The reasons are not completely clear, but tuberculosis epidemics likely had something to do with it. Force applied to the weakened joints of patients suffering from tuberculosis, a growing problem in overcrowded cities, could seriously harm and even disfigure patients. Bodily adjustment also required close contact with diseased bodies, so many doctors sought to limit their contact with contagious patients. But even as doctors grew more reluctant to use manipulation, public demand for these services persisted. So into the vacuum created by the absence of regular doctors stepped folk healers and amateur bonesetters like Sarah Mapp. Known as "Crazy Sally," Mapp was a slovenly eighteenth-century Englishwoman perhaps as well known for her drunkenness as for her skill at setting bones. Mapp's talent earned her mention in songs and even the theater, where a comedy called *The Husband's Relief, or The Female Bone-setter and the Worm Doctor* was based on her life.[7]

Bonesetters weren't new—nor were they all slightly loony drunks memorialized in verse—but they almost certainly found a larger patient base with the abdication of regulars from manual manipulation. Bonesetters did not just set broken or dislocated bones. They also helped with pains in the muscles, ligaments, and joints. These village bonesetters had undoubtedly passed on the tradition for centuries, long before formal recognition by the medical profession, but they now took a far more visible place in society for people of all classes. Many poor people had long relied on bonesetters for medical care. In England, Friar Thomas Moulton's popular medical manual *The Mirror, or Glass of Health* included sections on bonesetting and went through at least seventeen editions in the sixteenth century alone. A century later, Robert Turner published a revised and enlarged edition in London, known as *The Compleat Bone-setter*, aimed at a general user.[8] While some people learned from books, more still learned under the supervision of an accomplished master. Bonesetting skills often passed through families like other skilled trades. The homespun nature of bonesetting and its informally trained practitioners likely caused many regular doctors to associate the practice with the ignorant lower classes and to thus deem it beneath their dignity.[9]

But regular medical therapy offered few alternatives, so bonesetters found some success in adjusting deformities that doctors failed to treat. Nineteenth-century British surgeon James Paget suggested that doctors would do well to observe the techniques of the bonesetters, but he stopped far short of endorsing their methods, attributing the bonesetters' success more to luck than actual medical skill.[10] Manual manipulation soon fell out of the skill set of regular practitioners. American regulars tended to mirror the attitudes of their European counterparts, and lacking the long medical history of European medicine, the United States never developed a respected practice of manual medicine. From the beginning, American regulars lumped bonesetting together with a whole range of quackish folk practices.[11]

Everyday Americans did not seem to share their opinion, however. Bonesetters found a place in the United States just as they had in Europe, providing medical care to people who could not afford or did not have access to a regular doctor. Perhaps the most famous American bonesetters were the Sweet family of New England, who ministered to several generations of the sick in Rhode Island, Massachusetts, Connecticut, and New York in the late seventeenth century. Benoni Sweet, believing the skill an innate gift, passed on the practice to his sons. The family gained considerable fame after Benoni's son Job Sweet set the broken or dislocated bones of French officers encamped in Newport, Rhode Island, during the American Revolution. After the war, Job reset the dislocated hip of Vice President Aaron Burr's daughter, Theodosia, an achievement that won him a roster of patients and allowed him to practice bonesetting full-time. His was the rare case, though, as most bonesetters, including the other Sweets, worked other jobs and set bones on the side.[12]

Andrew Taylor Still first discovered the benefits of manual manipulation as a child. Born in a log cabin near the Cumberland Gap in Virginia on August 6, 1828, Still was the son of a Methodist minister who dabbled in medicine, the dual minister-physician role so common to early America, particularly on the frontier. One day, suffering from a terrible headache, Still tied a rope about ten inches off the ground between two trees. He wrapped a blanket around the rope as a kind of makeshift pillow, lay on the ground with his neck resting across the blanket-draped rope, and fell asleep. When he woke, the headache was gone. Still did not make much of it at the time, but years later the event took on historic proportions as Still's first lesson in osteopathy.[13]

Still's family was constantly on the move. Following the line of American settlement, the Stills moved first to Tennessee and then to Missouri and later Kansas as Still's father rode the Methodist circuit and cared for the sick. Inspired by his father to enter medicine, Still studied medical books and opened his own practice in Missouri. In 1854, he joined his father in Kansas in an ill-fated attempt to escape rising tensions over the expansion of slavery in the West. The issue of slavery became unavoidable, though, following Still, an ardent abolitionist, to his new home.[14]

Working alongside his father, Still found himself growing increasingly frustrated over his inability to heal as he watched patient after patient succumb to disease. Standard medical therapy seemed to inflict more harm on patients than if he simply left them alone. Wondering if there was a better way, Still began digging up Indian graves to study human anatomy. He spent hundreds of hours examining and charting the placement and workings of each of the body's bones. He also experimented with new treatments, including manual manipulation.[15] His studies convinced him that "if Samson could slay the Philistines, or at least 3000 of them, with the jaw bone of an ass (one bone), . . . I could with over 200 bones of the human body, enter into combat and slay the greater part of the diseases to which the human race is subject."[16] Unsurprisingly, Still's neighbors found his grave-digging a little strange, and his church eventually excommunicated him for emulating Christ by the laying on of hands.[17]

Still lost his confidence in medicine completely after the Civil War when three of his children died in an outbreak of spinal meningitis. Devastated by the loss and the doctor's inability to save them through heroic methods, Still relinquished his faith in drugs and the doctors who administered them, vowing, like Thomson did before him in tragedy, to devote his life to finding a better way to treat disease. Still spent the next decade researching and experimenting. He maintained his medical license and continued to prescribe some drugs, but he turned more and more to various manual techniques for alleviating pain.[18] Recalling his childhood experience with headache relief, Still slowly began to conceive of a theory of health based on a normally functioning musculoskeletal system. Undaunted by his excommunication, Still credited God with providing the inspiration for his theory and, thus, saw himself fulfilling a divine mission in working toward a drugless and nonsurgical approach to disease based on touch. Mesmerists, too, believed in the healing power of touch. A century earlier, Mesmer had witnessed the potential of the human spirit to heal as he passed his hands over the bodies of his patients. If there was any idea that would attract a spiritually inclined healer like Still, this was it, and he soon began advertising himself as a magnetic healer. Of course, the combination of magnetism and manual manipulation did little to win Still acceptance from the regular medical community or from many of his patients, who were bewildered by his change of methods. So in 1874, Still moved to Kirksville, Missouri, seeking a fresh start.[19]

At first, Kirksville proved scarcely kinder to Still's brand of medicine. To win people over, Still became a medical circuit rider, traveling from town to town performing his manipulations on skeptical volunteers and advertising himself as "the Lightening Bone Setter." His physical appearance likely gave a poor first impression. Tall and bearded, Still often arrived in town with a walking stick in hand, wearing a dowdy felt hat, a wrinkled suit, and baggy pants stuffed into the top of his boots. Flung over one shoulder was a bag of bones. It was a look that fairly shouted convention-flouting loony—or maybe macabre hobo.[20] Still claimed that rumors about him in his early days made even children cross to the other side of the street to avoid the man called "an infidel, crank, crazy."[21] But any doubts about Still were soon overcome by his masterful ability to heal the sick.

To many observers, it seemed as though Still could see straight into the body and know just what bone to manipulate. In one town,

Still freed a hard-drinking blacksmith from his taste for liquor by re-aligning his ribs. In another, Still relieved an Irish woman of nagging shoulder pain and asthma by resetting several ribs and an upper ver-tebra. As word of Still's miraculous cures spread, people came from great distances to see him. Still's demonstrations became like revival-ist camp meetings. He denounced the evils of the regular medical pro-fession and left people shouting in wonder at his startling treatments. In his wake, he left a trail of casts, crutches, and surgical devices no longer needed by patients.[22] Even his rumpled appearance became an asset, representing to some admirers his lack of concern with material things. Still soon won over Kirksville and gave up his itinerancy to practice in town. Realizing he needed a more distinctive name for his form of therapy than bonesetting, Still coined the name "osteopathy" from os for bone and pathology, the study of the cause and effect of disease.[23]

Still conceived of the human body as an intricate, God-created machine that worked in harmony with nature. "Quit your pills and learn from Osteopathy the principle that governs you," declared Still. "Learn that you are a machine, your heart an engine, your lungs a fanning machine and a sieve, your brain with its two lobes an electric battery."[24] He rejected drugs as unnecessary and potentially harmful and claimed that their use demonstrated a lack of faith in the pow-ers of nature and "accus[ed] God of incapacity." Still believed the body was chemically self-sufficient, a human drugstore designed and stocked by God with everything it needed to be healthy and happy. He claimed that his travels had confirmed to him that "all the rem-edies necessary to health are compounded within the human body."[25] Surely "the Architect of the universe was wise enough to construct man so he could travel from the Maine of birth to the California of the grave unaided by drugs," asserted Still.[26] The doctor's job then was to serve as the body's mechanic, tinkering with the machinery of the body to ensure the proper functioning of God's perfect creation. In Still's scheme, doctors were never directly responsible for the cure but simply acted as intermediaries between the patient's self-healing mechanism and nature.

Still identified blood as the essential ingredient to health. The lu-bricant that kept the body running, blood ensured the well-being of its tissues and organs. The artery was the "father of the rivers of life, health and ease, and its muddy or impure water is first in all disease," wrote Still of a concept that became known as the Law of the Artery.[27] Misaligned bones exerted pressure on the blood vessels, diverting and even blocking their life-giving current to the organs and causing disease and deformity.[28] He denied the existence of diseases as separate entities, seeing instead a collection of symptoms that pointed to a vascular blockage at a point known as the "osteopathic legion." These lesions were small abnormalities that threw off the body's whole system and caused patients to feel pain and other symptoms that they mistakenly associated with the disease itself. A similar idea underlay homeopathy, Thomsonism, and humoralism. "There is no such disease as fever—typhus, typhoid, or lung—rheumatism, sciatica, gout, colic, liver disease, nettle rash, or croup on to the end of the list," wrote Still. "They do not exist as diseases, but separate or combined are only effects."[29] Still believed that the osteopathic lesion could account for all human complaints. Gout, for instance, resulted from lumbar displacements. Still based his conclusion, in part, on the high number of cases he found among merchants who frequently stretched their arms and backs to stock goods on high shelves, wrenching their lower backs out of alignment. Goiters, on the other hand, came from pressure on the blood vessels in the neck from vertebrae, ribs, or the clavicles.[30]

Blood was not the only cause of lesions; nerves, too, had to remain unobstructed. The nervous system fascinated and awed Still. While he was unsure of exactly what electrical force powered it, he was sure that the brain operated like an "electric battery" on the body. He suggested that the artery takes blood from the heart and deposits it in the cells of the nervous system, which "act to give life, motion and form to organs, muscles, and all parts of the body."[31] So interference with nerve functioning also produced an osteopathic lesion. The blood and nerves worked in close collaboration. The rope swing Still had constructed as a child, he now determined, had cured his headache by putting pressure on the soft tissues in the back of his neck, relaxing the nerves and lessening the dysfunction while giving "harmony to the flow of the arterial blood to and through the veins."[32] While any misplaced bone could cause an obstruction, the spinal column at the center of the nervous system seemed especially liable to lesions given all of the stress, pressure, twists, and falls it endured in the course of daily living. As a result, osteopathic treatment tended to focus on the vertebrae and ribs.[33]

Still located lesions by touch, but also by taking a standard patient history. Feeling the body for problems, osteopaths diagnosed the affected organ and deduced the vessels and nerves involved. Still needed no specialized equipment or devices to carry out his manipulations. He pressed patients against chairs, walls, tables, and doorframes.[34]

Still drew careful and firm distinctions between osteopathy and massage, which many of his critics assumed he practiced. Osteopaths did not knead, rub, or tap patients. They were "physicians," asserted Still, who adjusted "bone, cartilage, ligament, tendon, muscle, or even ... the fascia which enfolds all structures."[35] As evidence of the distinction, one only had to read his description of the treatment he gave an old woman suffering from a "crooked neck and a stitch in the muscles." Still set one foot against the plank of a fence for leverage, while the woman rested against his knee. He placed one hand on her neck and the other on her head. He then gave her head a twist that reportedly corrected the lesion instantly.[36] With the lesion removed, the blood and nerve energy could flow freely, and the body recovered its health automatically under the ancient principle of *vis medicatrix naturae*, or the healing power of nature.

Still's original theory of disease was highly speculative, based only nominally in anatomy, but patients did not seem to care. Far more important was that it seemed to work. And trainloads of people flocked to his Kirksville infirmary seeking his help. Unable to treat all of the patients seeking his services, Still decided to open a school to teach others his system. He secured a charter from the state of Missouri and opened the American School of Osteopathy in Kirksville in October of 1892. Twenty-one students enrolled in the first class, six of them women. A state charter allowed Still to grant degrees of medical doctor, or MD, but seeking to visibly demonstrate osteopathy's distance from regular medicine, Still decided to grant his own degree, the DO, or doctor of osteopathy. Students earned the degree by attending two five-month sessions of training in manipulation and anatomy. The addition of Dr. William Smith, a respected Scottish regular doctor trained at the University of Edinburgh, to the faculty as a professor of anatomy lent the school legitimacy and the imprimatur of regular medicine. Because osteopathic methods were difficult to explain in words, Still stressed the importance of observation and hands-on learning.[37] Many students recalled afternoons in the infirmary with the "old doctor," as Still was affectionately known, working on patients. "We would hold the patients in position while Dr. Still

worked upon them, explaining to us as he treated why he gave this
movement in one place, and a different movement in another," wrote
Arthur Grant Hildreth years later.[38] Still took pride in making his
system available to anyone who wanted to learn, including members
of the lower classes, who often lacked a formal education and could
not afford the tuition. Rather than turn them away, though, Still welcomed them as a way to demonstrate his system's altruism and to
spread the word about osteopathy.[39]

Women found a particularly warm welcome in the American
School of Osteopathy, which advertised for female students and practitioners with blatant flattery. In 1895, the *Journal of Osteopathy* declared that "the science of osteopathy should particularly appeal to the
intelligent and ambitious women who desire a noble life-work which
will prepare them for a future free of pecuniary concern."[40] It was a
message squarely in line with the tenor of the late-nineteenth-century
women's rights movement, which embraced women's economic independence as a means to equality.[41] Still's passion for women's rights
was so strong and so genuine that he frequently suggested the US
Constitution needed an equal rights amendment to grant and assure
the rights and privileges women clearly deserved. Still held his female
students to the same standards as the men. The school catalog clearly
stated there would be "no distinction as to sex," and Still assured any
doubters that all his women graduates were "as well worthy diplomas
as any gentlemen who ever entered."[42]

Still welcomed women, in part, from a desire to reform obstetrical
care, an oft-repeated rallying cry among nineteenth-century irregulars. He particularly wanted to remove forceps from the birthing room
because he believed they lacerated women and caused "many fools and
idiots among children to-day."[43] Still had performed osteopathic de-
liveries himself, placing the mother in a semi-upright position and using manipulations, particularly of the pelvic bones, to make the labor
brief and as pain-free as possible, but he felt women might perform
these duties more effectively and empathetically. One of Still's early
graduates, Alice Patterson, became head of the American School of
Osteopathy's Department of Obstetrics and Gynecology, which had
its own infirmary. Patterson later moved to Washington, DC, and
built a successful osteopathic practice of her own.[44]

Among the many who came to Kirksville to learn osteopathy was
Daniel David Palmer, though he would later deny any contact with

Still. The similarity of osteopathy and chiropractic led some to charge that Palmer's system was simply a cheap imitation, an accusation that Palmer strenuously denied and that likely led him to refute any connection or exposure to Still. Osteopaths were only too happy to deny an association with Palmer as well, since if there was anything an osteopath hated more than a regular doctor, it was a chiropractor. Palmer recognized that the two systems shared similar features, but he rejected osteopathy's focus on the blood. Instead, he believed the nerve force was essential to health.

Born in a log cabin in Port Perry, Ontario, Canada, on March 7, 1845, Palmer was the son of a man who worked variously as a shoemaker, grocer, teacher, and postmaster. When his father's business failed in 1856, the family moved to the United States for a new start. Palmer and his brother Thomas dropped out of school and stayed behind in Canada to work, finally joining their family in Iowa in 1865. The young Palmer became a teacher in Muscatine, Iowa, and taught at several more schools before purchasing ten acres of land on a hillside above the Mississippi River just north of New Boston, Illinois. He raised bees, planted fruit trees, and began a new career as a horticulturalist, even developing a variety of raspberry known as "Sweet Home" that found a national market. Palmer's bees perished in the harsh winter of 1881, so Palmer sold the land and rejoined his family, now living in the Iowa town of What Cheer. He opened a grocery store that also sold goldfish, but competition forced him out of the grocery business and back into the classroom.[45]

But teaching, while practical and nearly always in demand, did not fire Palmer's passion. Spiritualism had first interested Palmer in the 1870s, but he soon shifted his attention to magnetism, the reverse course of many mesmerists, who subsequently became spiritualists earlier in the century. Palmer's interest stemmed in large measure from local magnetic healer Paul Caster in Ottumwa, Iowa, who had impressed Palmer with his reputation, his bustling practice, and perhaps most important of all, his massive fortune. After Caster's death, his son J. S. inherited the business and took the practice to Burlington, Iowa, in 1881. Palmer followed, hoping to ride the young Caster's coattails to monetary gain. He read books on magnetic healing, fascinated by the idea of drugless cures, and he became convinced that he possessed the gift of healing—that he could literally pour his own "vital magnetism" or life force into diseased patients to effect a cure.

He placed advertisements for his healing services in local newspapers. That Palmer lacked a formal education, not to mention actual training or experience in magnetism, was no barrier to medical practice. The competition in Burlington proved too intense, however, and Palmer moved to Davenport, Iowa, in 1887 to establish his own magnetic healing practice.[46]

Palmer opened his Magnetic Cure and Infirmary in the Ryan Building on the corner of Second and Brady streets with an aggressive advertising campaign. "Where can you get cured quicker and for less money, and without making a drugstore of yourself? It may not be popular to be cured without medication, [but] who cares so [long as] the sick will get well?" read Palmer's ad in the 1888 *Davenport Directory*. His "vital healing" services cost one dollar but were offered free to the poor.[47] Palmer treated everything from rheumatism and neuralgia to indigestion, sore throats, and toothaches using his hands to draw away the pain and disease from the problem area with a sweeping motion. He then stood aside and shook the illness from his hands and fingers, as if shaking off droplets of water.[48] Palmer's business flourished. His location by the Mississippi River allowed him to draw a client base from all over Illinois, Minnesota, Iowa, and Wisconsin. With his deep, penetrating eyes, feisty, self-assured manner, and scruffy bush of a beard just this side of menacing, he cut a commanding figure, as the original magnetist Franz Anton Mesmer had more than a century before. Palmer's was a personality far larger than his short and stocky five-foot-four-inch frame.[49] Many patients were lured to his office by his widely distributed ads touting miraculous cures: Jane Wilson of a decades-long sore throat; Ella Post of malaria.[50] By the 1890s, Palmer was seeing ninety to one hundred patients daily, and in 1895 recorded profits of $4,669 at a time when the average regular doctor made less than $1,500 annually.[51] His space had also grown from its original three rooms to forty-two by 1891, decorated with mounted animal heads and a glass-walled cage, home to four live alligators.[52]

Palmer's success convinced him of the validity of drugless approaches to healing and the importance of the spine, nerve power, and the doctor's touch to wellness, but he began to wonder about the relationship between the body's structure and its physiological function. These questions all led up to his September 18, 1895, encounter with janitor Henry Lillard and the adjustment that changed everything for

Palmer. It should be noted that Lillard remembered the events of that night a little differently than Palmer. Lillard recalled laughing with a friend in the hallway. The conversation, loud enough for Palmer to hear it, drew Palmer from his office to join in the banter. One joke struck Palmer as so funny that he slapped the janitor on the back with a book. A few days later, Lillard reported that he thought his hearing had improved. Only then did Palmer begin to explore manipulation as medicine.[53] Whatever happened, that day proved pivotal to Palmer, who declared a connection between Lillard's back and his deafness, and he soon shifted his attention from magnetism to manipulation.

Over the following months, Palmer experimented with what he called "hand treatments" on other patients with success. Realizing he needed a better name for his system, Palmer turned to Davenport minister and patient Samuel Weed for help. Weed suggested "chiropractic" from the Greek *cheir* meaning "hand" and *praxis* for "practice," meaning roughly "done by hand."[54] With a name, he also needed a theory to explain what he had discovered through experimentation. What he came up with married the vitalism of magnetism to the mechanical aspects of bonesetting.[55]

Palmer reasoned that all diseases resulted from some kind of spinal "impingement, a pressure on the nerves" that enervates the organs. Normal nerve tension, which he called tone, produced a perfect state of health, but if some bone, most often in the spine, imposed on nerves passing through it, they became too slack or too tense, resulting in disease. This point of pressure was called a subluxation. The idea of disease resulting from nerve dysfunction would make sense even to regulars. In the eighteenth century, Scottish physician William Cullen, the same man who had inspired homeopath Samuel Hahnemann, had theorized that disease resulted from a decrease of "nervous energy." Benjamin Rush modified Cullen's theory, claiming that disease came from both an increase and a decrease in nervous energy, and popularized it among American regulars. It was Palmer's interpretation of how that nerve dysfunction originated that made chiropractic unique.[56]

Using the magnetic idea of an internal physical force, Palmer explained that every living being possessed an eternal power known as "Innate Intelligence," or just "Innate," which animated every function of the body. This Innate circulated through the nerves, so a subluxation that caused impingement could disrupt its ability to govern the body and cause illness.[57] Since the nerves branched out from the spine, Palmer focused much of his attention on the alignment of the vertebrae. Palmer came to believe that 95 percent of diseases originated in the spine, so it was the chiropractors' job to facilitate the flow of nerve force, and the all-important Innate, through physical adjustments. Drugs were unnecessary because they did not solve the actual structural problem, and they might actually cause more problems with their harsh effects. Healing required nothing more than a resetting that, once accomplished, like osteopathy, allowed the body to restore itself.[58] "The Chiropractor removes the obstacles to nature's healing process," Palmer proclaimed.[59]

It also did much more than just return people to health. Palmer believed that his system could usher in the dawning of a new age by answering age-old questions about the meaning of life, disease, and death. Crime, poverty, and suffering were all diseased conditions that could be cured through the free flow of Innate. Palmer frequently referred to how the impingement of nerves created a lack of ease or "dis-ease" that was the cause of all human problems. Sounding like the spiritualist he once was, Palmer believed that chiropractic would "give us a conscious connection with that unseen life which is believed in by all nations," allowing humans to stop fearing death "because the life beyond the veil will be comprehended and known to us."[60] For a time, Palmer and his son, Bartlett Joshua Palmer, or B. J., as he was commonly known and who would eventually assume leadership of the profession, even considered classifying chiropractic as a religion rather than a new healing system due to its potential impact on humanity.[61] In the end, they decided to stick with medicine, reflecting their belief that chiropractic stood on sensible middle ground between the spiritualism of religion and the materialism of science. At a time when American culture was uncertain about the appropriate relationship between science, which was on the rise, and religion, which appeared to many to be losing its authority, chiropractors argued that they alone had discovered the perfect balance between them in a philosophy that dealt with "manifestations of the spiritual through the material physical body."[62]

Still, too, saw God in osteopathy. "God's greatest gift is Osteopathy," wrote Still. "God is the Father of Osteopathy and I am not ashamed of the child of his mind."[63] For the son of a Methodist minister who also practiced medicine, Still's conflation of osteopathy and religion is, perhaps, none too surprising. Still saw the human body as worthy of awe and devotion, an intricate piece of machinery divinely designed. Adjusting the body became a form of devotion for him.[64] "My highest and most profound worship is when I take up any part of the human body or any part of nature, and after examining it under the microscope, I give credit for all perfection to the great Architect," proclaimed Still in a 1903 speech.[65] Both Still and Palmer trusted in nature's healing power because they saw the beauty and complexity of nature as something only God could have created. Each of their systems was an attempt to harmonize the spiritual with the physical.[66]

Chiropractors discovered subluxations in the same manner as their regular and osteopathic peers: with a patient history. Like osteopaths, chiropractors did not believe that the symptoms of the disease were the disease; they were, instead, secondary manifestations of the problem. After locating the afflicted area, Palmer instructed practitioners to consider the nerves connected to that area and to then trace those nerves back to the part of the spine from which they emanate. Confirmation of the subluxation came by touch.[67] Specific ailments corresponded to individual vertebrae, so there would never be more than one impingement per disease. Smallpox, for instance, came from the fifth cervical vertebra, while heartburn emanated from the fifth thoracic.[68]

The removal of the subluxation through manipulation was officially known in chiropractic as an *adjustment*, a term osteopaths used as well, though not formally. Adjustments began with the patient lying face down on the adjusting table, a bench with a hole in the middle over which the chiropractor would position the blocked part of the body. The chiropractor would then stand on the side of the body where the vertebrae had been displaced. Resting the heel of his right hand against the vertebrae while wrapping his left hand around his right wrist, the chiropractor would apply enough pressure to move the vertebrae back into place. Palmer stressed that great force was not generally required, though it was up to each chiropractor to determine how much force was enough.[69]

At first, Palmer kept his system to himself, fearful of potential competitors and imitators. But a brush with death in a train accident in 1897 compelled him to share his system so that his great discovery did not die with him. He took on an apprentice and taught him enough of the basics of chiropractic technique that he could heal Palmer's injuries from the accident. This informal apprenticeship system was quickly replaced with a formal school, the Palmer Chiropractic School and Cure in 1897. Like osteopathy, chiropractic adjustments were not easy to explain in words but better learned through observation and experience. That first year, the school graduated its first student, who also happened to be a homeopath. Enrollment tripled the next year and had increased to five by 1901. In 1902, Palmer's own son B. J. enrolled. Many of these early students were regular doctors looking to add a new element to their practice. Women were also welcome, and many of the women who matriculated did so with their husbands, as Palmer offered a tuition break for spouses. Mae Parsons entered chiropractic with her husband not "seriously intending to practice," but once she learned more, she "became greatly interested."[70] One of the first women to graduate was Minora Paxson, who went on to coauthor the first chiropractic textbook. Another, Julia C. Bowman, set up a "Chiropractic Cure" on Hennepin Avenue in Minneapolis in 1899. Palmer's liberality only extended so far, however. Despite the importance of Henry Lillard, a black man, to the foundation of chiropractic, African Americans were not welcome at the Palmer School, or at most of the other chiropractic schools that soon opened, until the mid-twentieth century.[71]

And there were many more schools. The American School of Chiropractic was opened in Cedar Rapids, Iowa, in 1902 by two Palmer graduates. Schools also opened in Minnesota and Oklahoma, and in 1903, Palmer himself founded a school in Oregon. By the 1910s, schools conferring the degree of DC, doctor of chiropractic, had opened around the country, with particularly heavy concentrations in the Midwest and on the West Coast. Many were short-lived, closing after a few years or even a few months. Chiropractic's leaders regularly acknowledged the poor quality of many of these schools. At a lecture in Oklahoma City, Palmer lamented that "I teach the science to one person and that person teaches it to another . . . until chiropractic is in the hands of the third or fourth person [and] is hardly recognizable as chiropractic."[72] Even Palmer's own school was not safe from criticism. Oakley Smith recalled that the "first thing I learned was that there was no instruction to be given. There were no blackboards, no textbooks, no notes, not a single lecture. For six days I witnessed the giving of a number of treatments. That was the sum total of information that was transferred in exchange for tuition paid." At the end of the week, Smith was told he had learned all that he needed and that he "should do the treating thereafter."[73] Rather than ignore or deny the problems, though, chiropractors took steps to eliminate the abuses at their educational institutions, particularly diploma mills that issued degrees to anyone who could pay.[74]

Smith's negative review did little to hinder the growth of the Palmer School in Davenport, Iowa. The institution prospered under the charismatic and egotistical leadership of Palmer's son B. J., who had purchased the struggling school from his father in 1906. B. J. paid off his father's debts and purchased more land and buildings for the school. He then proceeded to shut his father out, even allegedly hitting his father with an automobile after Palmer refused to leave during the school's 1913 homecoming parade. B. J. announced himself as the "Developer" of chiropractic and his Palmer school as the "Fountain Head" of the field. He also shifted the system's focus from the divine to the more practical task of relieving daily pain through adjustments. Though he did not abandon the spiritual aspects completely, B. J.'s emphasis on the brain as the real seat of the body's power rather than Innate Intelligence in the nerves angered and embittered Palmer, who accused his son of robbing him of credit and financial reward for chiropractic.[75]

Short of stature and filled with the same impetuous self-confidence as his father, B. J. possessed an administrative and business-oriented mind that allowed him to ably recruit both staff and students to the school and to expand the entire chiropractic field. Students learned not only the skills and theories of chiropractic but also how to be good businessmen, a skill B. J. believed essential to success and prosperity in medicine. It was a prescient move, as today more than sixty regular medical schools offer combined degree programs in medicine and business for much the same reason. At a chiropractic convention in Butte, Montana, B. J. explained that his school operated "on a business and not a professional basis. It is a business where we manufacture chiropractors. They have got to work just like machinery. A course of salesmanship goes along with their training. We teach them the idea and then we show them how to sell it," B. J. proclaimed.[76] Students developed their business acumen in a one-month "Salesmanship" course that intensively studied the topics of "Personal Magnetism," "Business Relations," "Advertising," "Selling the Patient," and "Keeping Yourself

Sold." To promote chiropractic, B. J. taught, lectured, and published constantly. He also saw the potential of commercial radio far in advance of other businessmen. In 1910, he established Davenport station WOC, whose call letters stood for "Wonders of Chiropractic," one of the first and most powerful radio stations in the country. B. J. used the station, listened to by more than a million people, to promote the benefits of chiropractic care and to "establish Good Will for Chiropractic." The station was not solely the marketing mouthpiece for chiropractors; it also broadcast news, sports, music, and farm reports. In the 1930s, the station hired a promising young Illinois sportscaster named Ronald Reagan. Under B. J.'s leadership, the Palmer School grew from twenty-one students in 1906 to more than two thousand in 1920. It was the largest medical school of any system of healing, regular or irregular, anywhere in the world.[77]

The osteopathic education system grew rapidly as well. The last five years of the nineteenth century saw schools opening in Anaheim, Minneapolis, Denver, San Francisco, Milwaukee, Boston, Des Moines, and Chicago. Graduates set up practices throughout the United States as well as abroad in Canada, Mexico, Britain, Ireland, and China. Not all of these schools were of the highest quality, as the rapid expansion of the field drew entrepreneurs out to make a buck from various educational schemes.[78] Serious osteopaths worried about the damage these incompetent osteopaths might cause the fledgling field. Still was frequently moved to tears by stories of osteopathic charlatans preying on innocent patients or claiming osteopathic expertise. "They are drunken scoundrels, the very trash of your town," raged Still, who "are no more fit [to practice] than a donkey is to go in a jewelry-shop."[79] And then there were, of course, the biggest imitators of them all, the chiropractors, who sullied the good name of manual manipulation. Regulars seized on osteopathy's inferior schools as evidence of the profession's mercenary rather than selfless motives to heal. They published articles ridiculing the incompetency of osteopaths and their education system. The fact that regular medicine had its fair share of diploma mills and poorly run schools did not seem to temper their criticism. Rather than refute these accusations, osteopathy's leaders, like those in chiropractic, worked to upgrade and correct abuses.[80]

Many of the people who enrolled in osteopathic and chiropractic schools came from the lower classes. Too poor to afford regular medical school, which raised tuition in the late nineteenth century, many working-class Americans came to Palmer and Still seeking the promise of the American Dream, social mobility and economic independence. Osteopathic schools had historically maintained lower admission standards than regular medical schools, in part as a means of remaining accessible to poor students. In the 1920s, George Laughlin, president of the Kirksville College of Osteopathy, argued "that requiring two years of prior college work was hurting the underprivileged since they could least afford the additional schooling."[81] This commitment to accessibility had the unintended effect of creating an impression of osteopathy today as somewhat of a "back door" into medicine, a way for people who could not get into regular medical schools to become doctors.[82] Both osteopathy and chiropractic also recruited practitioners from the ranks of satisfied patients, which Still and Palmer touted as the ultimate validation of their systems. Relief from what was for many a pain-filled life often prompted a powerful and dramatic conversion experience to a new way of life, just as it had for many of the founders and followers of other irregular health systems. Chiropractic, in particular, drew converts from those discontented with medicine or simply the course of their lives. Many had no medical experience save for a positive encounter with chiropractic adjustment. In other cases, teachers, lawyers, and ministers came to chiropractic seeking the fulfillment lacking in their current jobs. The maturity of these early chiropractors may have helped them withstand the persecution that a chiropractic career, particularly in the initial years, often entailed.[83]

Professional journals and associations followed the educational expansion of chiropractic and osteopathy. The *Journal of Osteopathy* began in 1894, and three years later, in 1897, the American Osteopathic Association (AOA) organized in Kirksville with the intention of improving educational standards, imposing sanctions on incompetent osteopaths, and raising the profile of osteopathy as a profession.[84]

Chiropractors embarked on a similar professionalizing course. The first chiropractic journal, the appropriately named *Backbone*, debuted in 1903. The *Chiropractor*, a Palmer publication, began the following year. In 1905, the American Chiropractic Association organized in Cedar Rapids, Iowa, and the following year B. J. Palmer started the Universal Chiropractors' Association.[85]

These professionalizing tendencies differentiated chiropractic and

osteopathy markedly from the irregular systems that had arisen before. American medicine, not to mention American culture, had
changed. Experts and expertise increasingly mattered as people in every field banded together into professional organizations. While the
democratic impulse still animated Americans toward common sense
and resentment of elite knowledge and power, American culture in
the late nineteenth century increasingly deferred authority in some
fields, particularly science, to specialists. Irregulars could not rely on
the populist sentiment that had sustained them in the past.[86]

But even as they recognized the realities of the new medical marketplace, osteopathy and chiropractic were not without internal dis-
sensions that could potentially damage their growth. Osteopaths
wrestled over the scope of their practice, particularly in regard to
the range of therapies they should employ and the types of diseases
and conditions they should treat. Two groups vied for support and
control: those loyal to Still and his manipulative theory, known as
"straights," and those who doubted that manipulation could really
cure everything and blended osteopathy with regular and other irregular medical therapies, known as "mixers." Surgery presented the
first challenge. Those who believed in manipulation alone saw no
reason to add surgery to the osteopathic curriculum. Andrew Taylor
Still, while disgusted by regular medicine's overeagerness to reach for
the knife, felt surgery had some place after all other options had been
exhausted. It was the doctor, not the surgery, that was the problem,
he reasoned.[87] "We accept . . . surgery also as of great use and benefit
to mankind," wrote Still. "But when should the knife be used? Never,
until all nerves, veins, and arteries have failed to restore a healthy condition of the body in all its parts and functions."[88] But if osteopathy
was truly to compete with regular medicine and even other irregulars
like homeopathy, the mixers argued, it had to provide the same range
of services to patients. Still added surgery to the curriculum of his
school in 1897, in part, out of hope that osteopathy could bring some
reform to a field he thought too quick to send patients to the operating table. The conflict over inclusion of drugs was a far bigger and
longer fight. Unlike surgery, Still saw no use for drugs, and he continued to attack them as an assault on the body's natural healing power
and an insult to the wisdom of God. He managed to keep most of his
followers, who greatly respected his leadership even as they sought
modifications of his theory, in line during his life. But the struggle be-

tween straights and mixers over drugs simmered beneath the surface and eventually transformed osteopathy into its modern form.[89]

Early chiropractors argued endlessly over adjustment techniques, equipment, and even aspects of Palmer's theory itself. Many chiropractors developed their own way of manipulating subluxations. Others introduced a broad range of therapies to supplement physical adjustment, such as massage, electrical stimulation, and water therapy. Those methods that involved mechanical devices struck some pure chiropractors as particularly egregious, violating the meaning of a science whose name meant "done by hand." B. J. Palmer discovered this himself in 1923 when he attempted to introduce the Neurocalometer, a device that could supposedly find subluxations by detecting changes in nerve transmission along the spine. The device deeply divided chiropractors and further fractured the movement.[90] Many of the chiropractic schools, associations, and journals that formed operated as organs of these various splinter groups. The first chiropractic textbook was not published by Palmer but by some of his students who had set up a competing school in Cedar Rapids, Iowa. The authors not only neglected to credit Palmer, they also claimed the brain, not the nerves alone, was the source of all nerve function in the body, a position that Palmer's son B. J. gradually adopted.[91] B. J. himself also altered chiropractic theory and introduced new official chiropractic terms to maximize chiropractic's differences from osteopathy. Instead of a diagnosis, chiropractors made an "analysis"; an "adjustment" instead of treatment; and never "manipulation," the word most osteopaths used to describe their therapy.[92] Some chiropractors felt their techniques were so different from Palmer's as to be an entirely different medical system. One known as neuropathy blended chiropractic, osteopathy, and ophthalmology, while another called naprapathy was a form of manual medicine based on problems with the ligaments and connective tissues rather than nerves; both were started by Palmer graduates.[93]

Some chiropractors ignored the spiritual aspects of Palmer's theory altogether, applying his system to the nagging back troubles for which regular medicine had little to offer. This frustrated and angered Palmer, who saw his system as a way to alleviate the world's ills and illuminate life's mysteries, and not simply a method of relieving chronic back pain. Those who thought so, declared Palmer, were "unprincipled shysters" and "kleptomaniac scavengers."[94] But for people suffering from lumbago and sciatica, the most common nineteenth-century back ailments, the mysteries of life took a backseat to the relief of debilitating pain.

People had searched for and tried various back remedies for centuries. For "An old Stubborn Pain in the Back," John Wesley's eighteenth-century *Primitive Physick* suggested steeping the "root of Water-Fern in Water" and rubbing it over the affected area. Rheumatism, the old word for musculoskeletal pain, could be helped in a variety of ways, from wrapping the back in molasses-smeared bandages to living on fresh "Milk Whey" and white bread for fourteen days.[95] Many regular doctors prescribed opium for the pain, taken as laudanum or morphine or mixed in powders or elixirs. They also bled and made shallow cuts in the skin to reduce inflammation in the part of the body in pain. In the late nineteenth century, electrical devices became popular pain relievers. Dr. Scott's Electric Flesh Brush was "WARRANTED TO CURE" a panoply of illnesses, from rheumatism and "Diseases of the Blood" to those "Back Aches peculiar to Ladies." The brush produced an electromagnetic current through its bristles and came with a silver compass to test the potency of the charge.[96] Electrical devices are still popular today. One, known as a TENS (transcutaneous electrical nerve stimulation) unit, stimulates the low back and other painful areas and is sometimes prescribed by regular doctors despite conflicting evidence of efficacy.[97] As the range of these treatments suggests, no one had a clue how to relieve back ailments. That failure gave chiropractic an opportunity to fill a very real physical need. Palmer's disapproval did little to dissuade some chiropractors from focusing entirely on the technical rather than spiritual aspects of the system. A Dr. Metzger in Anaconda, Montana, even predicted that one day instead of asking others how they were, the daily greeting would be replaced with "How's your spine?" This focus helped chiropractic gain a devoted following.[98]

Part of the appeal of both osteopathy and chiropractic to many Americans was the simplicity of their theories. This was nothing new. Irregulars had long championed straightforward and accessible medicine. The idea of disease as an obstruction in need of correcting made intuitive sense to followers. But simplicity was also becoming increasingly anachronistic. Scientific discoveries in the late nineteenth century, most notably the germ theory of disease, convinced many medical researchers and regular doctors that disease could not be explained by one universal cause, especially one that accounted for both the body and the spirit as Palmer and Still believed their systems did. Manual manipulation also struck many regulars as too crude to address the wonders and intricacies discovered in the lens of a microscope. The regular medical profession had a vested interest in complexity, though. Medicine had to be beyond the comprehension and skill of the general public to command respect and prestige. Simple explanations undermined the authority and expertise of doctors.[99]

Osteopaths did not ignore or stand defiant in the face of new scientific discoveries. By the early twentieth century, most accepted that germs caused disease, though they interpreted the finding through an osteopathic lens. The health of the body's structure determined the viability of germs in the body, reasoned osteopaths. Germs thrived where the blood pooled and slowed: at osteopathic lesions, in other words. Manipulation stimulated the body's natural resistance by restoring the free flow of blood, which would overcome the infection.[100] How to combat and prevent infection became the determined preoccupation of regular doctors in the first decade of the twentieth century. They searched for effective, germ-killing drugs, an investigation that only heightened tensions among osteopaths over the admissibility of drugs into osteopathic education and daily practice.

Chiropractors, on the other hand, had a more complicated relationship with the germ theory. While most did not outright reject the existence of germs, chiropractors believed that regular medicine overemphasized germs—just like drugs and surgery—and that the true cause of disease was not outside, where germs lived, but inside the body. This idea left germs in a rather nebulous place in chiropractic theory. "Chiropractors have found in every disease that is supposed to be contagious, *a cause in the spine,*" wrote B. J. Palmer. "There is no contagious disease. . . . There is no infection. . . . There is a cause internal to man that makes of his body in a certain spot, more or less a breeding ground [for microbes]."[101] Chiropractors did believe that hygiene was important to health, just as regular medicine had come to believe thanks to the hydropaths by the late nineteenth century, though chiropractors likely saw it as a way to promote overall health rather than as a means of controlling and containing the spread of germs and thus disease.[102] Because they emphasized nature and viewed disease as an internal process, chiropractors also tended to reject medical devices and gadgets like electric massagers because the introduction of these technologies suggested that nature was inadequate to the task of healing. Chiropractic ambivalence about the germ theory of disease continued well into the twentieth century, coming to a head in the 1940s with the introduction of antibiotics, which made germs harder to ignore. Although this led to a decline in chiropractic opposition, some chiropractors to this day do not accept that microbes can cause disease. The idea of disease caused and cured from inside or outside the body still constitutes a real philosophical difference between chiropractic and regular approaches to health care.[103]

While many Americans frequented chiropractors and osteopaths for philosophical reasons, many others went out of necessity; they were the only doctors in town. Since colonial times, regulars had been concentrated in more populous areas of the country, leaving rural and frontier communities to fend for themselves. By the early twentieth century, advances in medical science began dividing medical practice into subspecialties. Doctors no longer served as clinician and surgeon treating all diseases and all patients as they had for centuries. Many regulars moved to hospitals and medical institutions in urban areas to practice where the money and patient pool offered greater opportunities and benefits, often leaving rural communities without medical care. Both chiropractors and osteopaths benefited from this shift. They earned their first and most loyal followers in the rural Midwest and other small towns around the country, where they found a grateful clientele whose care absolutely depended on the survival of these systems. They also thrived in urban areas by offering a distinctive treatment that had no counterpart in regular medicine, creating a patient population dependent on their services.[104] It certainly did not hurt that osteopathy and chiropractic tended to cost less than regular care as well.

Like most of the irregulars before them, osteopathy and chiropractic also legitimated all diseases as worthy of consideration and care, and they promised hope for all. Regular medicine often designated patients, particularly those suffering from chronic illnesses, as hopeless, or worse, as hypochondriacal. In osteopathy and chiropractic, nothing was impossible, nothing incurable. Each had a theory that provided a clear and coherent explanation for a range of sometimes confusing and conflicting symptoms that comforted patients in search of answers.[105]

And they did report great success in their treatments. Like those using hydropathy, most osteopathic and chiropractic patients were not generally acutely ill but suffered from chronic problems. These patients could generally get around, albeit painfully at times, and practitioners reported positive results with many patients who had given up on ever feeling better.

Regular medicine had plenty of biting criticism and ridicule for these new systems of manual medicine. Mark Twain rather precisely summed up the situation when he declared that asking a doctor what he thought about osteopathy was like "going to Satan to find out about the Christian religion."[106] Regulars disparaged not only the quality of osteopathic schools but also what they saw as its graduates' blind subservience to a poorly educated, hopelessly vague, and mystical leader. Osteopaths were guilty of "claiming impossible things and doing harmful ones." Any good that resulted from osteopathy was simply luck or the power of suggestion. "Happy is the charlatan who happens to be at hand when the triumph of the recuperative power takes place, and thrice happy is he when a reputable man who knows nothing about such things can be persuaded that mere coincidence is the brilliant demonstration of a new art of healing," proclaimed a 1905 *New York Times* editorial.[107] Regular physician Richard Newton declared osteopathy "a complete system of charlatanism, empiricism and quackery calculated and designed to impose on the credulous, superstitious and ignorant, and fraught with danger."[108]

Most Americans were at least willing to give osteopathy a chance, and the system received mostly favorable reviews in popular magazines and newspapers. In 1895, John R. Musick wrote a history of osteopathy for *Godey's Magazine* that included a record of its successes. He condemned regulars for dismissing it out of hand and suggested that they did so out of fear of new ideas. Still's theory "has certainly achieved much success in the past, and is worthy of careful investigation before it is condemned," Musick concluded.[109] Among osteopathy's most prominent supporters was Mark Twain, who after humorous run-ins and experiments with several other irregular health systems seemed to have found the system he'd been looking for and became an outspoken advocate of Still. Twain even testified at a hearing before the New York Assembly Committee on Public Health in 1901 in favor of a bill to license osteopaths. In trademark Twain fashion, he kept the room laughing with a speech that blended a plea for personal liberty with self-deprecation. "Now I am always wanting to try everything that comes along. It doesn't matter much what it is, I want to try it. And so I went to [osteopath] Mr. Kelgrin, was treated by him in London, and later on in Switzerland, and he did me a lot of good," said Twain, "although I must admit that my education doesn't qualify me to say just when I am in good health. But I should like to have the right to experiment with my own body to my heart's content. I don't care whether it is to my own peril or anybody else's."[110] Osteopathy also counted President Theodore Roosevelt, General Dwight Eisenhower, and businessman Howard Hughes among its supporters.[111]

Chiropractors mostly eluded the attention of regulars, at least at first. Perhaps they were too focused on osteopathy. But by the early twentieth century, reports of patient deaths due to "neck twisting," vertebral "dislocations," and other disfigurements were a regular feature in regular medical journals. B. J. Palmer's pretensions and showmanship captivated followers and became fodder for critics. "Chiropractic is a religion, it is the worship of B. J. Palmer," wrote Charles Warner. "Palmer encourages the idea by wearing his hair and beard to resemble Christ; and by having his pictures taken in a pose to imitate Christ in the painting 'Christ Before Pilate.'"[112] Regulars also delighted in sending barely literate letters requesting admission to chiropractic schools and publishing the results. In 1923, the *Journal of the American Medical Association* reprinted a letter supposedly from a young Texas widow seeking to enroll at the Carver Chiropractic College in Oklahoma City. "Sirs, Mister Kirpatic School, I want to rite letter an see if I can be kirpatic dr. if you can make a kirpatic dr. for how much money I got about 2 thousand dolers that my husband got wen he died." The Carver school responded with condolences to the widow and commended her interest in chiropractic. They offered her immediate admission and praised her decision to spend her money on "a real life's work."[113] Perhaps the most famous condemnation of chiropractic, though, came from Morris Fishbein, editor of the *Journal of the American Medical Association* and well known for his quack-busting crusades. Though no friend to osteopathy, Fishbein saw chiropractors as far worse, a "malignant tumor on the body of osteopathy. . . . Osteopathy is essentially a method of entering the practice of medicine by the back door. Chiropractic, by contrast, is an attempt to arrive through the cellar. The man who applies at the back-door at least makes himself presentable. The one who comes through the cellar is besmirched with dust and grime: he carries a crowbar and he may wear a mask."[114]

As much as regulars disparaged chiropractors, though, osteopaths might have hated them even more. They were certain that Palmer had simply copied Still's ideas and methods. Rumors of Palmer having visited Still in Kirksville proliferated. As proof, osteopaths pointed to Palmer's signature in Still's guestbook. Palmer denied ever being in Kirksville and claimed the signature was a fraud.[115]

While many Americans found much to like in chiropractic, it struggled to receive praise in the press. Many magazines and news-papers took an extremely negative view toward chiropractors and their philosophy, sounding every bit like regular doctors. In *Harper's Weekly* in 1915, journalist George Creel recalled visiting a chiropractor with a made-up problem needing treatment. The chiropractor cracked and popped Creel's neck and spine to the point that Creel felt "he had done his worst." Creel was wrong, though. "He turned me over on my face again, and in a few seconds I felt an awful pressure on my spine, first one spot, then another," described Creel. When Creel got home, he looked at his back in the mirror and saw "a large black spot the size of a grape fruit. Only heaven knows what would have been my present state had I not been in perfect health and strength when I took the treatment."[116] These types of stories often appeared in newspapers that also featured ads for chiropractors promising free consultations or "no cure, no pay" policies as a measure of good faith. Some chiropractors boldly asked for patients who seemed incurable. A Dr. Offerman in St. Paul, Minnesota, advertised, "When others fail come to me . . . don't give up. I will guarantee a cure. Remember that curing disease after all others have failed is my specialty."[117]

More than words, regulars tried to use the law to destroy, or at the very least restrict, osteopathy and chiropractic. The primary is-sue hinged on whether either actually qualified as a form of medi-cine. Many states narrowly defined medicine as prescribing drugs, so drugless systems like chiropractic and osteopathy were not medicine and therefore could not be regulated or subject to laws for practicing "medicine." But that did not stop regulars from claiming otherwise. Still's own son, Charles, who had achieved success treating victims of a diphtheria outbreak in Minnesota, was the first osteopath to come to the attention of the state health authorities. In treating the disease, Charles likely followed his father's instructions to "bring the clavicles and sternum far enough forward to take off any pressure that exists, in order to let venous blood and other fluids return to the heart" and to keep patients in a clean, well-ventilated room. As an infectious bacterial disease, diphtheria was likely little helped by Charles's manipulations. His patients may have had mild cases, and they probably recovered on their own; most fatalities from the disease occur in children under five. Working in such close proximity to his patients, Charles was fortunate to escape without contracting diphtheria himself, though he could not escape the law. Charles was arrested and charged with practicing medicine without a license. The case against him was dropped, however, as the number of people seeking his care grew so large that it became hard for the state to deny his effectiveness. Not every osteopath was so lucky, and many others faced trials in the 1890s.[118]

Chiropractors had to watch out not only for regulars but for osteopaths, too. Some hid their DC diplomas and practiced behind closed shades and locked doors. Many chiropractors did go to court for practicing without a license, but few were convicted. Those who were usually went to jail willingly as a demonstration of their dedication to medical freedom. One of the first to be jailed was Palmer himself, who was arrested in Davenport in 1905 for violating medical practice laws. The case hinged, in part, on claims made by Palmer in his journal, the *Chiropractor*, in which the state claimed that Palmer professed to cure all kinds of diseases with his unlicensed healing method. The jury found him guilty, but Palmer's refusal to pay the $350 fine led the *Davenport Democrat & Leader* to report, "He will stick with chiropractic to the end [and] offer himself as a martyr" by going to jail. In the end, Palmer only served twenty-three days of his 105-day sentence after his wife paid the fine.[119] Following Palmer's lead, the Federated Chiropractors of California launched a "Go to Jail for Chiropractic" campaign in the 1920s that helped to infuse chiropractors with a sense of martyrdom mixed with heroism. Arrests sometimes proved good for business. Publicly sacrificing oneself in defense of medical freedom against the tyranny of regular medicine was a winning storyline for many Americans.[120]

Although many received pardons and acquittals, osteopaths and chiropractors knew that depending on the favor of juries, particularly as regular medicine campaigned to have both prohibited by state legislatures, was a dangerous course. Besides legal action, regulars denied them membership in local medical societies and refused to allow them admission to university and public hospitals. Medical societies also prohibited regulars from any kind of professional cooperation, tactics they had previously employed against homeopaths, hydropaths, and other irregulars. Osteopaths and chiropractors responded with a very different course of action than their predecessors, though. Rather than fight the enactment and enforcement of licensing laws, as the Thomsonians had done in the 1830s, they fought to be licensed themselves.[121]

Osteopaths took a pragmatic course, fighting for full rights in some states and partial rights in others depending on their resources, support, and, of course, how much resistance they faced from regulars. In 1896, Vermont became the first state to license osteopaths, a move that led Dr. Robert T. Morris of the New York County Medical Society to label Vermont "the garbage ground of the profession."[122] Osteopaths often gave demonstrations and free manipulations to legislators to win support in key states. North Dakota and Missouri soon followed Vermont's lead, and by 1901, fifteen states had granted osteopathy legal standing. A little more than a decade later, osteopaths could lawfully practice in forty states. Not every state was so easily won, however; Mississippi, the last holdout, finally consented to license osteopaths in 1973.

Osteopathy also expanded its college curriculum in the early twentieth century to include surgery, obstetrics, and even, most controversially, drug therapy.[123] Many state legislatures insisted that if osteopaths were to be licensed to provide surgery, they should be required to study all of the same subjects as regular doctors, including drugs. Osteopathy yielded to the pressure, though not without considerable pain and torment to Still, who urged his supporters to not be "trampled in the mud" by regulars but to "hold up the pure and unadulterated osteopathic flag."[124]

Chiropractors suffered far more arrests and abuse than osteopaths because winning licensure was a slower process. In 1913, Kansas became the first state to license chiropractors, and the total had climbed to twenty-two by the early 1920s. Twenty-five more states had passed licensing laws by the end of the 1920s, leading journalist H. L. Mencken to complain of "a chiropractor at every cross-roads, and in such sinks of imbecility as Los Angeles they are as thick as bootleggers."[125] It would be decades before the chiropractic battle for licensure ended, though.

After licensure, improving education was the priority for both osteopaths and chiropractors. Osteopaths concentrated on keeping pace with the requirements and standards of regular medical schools so that by the 1930s, the curriculum of regular and osteopathic schools looked nearly identical; by the 1950s, most osteopaths had become more or less the equals of regular medicine practitioners.[126]

At the same time, osteopaths insisted on maintaining a separate identity, something homeopathy had failed to do. They were not MDs, as homeopaths had considered themselves, even though osteopaths legally had the right to use that title; they were DOs. Osteopaths maintained their own schools, hospitals, professional journals, and associations and asserted that the quality and scope of their care was comparable if not superior to regular medicine. They resisted joining regulars as a therapeutic option within regular medicine, understanding, as other irregulars had not, that the allure of ostensible acceptance would likely lead to their demise as the actual distinctions between osteopathy and regular medicine blurred. Osteopathy became, in essence, a parallel profession to regular medicine with a similar range of institutions and periodicals.[127] In fact, many doctors today wonder why osteopathy persists and question its reason for being. But many regulars are perhaps unaware of osteopathy's history and its rise to prominence at a time when no medical system, regular or irregular, dominated. While manual manipulation plays a smaller role in osteopathy than it did at first, many osteopaths still use it in their practices, particularly those in solo practice. Proficiency in manipulation does require practice and time, things that osteopaths practicing in regular institutions often do not have due to the constraints of the modern medical system.[128]

Most critically, osteopaths survived by locating a medical need and defining their own niche. Many served small towns and rural areas where they were often the only doctors in town. The geographic scarcity of doctors in some regions led both federal and state governments to appropriate funds for the training of osteopaths as one strategy for solving the primary care shortage in rural areas. Osteopaths also did not actively pursue new medical research and subspecialties as quickly as regulars. This was, in part, because outside of the developing regular medical system, osteopathy lacked the resources for schools, equipment, and training. They focused, instead, on primary care and took advantage of the growing need for general practitioners in the 1940s as more regulars choose to specialize in fields like surgery and psychiatry. Barred from providing medical service and exempt from the draft in World War II, osteopaths who had not volunteered for other war duties provided much-needed medical care on the home front. With roughly forty-five thousand regular doctors in the military defense force, many Americans who might not otherwise have been exposed to osteopathy gave it a try. Many regulars returned from the war and found they had lost their patients. Osteopathy, in essence, gained legitimacy by stepping into the primary care vacuum left by regulars, even if many patients did not know the difference between the two forms of medicine (a problem that persists to this day). With these shifts, regular doctors found themselves dependent on an irregular system as a source of referrals for their own specialty practices, a seemingly unimaginable outcome of the more than century-long struggle between regular and irregular healers.[129]

Even so, osteopathy traded ideological purity for survival. In the 1930s, many osteopathic schools began referring to their practice as "osteopathic medicine," with increasing emphasis on the word "medicine," to gain more financial backing. They may also have hoped to "pass" as regular doctors without the necessary theoretical qualifiers to attract more clients. Rather than stress their differences from regular medicine as they had in Still's time, osteopaths emphasized the quality of their care. They also relied less and less on manipulation as the primary mode of treatment. Today, many osteopathic medical schools still teach manual manipulation but regard it more as an option rather than as the only treatment. In deemphasizing manipulation, osteopaths tried to counter the accusations of regulars that osteopathy was a quackish cult. It seemed to work. In 1969, no longer able to easily justify their exclusion on the basis of education or quality of care, the AMA opened its membership as well as internships and residencies to osteopaths.[130]

Those patients who sought manipulative relief for chronic musculoskeletal problems continued to turn to chiropractic for help. Chiropractors' devotion to low-technology adjustment as their therapeutic method kept them on the fringes of regular medicine at a time when medical care was growing increasingly complex and technological.[131]

Palmer's belief that he had discovered a higher form of medicine, "the antithesis of medicine," in B. J. Palmer's words, significantly influenced the direction of the profession and its overall unwillingness to absorb the theories and therapies of regular medical science. Osteopaths, by contrast, tended to view themselves as reformers rather than crusaders of an entirely new health paradigm, so perhaps their accommodation and cooperation with regular medicine was more predictable.[132] To function within regular medicine, chiropractors would have to gain patients through referrals from regular doctors rather than reaching out to patients directly. Chiropractors proved unwilling to relinquish their autonomy, a position strengthened by osteopathy's move into primary care. Treatment of musculoskeletal conditions, particularly back pain, was left almost solely in their hands. While a far more diminished role than many chiropractors aspired to and that Palmer had envisioned for his science, this focus gave chiropractors authority in an arena where regular medicine had little to offer and allowed them to remain independent.[133]

In recent years, manual medicine has made some inroads into regular medicine, as regular doctors have recognized the benefits of osteopathic manipulation for specific cases. Some hospitals have even integrated it into overall patient management because it scores well in client satisfaction.[134]

Osteopaths themselves are osteopathy's most significant and visible influence on regular medicine today. Many now practice and interact on equal terms with regular doctors. But the parallel profession path has its problems, as many patients cannot distinguish between the two types of medicine, and osteopathy has struggled to maintain and assert its identity. The time and bureaucratic constraints of the modern medical system make it challenging for osteopaths to practice manipulation and to take the detailed patient histories that Still required. Many regulars, too, continue to view osteopathy as inferior and see its schools as an easier and substandard path to becoming a doctor.

Chiropractors, on the other hand, have remained a marginal profession, not quite accepted but not as far to the fringe as holistic health movements like naturopathy and even homeopathy in its modern form. Unresolved conflicts and tensions between chiropractors and regulars continue to color relations between the two and perhaps bear the most resemblance to the strife that characterized nineteenth-century medicine. Some regulars still feel that chiropractic adjustments pose potentially serious health risks. Several reports have linked chiropractic manipulation of the neck to stroke.[135] Many regulars would prefer that chiropractic-like adjustments be provided by physical therapists under their supervision or at least within the confines of a regular medical institution, a position chiropractors reject. Chiropractors today seem to have socially and psychologically accepted their outsider status, finding unity in a role as an extremely popular but "oppressed minority" within the dominant medical system.[136]

Perhaps that's just the way the elder Palmer and his son wanted it. The two made much of the martyrdom of chiropractors who suffered at the hands of the law for their healing convictions. Conflict increased solidarity and gave chiropractic practitioners and their followers a sense of righteous indignation. Regular medicine "condemns every method, every procedure, every theory, idea or help to humanity that does not originate within and financially help to fill the pockets of its own ranks," declared B. J. "It cares not what you, as a patient, think."[137]

CHAPTER EIGHT

The Fall and Rise of
Alternative Medicine

On an October evening in 1893, homeopaths from the Hahnemann Medical College marched proudly down the streets of Philadelphia in the city's annual medical parade. Cheered on by the crowd lining the streets, the students carried canes and waved banners in the royal blue and burnt orange of their school, proudly displaying their motto: "In things certain, unity; in things doubtful, liberty; in all things, charity." Unity and charity were far from the minds of the medical students at the University of Philadelphia, Jefferson, and Medico-Chirurgical colleges, however. After learning that the Hahnemann students were to lead the parade, the regular students flatly refused to participate, claiming that to do so would insult "their health and dignity." And so the homeopaths from Hahnemann along with students from the Philadelphia Dental College marched down Broad Street alone to the taunts of their regular peers: "Sugar pill, sugar pill, / Never cured and never will. / Rickety roup, rickety roup, / Hahnemann, Hahnemann, in the soup." Led by a brass band and a squad of mounted police called in to keep order, the 250 defiant and proud homeopathic students called out their school cheer as they passed: "Rah, rah, rah, Hahnemann, Hahnemann, sis boom ah."[1] It was a sweet moment for homeopaths, and yet another reminder to regulars that after nearly a century, the fight to vanquish their irregular competitors was far from won.

But American medicine had changed substantially in that century. The discovery of germs, the advent of X-rays, and the growth of sterile surgery among other medical innovations began to shift healing away from individual Americans and the home and into the hands of trained experts working in hospitals. Knowledge about the structure and function of the body had finally reached the point where daily medical practice began to change. These developments could not have come at a better time.

The closing decades of the nineteenth century brought major upheavals to nearly every aspect of life. The horrors of the Civil War had shattered the peaceful vision social reformers had promulgated earlier in the century of humanity's perfection through right living and self-control. Americans still thought it was important to work toward the common good, but to survive and thrive now seemed to demand risk and self-indulgence rather than personal example and self-sacrifice. Many people, especially the newly wealthy, became philanthropists and donated money to causes as the nation's now well-developed consumer ethos encouraged people to believe that good works—like good health—could be purchased. Meanwhile, immigration brought millions of new people to the United States just as the nation's workforce shifted from predominantly rural and farm labor to urban and industrial work. Cities exploded. Advances in transportation and communication networks lessened geographical distances and reduced isolation. Technology also made work more productive and efficient. As a result, business boomed. Economic fortunes were made and lost overnight. At the same time, at least half of all workers barely made enough money to survive.[2]

To a nation in flux and looking for answers, scientific progress appeared to be a cultural cure-all. Science held the promise of order and efficiency at a time when the nation seemed to many Americans unable to cope with the disorder and complexities of modern life. In response, nearly all fields began adopting more systematic methods and making claims of specific knowledge and expertise. Medicine, law, journalism, education, and even child rearing increasingly set boundaries defining the scope of their subject and the prerequisites for practicing.

Regular doctors had tried to set these boundaries and stake their claim on medical practice throughout the nineteenth century but to little effect. Many Americans, aided by the loud shouts of irregulars, had dismissed their argument as more mercenary than scientific, a self-interested effort to dissuade people from seeking the services of competitors—and they likely had a point. But advances in medical science now began to change the healing landscape. No longer just rhetoric, regular medicine had new tools and knowledge at its disposal that offered a tangible hope of healing. Americans did not lose their attachment to self-reliance, but many problems now seemed bigger than any one individual could possibly grasp through common sense alone. In this culture, expertise became a trait of increasing popular value. The unwillingness of some irregulars, namely hydropaths, Thomsonians, and mesmerists, to distinguish between formally trained practitioners and those who came to the field through a calling or hands-on experience now made them appear backward and less well equipped to compete with this new class of professional healers.[3]

These scientific advances and cultural shifts fueled the revival of the medical licenses deemed undemocratic earlier in the century. In the 1880s and 1890s, most state legislatures reinstated licensing requirements at the instigation of regular medicine's state and local societies. Until late in the century, these medical societies had largely proved ineffective at lobbying for the profession, torn apart by internal struggles over theory, practice, and leadership. These organizations grew stronger and more effective with time, and they succeeded in convincing politicians that medicine demanded a basic competency in science. By the late nineteenth century, the image of the ideal doctor had expanded to include laboratory methods rather than bedside manner and observation alone. These licensing laws did not drive irregulars out of practice, however. Homeopaths and the eclectic heirs to Thomsonism were too well established and the homeopaths far too popular to be suddenly outlawed. Regulars only succeeded in getting the licensing laws they wanted by allowing homeopaths and eclectics—the very groups they had originally organized to oppose— to be licensed as well. By the 1920s, many states had passed licensing statutes that covered newer irregular systems too, though it would be many decades until osteopathy and chiropractic achieved legal protection in every state.[4]

Buoyed by the return of medical licensure, the American Medical Association took a far more active political role in the early twentieth century. While still concerned with berating and exposing irregular quackery, the organization also seized on widespread concerns about the dangers of urban life to campaign for sanitation laws, public hospitals, and the creation of a national health bureau to implement and coordinate public health programs. They supported diagnostic tests for cholera and vaccination for diphtheria and required reporting of tuberculosis and other infectious diseases to city and state officials. Associating themselves with these concerns helped to forge an image of regular medicine as a proponent of social welfare and community health at a time when public health had itself because a distinct field of medicine out of concern over urban life. Improving public health could only improve the status of regular medicine in the eyes of patients and the government. The AMA fought to exclude irregulars from this new arena of health care by lobbying to prevent them from serving on medical councils and city boards of health and in public hospitals, efforts in which they mostly succeeded. Irregulars protested what they saw as political moves by regulars to monopolize public health and to destroy competition on the national level. Regular medicine's enthusiastic embrace of sanitation and hygiene was an especially paradoxical outcome for the hydropaths who had pioneered the principles and practices that underlay these public health campaigns.[5]

Regulars also pushed for educational reforms in the nation's medical schools. At the recommendation of the AMA, the Carnegie Foundation for the Advancement of Teaching sent high school principal Abraham Flexner to evaluate the ability of regular, eclectic, homeopathic, and osteopathic schools in the United States and Canada to produce doctors trained in regular methods. The famous Flexner report of 1910 revealed the sorry state of medical education. Flexner wrote complete analyses of each school. Of the 155 he visited, he recommended that 120 schools should close. Flexner declared the majority of the regular schools "utterly wretched" and "hopeless affairs" and discounted all irregular institutions as "worthless" and "fatally defective." He found most schools to be proprietary or commercial medical enterprises with minimal academic standards and little or no connection to the hospitals and laboratories that had increasingly become central to the provision of care. In the competitive rush to attract students, many proprietary medical schools, regular and irregular alike, had shortened terms and eliminated staff (or never hired them in the first place) to maximize profits. Although he had few kind words for regular schools, Flexner saved his particular scorn for irregulars. He warned that opening the profession to anyone who wanted to be a doctor endangered the well-being of society and the nobility of a profession dedicated to service.[6]

The Flexner report quickly achieved mythic status for catalyzing the reform of medical education in the United States, but its methods and conclusions, particularly concerning irregulars, do raise questions. Who could be surprised that irregular schools did not turn out *regular* physicians? That was not the goal of an irregular medical education. Flexner was also accompanied in his survey by regular doctor Nathan P. Cowell, secretary of the Council on Medical Education of the AMA. Hardly a disinterested party with regard to the outcome of the report, Cowell's council had in fact set the standards Flexner used to assess the schools, and the AMA had never seen irregular schools as anything but counterfeit. That's not to say that the nation's medical education did not need improvement—better-trained doctors would result in better medicine—but the political and economic motivations of those behind the Flexner report provided just as much if not more motivation than any idealistic appeals to improve the quality of medical education.[7]

In the wake of the report, nearly half of the nation's regular medical schools closed. Many schools that admitted women and African Americans, which tended to be weaker and financially unstable to begin with, closed. Those that survived drastically upgraded standards. Flexner had recommended that all medical schools require entrants to have a college degree and encouraged the adoption of a four-year medical curriculum. As encouragement, he persuaded the Rockefeller Foundation to make grants to those schools he hand-selected as worthy of investment. He chose mostly long-established institutions in the East as well as a handful in the South, Midwest, and West. Rockefeller's contributions stimulated other donations to support medical education.[8] Many irregular schools also improved their curriculum to match the new standards of regular medicine. While some of these irregular schools carried on, many failed, done in by the high costs of upgrading facilities and hiring high-quality staff. The net effect of the Flexner report was to widen rather than narrow the gap between the best and worst schools.[9]

Not every irregular kowtowed to Flexner's findings. Chiropractors, in particular, protested his recommendations. They argued that the adoption of Flexner's educational standards would exclude worthy but financially strapped students from becoming doctors. In the past, a lower-class person could become a doctor through hard work and desire. Under Flexner's plan, he or she would stand little chance because of the costs of obtaining both a college and medical education.

The chiropractors did have a point. Requiring college degrees for medical school admittance excluded a majority of the population: more than 90 percent of Americans did not have bachelor's degrees even by 1920. Longer and more costly training made medicine more exclusive and less accessible to minorities, women, immigrants, and working-class Americans.[10] Flexner, for his part, likely thought curbing enrollment a laudable goal of educational reform. He warned that awarding too many medical degrees only suppressed salaries and limited the field's ability to attract the best students. "It is evident that in a society constituted as our modern states," wrote Flexner, "the interests of the social order will be served best when the number of men entering a given profession reaches and does not exceed a certain ratio."[11] Raising standards was an effective means of reducing the number of doctors and increasing the social and economic status of the profession. Unlike many of his peers who believed female doctors would also lower medicine's status, Flexner actually supported coeducation in medical schools, though he rather myopically editorialized, "[N]ow that women are freely admitted to the medical profession, it is clear that they show a decreasing inclination to enter it."[12]

The path was hardly free and clear for women. Flexner speculated that fewer women entered medicine either due to a drop in demand for women doctors or less interest among women in becoming doctors. Neither was true. The closure of irregular medical schools and close alignment of others with regular medicine had a particularly detrimental effect on the women who achieved professional medical careers in irregular health care. Middle- and upper-class women had made great strides in the late nineteenth century, comprising 10 percent or more of enrollment at regular medical schools. While many attended female-only medical colleges, women still made up nearly 20 percent of the medical profession in eastern cities like Boston, New York, and Baltimore by 1900. But lacking adequate financial support, especially as medicine became more technologically sophisticated, many of these schools closed in the late nineteenth and early twentieth centuries. The result was a sharp decline in female medical students even before Flexner issued his report. Coeducation remained an option, and one that many women themselves wanted, but regulars did not make it easy.[13] Oliver Wendell Holmes acknowledged that women brought something unique to healing, but he stopped short of endorsing women's professional participation in his field. "I have often wished that disease could be hunted by its professional antagonists in couples—a doctor and a doctor's quick witted wife," wrote Holmes. "For I am quite sure there is a natural clairvoyance in a woman which would make her ... much the superior of a man in some particulars of diagnosis." Holmes was sure that "many a suicide would have been prevented if the doctor's wife had visited the day before it happened. She would have seen in the merchant's face his impending bankruptcy while her stupid husband was prescribing for his dyspepsia and endorsing his note."[14]

Regular medical schools routinely failed to provide opportunities to women and habitually limited the number of women they would even accept at a token 5 percent until the mid-twentieth century.[15] School administrators justified excluding qualified women by claiming that most would give up their medical practices after marriages, so they were not worth the investment. Even those men who seemed to support women's participation in the field betrayed certain biases about women. John Dodson, dean of Rush Medical College in Chicago, praised his school's female students as "a credit to themselves and to us" but concluded that "no matter how superior these students may have been in their college work," they "cannot but do otherwise than rejoice when matrimony claims them." A medical education also cost more as schools passed the expense of new equipment and faculty, expanded facilities, and lengthened training time on to students. Many women who had once financed their medical education by working could no longer afford to do so.[16] At the same time, the propriety of men and women studying the human body together in the same room remained a potent and divisive issue.[17]

It seems not far-fetched to say that women's involvement in irregular health systems from the very beginning provided all the evidence some regular doctors needed to dismiss it. In 1893, Harvard professor Edward H. Clarke warned that excessive intellectual activity diverted a woman's limited supply of energy from reproduction to the brain, which threatened not only her health but also that of her family and society. It was true that women could pursue the same educational course as men, Clarke declared, but "it is not true that she can do all this, and retain uninjured health and a future secure from neuralgia, uterine disease, hysteria, and other derangements of the nervous system." Worse, women engaging in men's work "unsexed" themselves by taking on male roles, and thus supposedly male traits, rendering them unable to have the children that would sustain civilization.[18] Medical texts touting the terror of women's equality and autonomy flourished. Many used scientific and medical language to rationalize women's exclusion from active public and professional roles. Dr. Alfred Stille, in his presidential address to the American Medical Association in 1871, declared, "Certain women seek to rival men in manly sports, and the strong-minded ape them in all things, even in dress. In doing so, they may command a sort of admiration such as all monstrous productions inspire, especially when they tend towards a higher type than their own."[19] The reverse was also true, though: those men who performed the same tasks as women lost their masculinity. Dr. Stille warned that "a man with feminine traits of character or with the frame and carriage of a female is despised by both the sex he ostensibly belongs to and that of which it is at once a caricature and a libel."[20] Working with women or spending too much time in the feminizing clutches of mothers, teachers, and wives sapped a man's masculinity. These societal assumptions could not help but influence perceptions about irregular health systems, particularly those like hydropathy and homeopathy where women took active leadership roles. With women in charge, irregular health was marked as both dangerous and ridiculous.[21]

Even with these barriers, women did not stop practicing medicine. Osteopaths, chiropractors, and Christian Scientists welcomed women into their professional fold. Other women, particularly homeopaths, organized locally and focused on lay practice through the first half of the twentieth century. Still more entered regular medicine in nursing and social work, careers that closely aligned with cultural assumptions about women's more caring nature, and as such were structurally subordinated to the mostly male doctors.[22]

The AMA's gains and control of public health along with the quickening pace of medical advances in the first decades of the twentieth century significantly challenged the strength of irregular medicine. The introduction of the first antimicrobial drugs, known as sulfonamides, in the 1930s presented a significant breakthrough in the fight against infectious disease and paved the way for the antibiotic revolution in medicine. The mass production of penicillin in the 1940s nearly eliminated diseases that had plagued humans for centuries, including syphilis, meningitis, and rheumatic fever. Streptomycin in 1945 dramatically reduced cases of tuberculosis and plague. Even better, these drugs were some of the first nonhomeopathic remedies to cause few side effects. Americans clamored for these "wonder drugs," and doctors dispensed them with what historian James Whorton has called "antibiotic abandon."[23]

The 1950s and 1960s saw the introduction of even more antibiotics, vaccines for polio and measles, the CAT scan, heart and kidney transplants, and coronary bypass surgery. In 1953, James Watson and Francis Crick announced their findings on the structure of DNA.[24] Controlled clinical trials became the gold standard for assessing the safety and efficacy of new therapies. As deaths from infectious disease dropped, regular medicine rose in public status, trust, and esteem.

Medicine also grew more bureaucratic, structured, and regulated throughout the twentieth century. That trend was already apparent to Mark Twain in 1900. "The doctor's insane system has not only been permitted to continue its follies for ages, but has been protected by the State and made a close monopoly," he wrote, calling it "an infamous thing, a crime against a free-man's proper right to choose his own assassin or his own method of defending his body against disease and death."[25] Twain had long supported free choice in medicine, even as he sometimes ridiculed the options, but that freedom became increasingly constrained as the century wore on. More medical care happened in hospitals, where regular doctors controlled access and tended to exclude irregulars from practicing in their wards. Specialty boards licensed and certified practitioners, and the federal government took a more active role in subsidizing medical research and approving drugs and therapies for public use. For regular doctors, these institutional and political structures eliminated many of the economic and political uncertainties that had plagued the profession in the nineteenth century. Competition with irregulars no longer provoked the same anxiety and financial peril, even if it seemingly did little to blunt professional handwringing over irregular practice.[26]

These structures of bureaucratic control, according to historian Charles E. Rosenberg, tightened the boundaries between regular and irregular doctors. Regular doctors tended to view the growing inflexibility of medicine as an affirmation of their system's scientific validity and stature. To regulars, the fight over public perception and for medical authority appeared finally won.[27]

Yet despite all of these advances in medical science, it was also becoming apparent that many of the wonder drugs were less than wonderful. Patients eager for the latest miracle drug they had learned about in newspapers and on television came asking for remedies and treatments by name. Under pressure both to cure disease and to satisfy their patients, some doctors overprescribed. Many people became addicted to the amphetamines and tranquilizers they took for anxiety, depression, insomnia, and other chronic ailments—a problem that persists to this day. The dangers became even more apparent during the thalidomide tragedy of the 1960s. The drug, marketed as a sedative, one of the most popular and widely used classes of drugs in the United States, was found to produce serious birth defects.[28] Suddenly, the drugs that had seemed so promising now seemed to many Americans to be more dangerous than good.

More than just the physical threat of these drugs, some also decried the breakdown of the doctor-patient relationship. Few could dispute that scientific and technical advances in medicine had improved the health of the nation and decreased the dangers of infectious diseases, but at what cost to personal health and individualized attention? Doctors gave drugs for everything, critics claimed, without listening to the particular ailments of their patients. The exam and patient history that had long defined the medical experience now took a backseat to the medicine bottle, surgical procedures, and test results. Regulars worked under growing structural and financial constraints that eroded the amount of time they could spend with patients, leading to a strained discussion of the specific problem rather than a longer conversation that took account of the context of the problem. As a result, some patients complained that their doctors paid them little attention and were unwilling to communicate with them about their health in a clear and understandable way.[29]

Regular medicine's increasing fragmentation into specialties also made medical care more expensive, even out of reach for many Americans. Doctors, who had already been concentrated in urban areas, accelerated their movement to city and university hospitals, leaving medical shortages in rural areas. That these specialists also made more money only encouraged this trend. Unlike before, though, the nation's hills and back roads no longer crawled with the herb doctors, midwives, itinerant folk healers, and bonesetters who had provided care where no other existed. Critics derided the medical profession as self-serving, elitist, and insensitive to the needs of patients for these holes in the system: a condemnation as familiar in 1960 as 1860.

Growing American disillusionment with regular medical practice and the high cost of care in the 1960s and 1970s led some to explore irregular medicine. Just as in the nineteenth century, broader cultural forces were at work. The Cold War, Vietnam, and atomic energy, among other social and political forces, made life feel uncertain and beyond individual control. In response, a counterculture emerged that rebelled against the authority of the government, science, and experts. Its members, mostly white and middle class like many of the nineteenth-century reformers, focused intently on tolerance, natural living, and individual rights. They embraced a simpler, more spiritual orientation to life that integrated the mind and body into well-being. These cultural trends burnished the appeal of irregular medicine. Americans rediscovered homeopathy and botanical remedies as well as a host of other therapies like naturopathy and the hydropathic Kneipp Cure. Health foods, exercise routines, and vitamins became topics of broad popular interest. To a new generation, irregular health-care approaches represented freedom, self-reliance, personal empowerment, and affordable care, the familiar chords that had stoked American health reform in the nineteenth century.[30]

Of course, most of these new alternatives were not new at all. Nor had Americans ever stopped self-dosing and using irregular medicine. It was certainly true that many popular nineteenth-century health systems were not as strong or as visible in the mid-twentieth century as they had once been. Many Americans did not even realize the significant historic challenge irregulars like homeopaths had once posed to regular medicine when they began to emerge again in the 1960s and 1970s. But these healers had never disappeared. The number of homeopaths, phrenologists, mesmerists, and botanic healers sharply declined in the early twentieth century, but osteopaths, chiropractors, and many other kinds of healers made up for the retreat of older systems.[31] In the 1920s, the Illinois Medical Society found that among six thousand Chicago residents, 87 percent reported using what regular medicine had taken to calling "cult medicine." A similar national survey carried out by the federal government between 1929 and 1931 found that irregular practitioners comprised 10 percent of all health-care visits.[32] And in 1965, homeopath Wyeth Post Baker released confidential reports from the Senate Finance Committee revealing that an estimated twelve million people used homeopathic remedies without the advice or consent of their doctors.[33] The tenacity of irregular health care's appeal to the general public alarmed regulars: many had assumed irregular medicine's demise decades earlier and had consigned its remaining users to a small fringe on the margins of society. These surveys told a different story. While it was mostly true that regular medicine had seized political and institutional authority in the twentieth century, at the level of daily practice and individual therapeutic choice, the ground remained highly contested.

The renewed interest in and popularity of irregular medicine in the 1960s led to the adoption of the words "complementary" and "alternative" to describe the systems that regulars had labeled "irregular," "unorthodox," "cultish," and "quackery" for more than a century. These terms better reflected how many Americans saw and used irregular therapies for centuries—as an accompaniment or substitute for regular medicine.[34] Calling something "regular" or "irregular" implied a common understanding of what constituted legitimate medical practice that many Americans (and many of their doctors) may not have shared even as they used these names to describe their healers. It's doubtful that nineteenth-century Americans saw their healers as "irregular" or as "quacks" in the negative way that we have come to understand the words. Based on how many people used irregular treatments and with what frequency they sought an irregular's help, irregular health was a regular part of daily life.

Irregular medicine also became known as "holistic" in the 1980s. Broadly speaking, holistic meant anything alternative and "natural" that took into account patients' mental status and their social and physical situation. Unique as the concept seemed, though, holistic principles could be found in medical practices as ancient as Ayurveda in India and Qigong in China as well as in hydropathy, mesmerism, Thomsonism, homeopathy, osteopathy, and even the humoral theory that underlay regular medicine. Until the mid-nineteenth century, prevailing therapeutics and understandings of disease assumed multiple causes. Environmental, emotional, moral, and social factors all determined sickness and its cure. Advances in physiology, chemistry, bacteriology, and pharmacology as well as medical technology in the late nineteenth century began to change regular medicine's perceptions of disease and what counted as medicine. The diagnostic precision and objectivity of scientific medicine promised one path to the truth, not multiple paths. Disease became less amorphous, recast as a specific thing with characteristic patterns and mechanisms best understood through laboratory analysis rather than social and environmental factors. Holistic treatments designed to treat the whole person rather than to attack any specific disease largely fell by the wayside in regular medicine while irregulars tried, with varying success, to incorporate the science without sacrificing their holistic approach.[35]

But in the 1970s, perhaps influenced by the resurgence of irregular health, some regular doctors began to show interest in holistic medicine. In 1979 a group of regulars organized the American Holistic Medical Association and announced themselves "dedicated to the concept of medicine of the whole person," which may "demand combination of both orthodox and non-damaging unorthodox approaches."[36] That some regulars accepted the idea of holistic medicine was not news by the late 1970s, nor had it been in the past, as many regulars had never taken the hard line against irregulars or their therapies that the AMA demanded. But the establishment of a professional organization of regulars dedicated to the integration of body, mind, and spirit certainly was. Even more arresting, these regular doctors envisioned a possible collaborative future for irregular and regular health. The organization's *Journal of Holistic Medicine* soon included a list of acceptable topics for publication in its pages, a list that included homeopathy. Rarely, if ever, had regulars discussed homeopathy as anything other than a fraud. Now it could be featured and studied in a regular medical journal? Not every regular was sold on the idea of holistic medicine, though, and many of its advocates met with the skepticism and sometimes harsh rebuke of colleagues.[37]

Public enthusiasm for holistic and alternative remedies only continued to intensify, though. Drugstores and health food stores began to carry nonprescription homeopathic remedies as well as other botanical remedies and mesmeric-like medical magnets in the 1980s. By the late 1990s, consumers could actually purchase homeopathic kits just as they had been able to in the past, and sales of homeopathic remedies grew 20 percent annually. Alongside these well-established remedies, though, came an explosion of products labeled "holistic" and "natural" that sought to cash in on the potential marketing bonanza, just as medical entrepreneurs had in the past. Dr. Arnold Rellman, editor of the *New England Journal of Medicine*, complained that the valuable message of the holistic movement was "ill served by those who seek quick solutions to the ills of mankind through the abandonment of science and rationality in favor of mystical cults."[38]

Then in the 1980s, concerns about the nation's rising health-care costs led to an even more remarkable endorsement of alternative medicine—one nearly unthinkable only a few decades earlier. In 1991, the US Senate Appropriations Committee instructed the National Institutes of Health to develop a research program in alternative medicine. Championed by Senators Tom Harkin of Iowa and Orrin Hatch of Utah, the Office of Alternative Medicine (now known as the National Center for Complementary and Alternative Medicine) was hailed by some as a victory for irregular medicine while others denounced it as tax dollars wasted on snake oil.[39]

Skepticism about government funding for alternative medicine has not stopped major academic medical centers from establishing integrative clinics combining irregular and regular health—Harvard, Yale, Duke, and the Mayo Clinic are among more than forty across the United States. Irregular medicine is more accepted in Europe, where a relatively large number of regular doctors either recognize or practice some form of irregular therapeutics. The emergence of these centers in the United States seems to indicate the willingness of regular medicine to consider or at least tolerate the merits of their competitors, an almost unimaginable idea less than a century ago. While a cynic could attribute integrative clinics to a heedless grab for precious research dollars, it's not hard to find true believers on the ground. Even outside integrative medicine clinics, many doctors now recommend meditation, discuss exercise habits, and emphasize good nutrition to patients. Among the nation's most widely read and popular doctors today are Deepak Chopra and Andrew Weil, regular doctors who champion integrative health. The Harvard-educated Weil emphasizes diet, botanicals, and mind-body techniques in his practice. Chopra uses the Indian Ayurvedic system and focuses on the spiritual nearly as much as the physical in his teaching. Millions of Americans read their books, watch them on television, visit their websites, and pay close attention to what they teach. Their followers are not ignorant or uneducated, the reflexive explanation some regulars have put forth to explain the popularity of irregular medicine. Several studies have shown that those Americans with more education, including 50 percent of those with graduate degrees, and a higher economic status are more likely to use alternative medicine than those less educated and less affluent. They share much the same demographic profile as the well-educated, middle- and upper-class white Americans who found irregular medicine so attractive in the nineteenth century. Many of these Americans turned to irregular medicine for help and found it effective. That personal experience goes a long way toward explaining the long history and popularity of irregular medicine in the United States, even if popular lore and historical thinking tends to tell a different story.[40]

Irregular medicine often gets blamed for the problems that were, in many ways, the problems of the larger nineteenth-century American culture in which they arose, practiced, and prospered. It's far easier to make fun or to hold up irregular health systems as a bizarre specimen of the past than to try to understand what they meant and the very real problems they sought to address and continue to address to this day.

Irregular health resonated with concerns about the moral implications of the inventions and technologies revolutionizing American society in the nineteenth century. The democratic spirit of the century coupled with the emerging capitalist marketplace fostered a climate conducive to the proliferation of reform movements seeking to change all aspects of life. Social movements tend to arise during times of unrest and change, as people become more open to new ideas because of problems they perceive with the status quo. Irregular healers tapped into cultural yearnings for simplicity and a way of life that emphasized hard work, self-improvement, and common sense. They advocated for direct competition and empowered patients to become arbiters of a healer's merit and efficacy.[41]

During their heyday, irregular healers amassed an impressive record of testimonial success and drew millions of followers. They had a pervasive influence on American cultural trends in areas ranging from egalitarianism and women's rights to philosophy, religion, literature, linguistics, and science. Stories about phrenological readings, homeopathic remedies, and trips to the water cure filled newspapers and magazines. Irregular therapies became part of storylines in novels and their jargon was used in everyday conversation. The very existence of irregular health, even if most regulars saw it as a profound negative, fostered an atmosphere ripe for contemplating new research and theories both within and outside medicine.

Regular medicine in the nineteenth century demonstrated an unwillingness to innovate and take risks. Irregulars, on the other hand, wanted something better and proposed new solutions to old medical problems. Irregulars suggested novel and creative theories about what caused disease and constituted healthy living at a time when medical advancement appeared stalled.

In hindsight, many questions can be raised about the legitimacy of the cures or experiences associated with some nineteenth-century irregular healers just as they can with regular medicine. Why would anyone believe that cold pure water—and nothing else—could cure everything as the hydropaths believed? Or for that matter that bleeding could relieve a fever?

Facing an explanatory void and without the tools needed to understand disease and human physiology, people developed theories and stories to make sense of the world. It's a perfectly human response. We want health to be predictable and our symptoms contained within reassuring frameworks that offer both meaning and action steps to resolution. Regular and irregular doctors alike conjured animal magnetism, spiritual essences, miasmas, and humors to make sense of a world barraged with illnesses that disabled, maimed, and killed. Just like today, Americans sought answers to their problems and the powerful medicine that comes from the comfort and reassurance of a promised cure.

Irregular medicine's gains and criticisms transformed regular medical practice. Most of heroic medicine's most violent measures gave way to new drug therapies after the Civil War. These therapies were in many ways, though, just as vigorous as those they replaced, at least until the advent of antibiotics in the twentieth century. It was not scientific advances that caused this change so much as the continual criticism and pressure doctors faced from irregulars and the general public. Not that they admitted as much. A few claimed that industrialization had changed the body's composition and that cures thus required new therapies. Others trusted more in nature while a still larger group abandoned their old ways without clear explanation.[42]

Irregular ideas did find their way into regular medicine. Regular doctors investigating the irregular theories they found so ridiculous and sought to prove wrong sometimes ended up discovering something new and useful in the process. Other aspects of irregular medicine were simply absorbed into the practices of regular medicine. Both tactics profoundly influenced the shape of modern medicine. Phrenology's suggestion that the brain consisted of a mosaic of functional organs pushed scientists to examine the organization of the brain and its relationship to the mind. Mesmerism's revolutionary discovery of the unconscious opened a new realm for human exploration and encouraged the scientific study of hypnosis. Both mesmerism and phrenology laid the foundation for modern psychology and psychiatry. Hydropathy's advocacy of good hygiene—exercise, diet, water, sanitation—provided the foundation for public health campaigns to improve urban living conditions as well as the core principles of health and nutritional campaigns to this day. Homeopathy challenged the idea that healing had to hurt and helped condition patients to expect medicines with few side effects; few Americans today would likely accept the vomiting, headaches, and crushing pain of standard nineteenth-century care. In all these cases, an irregular idea was refined, molded, and reshaped into something beneficial to regular medicine and integral to modern ideas of health and wellness.

No one pushed for preventative care and health hygiene as much as irregulars. Many sought to eliminate disease before it could even take hold rather than respond to disease, as was common in regular medicine. Irregulars viewed health as a goal to strive for and one that was attainable through certain actions and activities. Attention to diet, exercise, and other lifestyle concerns is now a standard part of a visit to a primary care physician, in part because many of the most costly and common chronic diseases today, including diabetes and heart disease, are at least somewhat preventable with lifestyle and behavior modifications.[43] Irregulars recognized this and incorporated it into their systems with far more attention and emphasis than regular medicine. It certainly helped that Americans liked having a system to follow that seemed to promise rich reward; the urge continues to drive the diet, health, and self-help industry today. In the nineteenth century, irregulars seized on this impulse more voraciously than regulars, crafting a health regimen that gave individuals control and self-determination in the face of broader uncertainty.

Despite protests to the contrary from both sides, regular and irregular medicine had much in common. Both employed distinctive treatments based on the subjective selection of symptoms. Both tended to be dogmatic in their assertions and to have bombastic leaders and spokespeople. Both had journals, medical schools, and professional societies. And both appropriated the authority of science before any therapy could be reasonably judged scientific, as the term is used today. Nearly everyone could agree that science was fundamental to medical practice, but before the twentieth century, science had many meanings and included a wide range of disciplines, such as philosophy, unlikely to be called scientific today. To do science generally meant to make observations and classify them in such a way as to discern natural laws. Regulars and irregulars acquired this knowledge by examining and treating thousands of patients. The multiplicity of meanings attached to science made it easier for people to claim scientific status and to benefit from its social and cultural authority.[44] Only in the 1890s did the laboratory techniques and clinical measurement associated with science today begin to make inroads into regular medical practice in the United States and to shape and limit the modern meaning of the word.[45]

Both regular and irregular medicine also recognized the importance of organization and leadership to success. Charismatic leaders like Samuel Thomson and Daniel David Palmer could grow movements and keep them together for a time, but many irregular systems were done in by internal struggles between those with different visions and strategies for the future. The democratic nature of the irregular health movements encouraged the multiple interpretations that come from broad participation but also brought with it all the difficulties of forging consensus and understanding. The uncompromising personalities of many irregular health leaders only made this more challenging. Despite their own internal differences, regular healers managed to create and sustain a unified front by the late nineteenth century, largely behind the increasing power of the American Medical Association, that allowed them to benefit from irregular medicine's disarray.

Regular doctors proved in many ways to be better chameleons than irregulars. They incorporated scientific advances as well as the most popular theories and therapies of their rivals and modified their treatments in response to criticism, all without relinquishing their fundamental beliefs. Take the germ theory, a discovery that both regulars and irregulars struggled to interpret through their philosophical frameworks. Until late in the nineteenth century, regulars tended to be skeptical of the germ theory's validity. Many ignored it and continued to credit disease to miasmas, atmospheric factors, and spontaneously generated pathogens. After much debate and accumulating evidence, regulars finally came to terms with germs by asserting that they had always believed disease came from outside the body even if they had previously not known the specifics of the actual entity that caused it. Accepting germs gave regulars a new basis for prescribing drugs and a powerful response to their antidrug opponents. Science now seemed to prove that drugs were, in fact, an effective means of destroying disease-causing germs, even though regulars still had no more idea which drugs worked against specific germs than they had before: those discoveries had not yet come.[46]

Even so, irregular medicine did not disappear. Its story is not of a comeback but of persistence. Part of that persistence must certainly come down to the story itself. Irregular healers told accessible and believable stories to win followers in the nineteenth century. People went to these healers because what they said made sense. Every symptom had a cause and a cure. Humans impose narratives on life because uncertainty is hard to accept. Irregular medicine today has in many ways a better story than regular medicine does. The very complexity of the body and scientific medicine doesn't make for the same neat linear narrative of cause and effect that humoral medicine once provided. There are many things that regular doctors just don't know or can't explain. Irregular medicine, on the other hand, tends to still tell a coherent story and offer a remedy and health program that is believable and easy to understand. This may in fact go a long way toward explaining irregular medicine's popularity and efficacy. Understanding the cause of your disease and your path to improvement goes a long way to healing. Belief is powerful medicine.

Our same desire for a story to make sense of the world may also explain the popular myth that obscures the history of irregular medicine. Regular medicine's rise to dominance by vanquishing irregular quacks with science makes for a simple and engaging narrative but also one that is deeply flawed. All of the evidence to the contrary is around us, in the countless ads for acupuncturists, storefront homeopaths, and in integrative medical clinics. If regular medicine won, why are there are still so many irregular healers?

That many types of irregular medicine have survived and even expanded in recent years can obviously not be explained by the usual story of deviance and public danger. Regular medicine's authority over healing remains far from complete. More than a third of Americans with chronic back pain, for instance, seek chiropractic rather than regular medical treatment, while between a quarter and half of all people suffering terminal illnesses seek alternative care at some point. Domestic medicine and home health manuals did not disappear with the rise of scientific medicine. Self-help, diet, and exercise books line store shelves and top best-seller lists. Even greater numbers of Americans turn to a proliferation of web-based medical advice and educational sites. Most people continue to treat and prevent illnesses themselves, without the help of doctors.[47]

American attitudes toward medicine have long been somewhat ambivalent. People tend to trust individuals—their doctor, whether regular or irregular—and scientific medicine to a degree, but they remain skeptical of the profession as a whole. More than a third of Americans report using alternative medicine regularly despite scientific studies that show again and again that most alternative therapies help patients no more than placebos.[48] But as medical historian James Whorton has said of homeopathy, "Whether or not homeopathy works, it fulfills a need in a lot of people."[49] The same could be said of nearly all healing systems.

Regular and irregular medicine today have reached a partial truce. Many regulars have abandoned their hostile attitude and seem more open to a variety of approaches to health and wellness. Irregulars, too, have mellowed, showing more interest in integrating rather than pursuing the overthrow of the regular system that had motivated them for most of the last two centuries. Perhaps both are listening more to their patients and following their lead. Most followers of irregular medicine today, as they did in the past, use a combination of regular and irregular therapies, forging their own individual integrative practices.

Irregular medicine has demonstrated considerable strength in some areas where regular medicine continues to falter. The twentieth-century scientific medical model trained doctors for quick and decisive action but left them less prepared for the long-term management and personal attention people often require. The constraints and pressures on a regular doctor's schedule can make patients feel that their doctor has no time for them or that they may be wasting their doctor's time if they talk too much. Irregulars, in comparison, tend to be more numerous and easier to access, and they often encourage long appointments. Most also work in more pleasant office spaces that help to put their patients at ease and lead to more positive medical encounters. Few people are likely to cite their doctor's office or local hospital as an inspiring, well-designed, comfortable place.

Scientific medicine tends to work best on easily pinpointed diseases and less well on illnesses lacking obvious physical causes, particularly those of psychological origin. Many people go to irregular healers for anxiety, chronic pain, and back problems, issues for which regular medicine currently has few easy answers.[50] Other patients, after an examination by a regular doctor, are told that nothing can be found wrong with them, but they continue to feel sick. These conditions are some of the most frustrating to deal with for both patients and their doctors. No patient wants to hear that his doctor does not know everything and no doctor wants to tell her patient that there's not much that can be done. Yet that's often what happens. Not surprisingly, patients are unhappy with this answer. They are suffering and want relief, so they are willing to try other therapies and other healers. Irregulars are often more willing to diagnose and treat symptoms and provide a more satisfactory explanation to the patient to address concerns and complaints.[51]

The placebo effect may play some role. The effects of placebo have been recognized for centuries. One of the first to describe its power was sixteenth-century philosopher Michel de Montaigne, who wrote, "[T]here are men on whom the mere sight of medicine is operative."[52] Oliver Wendell Holmes declared that patents receive the best medical benefit "through the influence exerted on their imaginations."[53] Nearly everyone, regular and irregular alike, understands that the placebo effect is real even if no one understands how it works. Studies have confirmed the efficacy of placebos in nearly every area of medicine, from pain alleviation and depression to inflammatory disorders and cancer. The effects can come from belief or expectations as well as subconscious associations between recovery and the treatment experience: a white coat, a doctor's office, and a handful of pills can convey tremendous healing power.[54]

Placebo has a bad reputation, though. When a treatment or drug is said to be "no better than placebo," the underlying message is that the benefits are all in your mind and not worth pursuing. And those patients that respond to it are often assumed, like followers of irregular medicine more generally, to be gullible and weak. But the placebo effect is far more than patients merely thinking they are better. It triggers something in the patient's brain that causes real physiological change and is influenced by multiple factors.[55] The sights, smells, touch, and sounds all tell a patient that a therapy is being performed. When a patient expects a treatment and then expects to feel better afterward, neurotransmitters are released that can help him or her feel better. Scientists are still not sure how that works. Perhaps placebo is one form of the ancient idea of the healing power of nature, *vis medicatrix naturae*.[56] Its effects are fickle, though, operating in different ways with large individual and cultural variations.[57] Nonetheless, placebo appears to have real therapeutic value.

But even so, many doctors, pledged to the health and well-being of the patient, are leery of using it because it may require some deception. Can it ever be right to prescribe placebo without telling the patient?

Many opponents of irregular medicine also argue that its reported benefits are nothing but placebo. If so, and that question remains open to debate, irregular therapies may excel at activating and deploying the placebo effect, even if that's not what the healer intended or believes about the treatment himself. Many aspects of irregular medicine correlate to effects associated with inducing placebo. A doctor who takes the time to listen, asks questions, and pays attention provides the good bedside manner that is often lacking for a variety of reasons in the modern medical system but has been shown to improve patient outcomes. Like regulars, irregulars also believe strongly in their treatments and administer them with confidence and reassurance. That alone can perhaps be enough to do a patient good.[58] It may even be possible that treatment by persuasive irregular healers may realize the full potential of the placebo effect in ways not possible in regular medical settings, making them an effective option for conditions that appear to respond best to placebo.

Placebo is alive and well in regular medicine, too. In 2002, patients suffering osteoarthritis who underwent a sham arthroscopic surgery reported just as much relief and improved mobility as those who had actually had their bony spurs and degenerated cartilage removed.[59] Pharmaceutical companies have struggled to develop new drugs that best placebo. Half of all new drugs developed today fail in late-stage clinical trials, unable to beat sugar pills.[60]

The placebo response itself, however, does not distinguish between regular and irregular medicine as its practitioners do. It may be triggered by a benign drug, a compassionate caregiver, a sugar pill, or a magnet. All that is required is that the patient have a realistic expectation of getting better.

Irregular health is not the province of hippies and hipsters either. Its politics are far more complex. Look only to the two senators who endorsed the study of alternative medicine at the National Institutes of Health: a Democrat from Iowa and a Republican from Utah. Sociologist Michael Goldstein believes that alternative medicine transcends the expected political divisions by drawing on ideologies from both ends of the spectrum. From the left, alternative medicine "opposes the dominance of professionals as well as excess profit-making in medicine," writes Goldstein, while also encompassing "a strong countercultural component whose roots are on the left. Yet, the strong focus on enhanced individual responsibility for health, along with an emphasis on nongovernmental solutions to health problems, often gives alternative medicine a distinctly rightward cast."[61] In other words, followers of alternative health systems don't fall neatly into categories, political or otherwise.

Alternative health care has long offered followers multiple strands of meaning by which individuals can understand themselves and their world. Every discipline, from history and political science to sociology, biology, and psychology, has its own preferred method of explaining human behavior and belief, and each of these theories may be right or offer some hope for at least some segment of irregular health's believers. We tend to look to individuals, not systems, for help and to put our trust in those who have demonstrated their facility in healing no matter the method. That's how irregulars gained power and adherents and a primary reason they have survived for centuries. People seek, and often find, in alternative medicine a more personalized, holistic, and less aggressive approach to healing that appreciates the relationships between mind, body, and spirit.

The truth is that Americans have used and sought out many forms of medical care for centuries. We don't want one rigid system with only one model of care. In medicine, as in everything else, choice is what we want and what we've always wanted, so the sense of novelty and "newness" attached to alternative health is far greater than deserved given its long history. But choice from the perspective of regular medicine is often seen as illegitimate, ignorant, and misguided, even though a true accounting of our nation's medical history shows that the dominance of one form of care is the historical anomaly.

Attacks on alternative medicine tend to focus exclusively on whether alternative medicine works according to the criteria of efficacy of modern scientific medicine. And while it's an important question, as regular doctors have significant safety concerns about many irregular therapies, it isn't the only question. Perhaps serious consideration should also be given to why these alternatives persist and what that says about medicine and what it can and cannot do. Medicine has made great strides in the last century, vastly improving public health and increasing life expectancy. But holes remain. When people have so little faith in scientific evidence that they go with their gut, then something is wrong. Irregular healers have demonstrated significant abilities to help people feel better whatever the mechanism—and it may be nothing more than a highly potent placebo. Reports and anecdotes of irregular success offer a tremendous database that may be low on scientific precision but is rich with ideas and possibilities to improve all aspects of medical care. As medical historian Owsei Temkin has noted, "Medicine is healing based on such knowledge as is deemed requisite. The fact that medicine in our days is largely based on science does not make other forms less medical."[62] The scientific case for the efficacy of irregular health may perhaps lie in the millions of people over hundreds of years who have found some measure of relief and comfort in its care.

There will likely always be boundaries between different types of healers, but those lines will shift and transform with new technology, new scientific discoveries, and cultural trends. Medicine, even in its modern form, is not a rigid structure but a culture in continual redefinition and negotiation. Even so, the chaos and contentiousness, not to mention unbridled enthusiasm and hopeful thinking, that characterized nineteenth-century medicine seems unlikely to surface again. But medicine will continue to change and evolve with human needs both existing and emerging. Simply disregarding irregular health and its believers rather than trying to understand them does nothing to advance what we all are seeking: a way to feel better.

Even in the nineteenth century, when cooperation between regular and irregular medicine seemed all but impossible, some doctors expressed hope for the future. In the 1850s, homeopath Walter Johnson implored his fellow healers to come together. "I think it sheer bigotry for any party to lay claim to exclusive possession of the truth," he wrote.

> Let us then join hands, and instead of degrading ourselves by contemptible bickering, devote our whole energies to the relief of suffering humanity, and earnestly hope for the dawn of that day, when the ephemeral systems which we now practice, shall be absorbed by a new revelation, and cease from affording a pretence [sic] for sectarian dissension.[63]

He was not alone. A regular by the name of Dr. Forbes proclaimed himself in 1846 "ready to grasp any proffered good in the way of healing, whoever may be the offerers, and wheresoever they may have found it."[64]

ACKNOWLEDGMENTS

Understanding the history of an idea is hard. But harder still might be tracing the path back to the beginning of your own ideas, particularly those that somehow move from a question to an entire book comprising several years of your life. For this, I thank Matt Jensen for introducing me to his field of medicine and for pushing me to take a look around with a questioning historical eye. Much to my surprise, I discovered that the history of medicine brought together some of my long-standing interests in women's history, utopian thinking, and oddball characters. Our conversations on medicine and nineteenth-century history formed the core of this book, as Matt questioned and challenged my assumptions, and offered me new insights and ideas that I never would have come to alone. Having the critical eye of an in-house doctor also proved invaluable as he disputed my claims and characterizations of regular medicine. For this, I thank him, and I apologize, since I'm sure my thankfulness frequently appeared as annoyance in the moment.

Thanks also to Christopher Hoolihan at the Edward G. Miner Library at the University of Rochester Medical Center and to the staff at Ebling Library at the University of Wisconsin-Madison for help in locating items new, old, and rare. Thanks as well to the librarians and archivists of the Wisconsin Historical Society and Memorial Library at the University of Wisconsin-Madison.

Thanks to my agent, Janet Rosin, for her excitement about this project when it was only half formed, and to the critical eyes of my editors, Helene Atwan and Crystal Paul, at Beacon Press.

Thanks as well to those friends who expressed (polite) interest and found themselves unexpectedly in a conversation about irregular medicine, particularly Anne Strainchamps, Mary Ellen Gabriel, Michael Edmonds, Nicole Miller, and Laura Kearney. Your comments and questions made me think and laugh, which added immeasurably to this book and the writing process.

INTRODUCTION

1. William D. McArdle, Frank I. Katch, and Victor L. Katch, *Essentials of Exercise Physiology*, 3rd ed. (Baltimore: Lippincott, Williams & Wilkins, 2005), 15–16.

2. Kimberly Harper, "Historic Missourians: John S. Sappington," State Historical Society of Missouri, http://shs.umsystem.edu/historicmissourians/name/s/sappington/index.html.

3. Charles Neider, ed., *The Autobiography of Mark Twain* (New York: Harper & Row, 1959), 64–65.

4. Ibid., 65–66.

5. Albert Bigelow Paine, *Mark Twain, a Biography: The Personal and Literary Life of Mark Twain* (New York: Harper & Brothers, 1912), 2:162.

6. Joshua Wolf Shenk, "Lincoln's Great Depression," *Atlantic* (October 2005), http://www.theatlantic.com/magazine/archive/2005/10/lincolns-great-depression/304247/.

7. Lora Romero, "Bio-Political Resistance in Domestic Ideology and *Uncle Tom's Cabin*," *American Literary History* 1, no. 4 (Winter 1989): 734.

8. Fernando Orrego and Carlos Quintana, "Darwin's Illness: A Final Diagnosis," *Notes and Records of the Royal Society* 22 (January 2007): 25; Maria H. Frawley, *Invalidism and Identity in Nineteenth-Century Britain* (Chicago: University of Chicago Press, 2004), 46.

9. Edgar W. Martin, *The Standard of Living in 1860: American Consumption Levels on the Eve of the Civil War* (Chicago: University of Chicago Press, 1942), 225–47.

10. Charles E. Rosenberg, "The Practice of Medicine in New York a Century Ago," in Leavitt and Numbers, *Sickness and Health in America*, 63.

11. Charles E. Rosenberg, "The Therapeutic Revolution: Medicine, Meaning, and Social Change in Nineteenth Century America," in Vogel and Rosenberg, *Therapeutic Revolution*, 8.

12. "Bloody Suckers: Leech Therapy," *Nature*, PBS http://www.pbs.org/wnet/nature/bloodysuckers/leech.html (accessed March 21, 2013).

13. Roy Porter, ed., *The Cambridge History of Medicine* (Cambridge, UK: Cambridge University Press, 2006), 56, 58, 109.

14. Duffy, *From Humors to Medical Science*, 15; Whorton, *Nature Cures*, 4–5.

15. Duffy, *From Humors to Medical Science*, 14–16.

16. Rush quoted in John Warner, *The Therapeutic Perspective: Medical Practice, Knowledge, and Identity in America, 1820–1885* (Cambridge, MA: Harvard University Press, 1986), 18; Whorton, *Nature Cures*, 6.

17. Wesley, *Primitive Physick*, 36, 84.

18. John R. Betts, "Mind and Body in Early American Thought," *Journal of American History* 54, no. 4 (March 1968): 791; Thurs, Science Talk, 30–31.

19. T. Gregory Garvey, *Creating the Culture of Reform in Antebellum America* (Athens: University of Georgia Press, 2006), 2, 33.

20. Ibid., 33; Haller, *Medical Protestants*, 31; Numbers, "Do-It-Yourself the Sectarian Way," 49.

21. Ralph Waldo Emerson, "Self-Reliance," *Essays: First Series* (Stilwell, KS: Digireads, 2007), 31.

22. Porter, *Greatest Benefit to Mankind*, 281; Starr, *Social Transformation of American Medicine*, 595; Eric H. Christianson, "Medicine in New England," in Leavitt and Numbers, *Sickness and Health in America*, 64; Whitfield J. Bell, "A Portrait of the Colonial Physician," in Leavitt and Numbers, *Sickness and Health in America*, 45–46.

23. Haller, *Medical Protestants*, 3; Cassedy, *Medicine in America*, 191; Reed, *Healing Cults*, 67–71.

24. Worthington Hooker, *The Treatment Due from the Profession to Physicians Who Become Homeopathic Practitioners* (Norwich, CT: John G. Cooley, 1852), 8.

25. Wrobel, "Introduction," in Wrobel, *Pseudoscience and Society*, 2–3.

26. "American versus European Medical Science Again," *Medical Record* 4 (May 15, 1869): 133.

27. Starr, *Social Transformation of American Medicine*, 65.

28. Charles Rosenberg, "The American Medical Profession: Mid-Nineteenth Century," *Mid-America* 44 (July 1962): 166, 168.

29. William Cobbett, "Comments," Republican Rush-Light 1 (1800), 49; "Doctors in Trouble," Eclectic Medical Journal 1 (1853), 132; Thomas Jefferson to Dr. Caspar Wistar Jr., June 21, 1807, in The Writings of Thomas Jefferson, vol. 10, Correspondence and Papers, 1803–1807, ed. Paul L. Ford (New York: G. P. Putnam and Sons, 1904–1905), 81–85.

30. Caroline de Costa and Francesca Miller, "American Resurrection and the 1788 New York Doctors' Riot," Lancet 33, no. 9762 (January 2011): 292–93.

31. Cohen, "Medical Social Movements," 32.

32. Duffy, From Humors to Medical Science, 12–17.

33. Matthew Baillie quoted in Porter, Greatest Benefit to Mankind, 266.

34. Starr, "Medicine, Economy and Society," 591.

35. "American vs. European Medical Science Again," 183; Ronald L. Numbers, "The Fall and Rise of the American Medical Profession," in Leavitt and Numbers, Sickness and Health in America, 225–26.

36. Thomson, New Guide to Health, 7.

37. Starr, "Medicine, Economy and Society," 591.

38. Caleb Ticknor, A Popular Treatise on Medical Philosophy; or, An Exposition of Quackery and Imposture in Medicine (New York: Gould and Newman, 1838), 17.

39. Oliver Wendell Holmes, Currents and Counter-Currents in Medical Science with Other Addresses and Essays (Boston, 1861), 27.

40. "Reviews," American Journal of the Medical Sciences 40 (Philadelphia: Blanchard and Lee, 1860): 469–70.

41. Hooker, Physician and Patient, 37.

42. Haller, American Medicine in Transition, 98–99; Whorton, Nature Cures, 6–7.

43. Thurs, Science Talk, 13–14, 20; Porter, Greatest Benefit to Mankind, 29, 40.

44. Morantz, "Women in the Medical Profession," 163–64.

45. Morantz-Sanchez, Sympathy and Science, 8–9; "Opposition to Women," Evening Bulletin (Philadelphia), November 8, 1869.

46. Morantz-Sanchez, Sympathy and Science, 168; Eve Fine, "Women Physicians and Medical Sects in Nineteenth-Century Chicago," in More, Fee, and Parry, Women Physicians, 256–57.

47. "African American Physicians and Organized Medicine, 1846–1968," American Medical Association, http://www.ama-assn.org/resources/doc/ethics/afamtimeline.pdf; "Dr. Rebecca Lee Crumpler," Changing the Face of Medicine, National Library of Medicine, http://www.nlm.nih.gov/changingthefaceofmedicine/physicians/biography_73.html; Haller, History of American Homeopathy, 56–57; Duffy, From Humors to Medical Science, 305–6.

48. Mary Gove Nichols, "Woman the Physician," *Water-Cure Journal* 11 (1851): 74–75.

CHAPTER ONE: EVERY MAN HIS OWN PHYSICIAN

1. Samuel Thomson, *The Constitution, Rules and Regulations to be Adopted and Practiced by the Members of the Friendly Botanic Society at Eastport, Pass.* [sic] *and Portsmouth, N.H. Together With the Preparation of Medicine and System* (Portsmouth, NH: 1812), 21–22.

2. E. E. Helm, "Untitled," *Botanico-Medical Recorder* 8 (January 18, 1845): 83.

3. Anonymous, "Ode to Lobelia," *Thomsonian Manual and Lady's Companion* 5 (June 15, 1839): 230.

4. Haller, *People's Doctor*, 33–34.

5. Flannery, "Early Botanical Medical Movement."

6. Haller, *Medical Protestants*, 9–10, 37.

7. Thomson, *New Guide to Health*, 16.

8. Ibid., 16.

9. Whorton, *Nature Cures*, 26; Haller, *Medical Protestants*, 38.

10. Rothstein, "Botanical Movements," in Gevitz, *Other Healers*, 30–32; Haller, *Medical Protestants*, 8–9; Susan M. Kingsbury, ed., *Records of the Virginia Company of London*, vol. 3 (Washington, DC: Government Printing Office, 1933), 237–38.

11. Haller, *People's Doctor*, 8.

12. Rothstein, "The Botanical Movements and Orthodox Medicine," 33; "Herbal Medicine," University of Maryland Medical Center, http://www.umm .edu/altmed/articles/herbal-medicine-000351.htm.

13. Rothstein, "Botanical Movements," 32–33.

14. Haller, *People's Doctor*, 10–11.

15. Numbers, "Do-It-Yourself the Sectarian Way," 49–51; Thomson, *New Guide to Health*, 38–43.

16. Haller, *Medical Protestants*, 38–39; John S. Haller Jr., "Samuel Thomson and the Poetry," in *Samuel Thomson and the Poetry of Botanic Medicine, 1810–1860*, Lloyd Library and Museum, http://www.lloydlibrary.org/Haller/haller-poetrychone.html (16 January 2012); "Dr. Samuel Thomson," *Boston Investigator*, November 15, 1843.

17. Thomson, *New Guide to Health*, 40.

18. John S. Haller Jr., "The American Hippocrates," Lloyd Library and Museum, www.lloydlibrary.org/Haller/hallerpoetrychone.html.

19. Rothstein, "Botanical Movements," 42–43; ibid.

20. Thomson, *New Guide to Health*, 42.

21. Ibid., 6.

22. Thomson, "Narrative of the Life," in ibid., 30–44.

23. J. U. and C. G. Lloyd, eds., *Bulletin of the Lloyd Library: Life and Medical Discoveries of Samuel Thomson and a History of the Thomsonian Materia Medica* 11 (Cincinnati: Lloyd Library, 1909), 32; Thomson, *New Guide to Health*, 56–58.

24. Haller, *People's Doctor*, 18–21.

25. "Cold," *Online Etymology Dictionary*, http://www.etymonline.com/index.php?term=cold.

26. Haller, *People's Doctor*, 20–21; Thomson, *A New Guide to Health*, 40–48.

27. Thomson, *A New Guide to Health*, 40–42, 48–52.

28. Haller, *People's Doctor*, 20–26; ibid., 62, 57.

29. Haller, *Medical Protestants*, 42–44; Thomson, *New Guide to Health*, 62–65.

30. Samuel Thomson, "Three Crafts," in Thomson, *Learned Quackery Exposed*, 12–15.

31. D. L. Terry, "The Botanic's Song of Liberty," *Botanico-Medical Recorder* XII (September 21, 1844): 364–65.

32. Flannery, "Early Botanical Medical Movement"; John S. Haller, "The Thomsonian System," Lloyd Library and Museum, http://www.lloydlibrary.org/Haller/hallerpoetrychtwo.html.

33. Samuel Thomson, "General Introduction," *The Thomsonian Materia Medica or Botanic Family Physician* (Albany: J. Munsell, 1841), 8; Alex Berman, "The Thomsonian Movement and its Relation to American Pharmacy and Medicine," *Bulletin of the History of Medicine* 25 (1951): 405, 406.

34. Whorton, *Nature Cures*, 30–31.

35. W. A. A., "Thomsonism," *Boston Medical and Surgical Journal* (January 16, 1839): 19, 24, American Periodicals, accessed September 5, 2012; Whorton, *Nature Cures*, 32.

36. Whorton, *Nature Cures*, 35–40.

37. Haller, *People's Doctor*, 16, 23.

38. Ibid., 33.

39. Samuel Thomson, "Calomel," in Thomson, *Learned Quackery Exposed*, 10.

40. Thomson, *Narrative of the Life*, 17.

41. Holmes, *Medical Essays*, 379.

42. J. Dickson Smith, *Rational Medicine and Thomsonism: An Essay* (Macon, GA: Telegraph Steam Printing House, 1859), 31–32.

43. Lebergott, "Wage Trends," 462.

44. Haller, *People's Doctor*, 33; Whorton, *Nature Cures*, 41–42.

45. Haller, *Medical Protestants*, 41.

46. Quoted in James Harvey Young, "American Medical Quackery in the Age of the Common Man," *Mississippi Valley Historical Review* 47, no. 4 (March 1961): 582–83.

47. Haller, *People's Doctor*, 146–47, 154–55.

48. "Thomsonian Dinner," *Hagerstown (MD) Mail*, May 24, 1839.

49. Whorton, *Nature Cures*, 38; Rothstein, "Botanical Movements and Orthodox Medicine," 46; Thomson, *New Guide to Health*, 134.

50. An Observer [Samuel Thomson], "Doggerel Verses; A Paraphrase on a Chapter in the History—Or, a Compend of the History of Mr. Aaron Dow," *Thomsonian Manual* 2 (September 15, 1837): 175.

51. Haller, *People's Doctor*, 37–38; Thomas Sewall, "On the Use of Arsenic in Cancerous Complaints," *New England Journal of Medicine and Surgery* 4 (April 1815): 111.

52. Haller, *People's Doctor*, 39.

53. Haller, *Medical Protestants*, 40.

54. "Public Notice," *Columbian Centinel and American Federalist* (Boston), August 6, 1825.

55. Rothstein, "Botanical Movements and Orthodox Medicine," 45.

56. Haller, *Medical Protestants*, 40.

57. Samuel Thomson, "To the Public," *Thomsonian Recorder* 2 (1833): 10; "Proceedings of the Convention of the Friendly Botanic Societies of the United States, Held at Baltimore," *Thomsonian Recorder* 3 (October 1834): 72–73.

58. Haller, *People's Doctor*, 148.

59. Haller, *Medical Protestants*, 52.

60. Thomson, *New Guide To Health*, 73–74.

61. Haller, *Medical Protestants*, 45.

62. Haller, *People's Doctor*, 52.

63. Ibid., 251.

64. Flannery, "Early Botanical Medical Movement."

65. Ibid.

66. Haller, *People's Doctor*, 46.

67. Thomson, *New Guide to Health*, 132.

68. Haller, *People's Doctor*, 83.

69. T. Hersey, *The Thomsonian Recorder* 2, no. 9 (February 1, 1834): 133.

70. Whorton, *Nature Cures*, 39; US Census, *Abstract of the Fifth Census of the United States, 1830* http://www.census.gov/prod/www/abs/decennial/1830 .html.

71. Thomson, *New Guide To Health*, 130–31.

72. Ibid.; M. Simpson et al., "Raspberry Leaf in Pregnancy: Its Safety and Efficacy in Labor," *Journal of Midwifery and Women's Health* 46 (March–April 2001): 51–59.

73. Stephen Lyng, *Holistic Health and Biomedical Medicine: A Countersystem Analysis* (Albany: SUNY Press, 1990), 182–87; Janet Farrell Brodie, *Contraception and Abortion in Nineteenth-Century America* (Ithaca, NY: Cornell University Press, 1997), 149–50.

74. Haller, *People's Doctor*, 125–27.

75. Ibid., 126.

76. "More Quack Murder," *New York Courier*, reprinted in *Daily National Intelligencer* (Washington, DC), June 2, 1885.

77. Daniel Drake, *The People's Doctors* (Cincinnati: The People, 1830), 59–60.

78. "Influence of Quackery on Health, Morals, &c," *Boston Medical and Surgical Journal* 39 (January 10, 1849): 471–80, American Periodicals, accessed September 5, 2012.

79. Thomson, *New Guide to Health*, 72; Haller, *People's Doctor*, 127; William G. Rothstein, *American Physicians in the Nineteenth Century: From Sects to Science* (Baltimore: Johns Hopkins University Press, 1992), 146–49.

80. Thomson, *Narrative of the Life*, 87–105; Whorton, *Nature Cures*, 43; Haller, *People's Doctor*, 129.

81. Benjamin Waterhouse and Robert D. Montgomery, "Communications," *Daily National Intelligencer* (Washington, DC), June 2, 1835.

82. Haller, *People's Doctor*, 123–24.

83. Berman, "The Thomsonian Movement," 405–28.

84. Rothstein, "Botanical Movements and Orthodox Medicine," 46.

85. J. P. Shepherd, "Communication," *Botanico-Medical Recorder* 6 (1838): 129–30.

86. Haller, *People's Doctor*, 159.

87. Whorton, *Nature Cures*, 45; John S. Haller, *Kindly Medicine: Physio-Medicalism in America, 1836–1911* (Kent, OH: Kent State University Press, 1997), 27–28.

88. Whorton, *Nature Cures*, 45.

89. Haller, *People's Doctor*, 90–93.

90. Alva Curtis, "Notes," *Thomsonian Recorder* 4 (1836): 188.

91. Samuel Thomson, "Please to Take Notice," *Thomsonian Manual* 1 (1836): 140.

92. Whorton, *Nature Cures*, 46–47; Haller, *People's Doctor*, 84–111.

93. Whorton, *Nature Cures*, 47.

94. Haller, *Medical Protestants*, 92.

95. Quoted in Alex Berman and Michael Flannery, *America's Botanico-Medical Movements: Vox Populi* (New York: Informa Healthcare, 2001), 120.

96. Whorton, *Nature Cures*, 46–48; Haller, *People's Doctor*, 103–5.

97. John S. Haller, *A Profile in Alternative Medicine: The Eclectic Medical College of Cincinnati, 1845–1942* (Kent, OH: Kent State University Press, 1999), 15–20.

98. Whorton, *Nature Cures*, 39.

99. Thomson, *New Guide to Health*, 7–8, 12–16.

100. Haller, *People's Doctor*, 1–4; O. S. Fowler, "Phrenological Developments of Dr. Samuel Thomson," *Phrenological Almanac* 13 (1845): 359–60.

CHAPTER TWO: THE ONLY TRUE SCIENCE OF THE MIND

1. Stern, *Heads and Headlines*, 55.

2. Ibid., 55–56; Ruth Clifford Engs, *Clean Living Movements: American Cycles of Health Reform* (Westport, CT: Greenwood Publishing Group, 2001), 71–72.

3. Untitled article, *Phrenological Journal* 68, no. 6 (June 1879): 288–92; Stern, *Heads and Headlines*, 55–57.

4. Fenster, *Mavericks, Miracles and Medicine*, 189–90.

5. Ibid., 190.

6. Ibid., 192.

7. Finger, *Minds Behind the Brain*, 122; Simpson, "Phrenology and the Neurosciences," 475–76.

8. Finger, *Minds Behind the Brain*, 123–24.

9. Simpson, "Phrenology and the Neurosciences," 476.

10. Finger, *Minds Behind the Brain*, 28–30.

11. George P. Landow, "Emanuel Swedenborg's Vision of Christ," Victorian Web, http://www.victorianweb.org/religion/swedenborg2.html; Finger, *Minds Behind the Brain*, 119–121; Finger, *Origins of Neuroscience*, 29–31.

12. Finger, *Minds Behind the Brain*, 126–27.

13. Simpson, "Phrenology and the Neurosciences," 477.

14. Finger, *Minds Behind the Brain*, 130.

15. Ibid., 126–27.

16. Ibid., 126–30.

17. Greenblatt, "Phrenology," 793–94.

18. Paul, *Cult of Personality Testing*, 7.

19. Robert E. Riegel, "The Introduction of Phrenology to the United States," *American Historical Review* 39, no. 1 (October 1933): 74.

20. Greenblatt, "Phrenology," 794.

21. Thurs, *Science Talk*, 25–26.

22. J. Collins Warren, "The Collection of the Boston Phrenological Society: A Retrospect," *Annals of Medical History* 3 (Spring 1921): 6; Dominic Hall, "James Roberton Returns," *CHoM (Center for the History of Medicine) News*, Harvard Medical School, https://cms.www.countway.harvard.edu/wp/?p=2439.

23. Nelson Sizer, "Remarks" in "The Semi-Centennial of Spurzheim," *Phrenological Journal* 76 (January 1883): 27–30.

24. Wrobel, "Introduction," in Wrobel, *Pseudoscience and Science*, 13.

25. Young, "Orson Squire Fowler," 121.

26. John van Wyhe, "George Combe (1788–1858): Phrenologist and Natural Philosopher," *Victorian Web*, http://www.victorianweb.org/science/phrenology/combe.html.

27. Tomlinson, "Phrenology, Education, and the Politics of Human Nature," 12–15.

28. Finger, *Minds Behind the Brain*, 131; Emerson quoted in Robert D. Richardson Jr. and Barry Moser, *Emerson: The Mind on Fire* (Berkeley: University of California Press, 1995), 100.

29. "Phrenology," *Ladies' Magazine* 6 (1833): 11.

30. Derek Hodson and Bob Prophet, "A Bumpy Start to Science Education," *New Scientist* (August 14, 1986): 26–27.

31. Young, "Orson Squire Fowler," 121.

32. Paul, *Cult of Personality*, 8.

33. Thurs, *Science Talk*, 29–31; O. S. Fowler, L. N. Fowler, and Samuel Kirkham, *Phrenology Proved, Illustrated and Applied* (Philadelphia: Fowler and Brevoort, 1839), 46–47, 56–59.

34. Young, "Orson Squire Fowler," 122.

35. Paul, *Cult of Personality*, 8.

36. Alice Dixon, "A Lesser-Known Daughter of Nantucket: Lydia," *Historic Nantucket* 41 (Winter 1993–94): 60–62; John B. Blake, "Lydia Folger Fowler," Notable American Women: A Biographical Dictionary (Cambridge, MA: Radcliffe College, 1971), 654–55.

37. Stern, *Heads and Headlines*, 166–68.

38. "How to Take Plaster Casts," *American Phrenological Journal* (1838–69): 87, American Periodicals, accessed January 10, 2012; Colbert, *Measure of Perfection*, 21–24.

39. Stern, *Heads and Headlines*, 29–31, 52.

40. Young, "Orson Squire Fowler," 122.

41. Thomas F. Gossett, *Race: The History of an Idea in America* (New York: Oxford University Press, 1997), 72–76; Colbert, *Measure of Perfection*, 24–29; Stern, *Heads and Headlines*, 55–58.

42. Young, "Orson Squire Fowler," 122.

43. Thurs, *Science Talk*, 29; Tomlinson, "Phrenology, Education, and the Politics of Human Nature," 2.

44. Young, "Orson Squire Fowler," 122; Stern, *Heads and Headlines*, 36–37.

45. Paul Collins, *The Trouble with Tom: The Strange Afterlife and Times of Thomas Paine* (New York: Bloomsbury, 2009), 97.

46. Colbert, *Measure of Perfection*, 21.

47. Ibid., 41–42.

48. O. S. Fowler and L. N. Fowler, *The Illustrated Self-Instructor in Phrenology and Physiology* (New York: Fowler and Wells, 1857), 128–29.

49. Tom Quirk, *Mark Twain and Human Nature*, 2nd ed. (Columbia: University of Missouri Press, 2011), 26.

50. William James, *Principles of Psychology* (1890; repr. ed. New York: Dover, 1950), 1:28.

51. Colbert, *Measure of Perfection*, 21–22.

52. Stern, *Heads and Headlines*, 38.

53. "Phrenology in the Montreal Post-Office—A Curious Story," *New York Times*, December 15, 1867, ProQuest Historical Newspapers: *New York Times* (1851–2007), accessed January 10, 2012.

54. "Modes of Wearing the Hair," *Godey's Lady's Book*, May 1855, American Periodicals, accessed January 10, 2012.

55. Stern, *Heads and Headlines*, 42–46; Lorenzo Fowler, *Marriage: Its History and Ceremonies* (New York: Fowler and Wells, 1847), 11–14, 128–53, 196, 216–18; O. S. Fowler, *Matrimony; or, Phrenology and Physiology Applied to the Selection of Companions for Life* (Philadelphia, 1841), 17, 24, 30.

56. "Use of Phrenology," *Godey's Lady's Book*, January 1833, American Periodicals, accessed January 10, 2012.

57. Paul, *Cult of Personality Testing*, 9.

58. Stern, *Heads and Headlines*, 19–20.

59. Nelson Sizer, "Character Studies: No. 10," *Phrenological Journal and Science of Health* (July 1894): 23.

60. Stern, *Heads and Headlines*, 133.

61. *Charles Dickens' Complete Works: The Adventures of Oliver Twist; American Notes; The Uncommercial Traveler* (Boston: Estes and Lauriat, 1881), 149; Thurs, Science Talk, 22.

62. "Appearance of President Johnson—Who Visit Him—What Men He

Appoints to Office," *New York Times*, May 21, 1866, ProQuest Historical Newspapers: *New York Times*.

63. "A.D. 3000," *Harper's New Monthly Magazine* 7 (January 1856): 151–52.

64. Herman Melville, *Moby Dick; or, The White Whale* (St. Botolph Society, 1892), 330, 52

65. Whitman reading quoted in Stern, *Heads and Headlines*, 102–4.

66. Arthur Wrobel, "Whitman and the Phrenologists: The Divine Body and the Sensuous Soul," *PMLA* (Modern Language Association) 89 (January 1974): 20–22; Nathaniel Mackey, "Phrenological Whitman," *Conjunctions* 29 (Fall 1997), http://www.conjunctions.com/archives/c29-nm.htm; Harold Aspiz, "Science and Pseudoscience," in *A Companion to Walt Whitman*, ed. Donald D. Kummings (Malden, MA: John Wiley, 2009), 227–28.

67. Perry Meisel, *The Myth of Popular Culture: From Dante to Dylan* (Malden, MA: John Wiley, 2009), 3.

68. Alan Gribben, "Mark Twain, Phrenology and the 'Temperaments': A Study of Pseudoscientific Influence," *American Quarterly* 24, no. 1 (March 1972): 55.

69. Wrobel, *Pseudoscience and Society*, 15; Minna Morse, "Facing a Bumpy History," *Smithsonian* (October 1997), http://www.smithsonianmag.com/history-archaeology/object_oct97.html.

70. P. Flourens, *Phrenology Examined*, Charles de Lucena Meigs, trans. (Philadelphia: Hogan and Thompson, 1846), 102; Finger, *Minds Behind the Brain*, 132–34.

71. Oliver Wendell Holmes, *The Professor at the Breakfast-Table* (Boston: Ticknor and Fields, 1868), 251.

72. Finger, *Minds Behind the Brain*, 129–32.

73. Stern, *Heads and Headlines*, 84.

74. Thurs, *Science Talk*, 33–36.

75. Greenblatt, "Phrenology," 790.

76. "David Ferrier," in *Mind Matters: Neuroscience and Psychiatry*, online exhibition, King's College London http://kingscollections.org/exhibitions/specialcollections/mind-matters/the-origins-of-modern-neuroscience/david-ferrier; Finger, *Origins of Neuroscience*, 53–55.

77. P. Thompson, T. D. Cannon, and A. W. Toga, "Mapping Genetic Influences on Human Brain Structure," *Annals of Medicine* 34 (2002): 523–26; Fenster, *Mavericks, Miracles and Medicine*, 189; Simpson, "Phrenology and the Neurosciences," 480–81; Finger, *Minds Behind the Brain*, 133–36.

78. Davi Johnson Thornton, *Brain Culture: Neuroscience and Popular Media* (New Brunswick, NJ: Rutgers University Press, 2011), 2–4.

79. Stern, *Heads and Headlines*, 125–28, 178–79, 244.

80. "Statistics from the Water-Cure Establishments," *Water-Cure Journal* (October 1851): 90–91; Young, "Orson Squire Fowler," 123.

CHAPTER THREE: QUENCHING THIRST, HEALING PAIN

1. T. L. Nichols, "Childbirth Without Pain or Danger," *The Herald of Health: Papers on Sanitary and Social Science* (London: Nichols & Co., 1881), 145; Silver-Isenstadt, *Shameless*, 130–33.

2. Silver-Isenstadt, *Shameless*, 74–75; Phinney, *Water Cure*, 72–73.

3. Cayleff, *Wash and Be Healed*, 20–21.

4. Ibid., 21, 186.

5. Legan, "Hydropathy," 74–76; Cayleff, *Wash and Be Healed*, 21.

6. Whorton, *Nature Cures*, 81; Cayleff, *Wash and Be Healed*, 22.

7. Whorton, *Nature Cures*, 81; Cayleff, *Wash and Be Healed*, 23.

8. Silver-Isenstadt, *Shameless*, 67.

9. Cayleff, *Wash and Be Healed*, 18–19.

10. Whorton, *Nature Cures*, 78.

11. Cayleff, *Wash and Be Healed*, 19–20.

12. "Practical Medicine: John Wesley, Methodism, Medicine," History of Medicine Collection, Southwestern University Library, http://www.southwestern.edu/library/Early-Medical-Texts/index.htm.

13. Benjamin Rush, *Directions for the Use of the Mineral Water and Cold Baths, at Harrogate, Near Philadelphia* (Philadelphia: Melchior Steiner, 1786).

14. Trall, *Hydropathic Encyclopedia*, 4.

15. Francis Graeter, "Treatment of Single Diseases: Weak Digestion, Debility of The Stomach," in *Hydriatics; or Manual of the Water Cure, Especially as Practiced by Vincent Priessnitz in Grafenberg*, 3rd ed., ed. and trans. Francis Graeter (New York: William Radde, 1843), 105–6.

16. Legan, "Hydropathy," 86–87; Whorton, *Nature Cures*, 80–81.

17. Legan, "Hydropathy," 86–87.

18. Silver-Isenstadt, *Shameless*, 66; Cayleff, *Wash and Be Healed*, 22; Judith Ann Giesberg, *Civil War Sisterhood: The US Sanitary Commission and Women's Politics in Transition* (Lebanon, NH: University Press of New England, 2000), 181.

19. Whorton, *Nature Cures*, 81; Marland and Adams, "Hydropathy at Home," 499–529.

20. Cayleff, *Wash and Be Healed*, 23.

21. Ibid., 19.

22. Whorton, *Nature Cures*, 82.

23. Cayleff, *Wash and Be Healed*, 20, 24; Legan, "Hydropathy," 80.

24. Trall, *Hydropathic Encyclopedia*, 277, 50, 446.

25. R. T. Trall, *The New Hydropathic Cook-Book; with Recipes for Cooking on Hygienic Principles* (New York: Fowlers and Wells, 1854).

26. Cayleff, *Wash and Be Healed*, 25; Legan, "Hydropathy," 81.

27. Whorton, *Nature Cures*, 83.

28. Legan, "Hydropathy," 82.

29. Ibid., 83.

30. "Phrenological Hydropathy," *Boston Medical and Surgical Journal* 34 (July 15, 1846): 485–86.

31. Cayleff, *Wash and Be Healed*, 15–16, 18.

32. Frontispiece opposite index, *Water-Cure Journal* 31 (1861).

33. Cayleff, *Wash and Be Healed*, 136, 109–12.

34. Mary Gove Nichols, *Mary Lyndon, or Revelations of a Life: An Autobiography* (New York: Stringer and Townsend, 1855), 146; Blake, "Mary Gove Nichols," 220–23; Jean Silver-Isenstadt, "Mary S. Gove Nichols: Making the Personal Political," in *Ordinary Women, Extraordinary Lives: Women in American History*, ed. Kriste Lindenmeyer (Lanham, MD: Rowman & Littlefield, 2000), 77–79.

35. Thomas L. Nichols, *Nichols' Health Manual* (London: Allen, 1887), 29.

36. Blake, "Mary Gove Nichols," 223; Silver-Isenstadt, *Shameless*, 1.

37. Phinney, *Water Cure*, 72.

38. "Elmira Water Cure," *Chemung County Historical Journal* 11 (December 1966): 1539.

39. Cayleff, *Wash and Be Healed*, 76–78.

40. Ibid., 83.

41. Mark Twain, "Medicine: Gurgle, Gargle, Guggle," *British Medical Journal* (July 8, 1857).

42. Phinney, *Water Cure*, 72.

43. Ibid., 73–75.

44. Lebergott, "Wage Trends," 462, 464.

45. Thomas Low Nichols, *An Introduction to the Water Cure* (New York: Fowlers and Wells, 1850), 16.

46. Legan, "Hydropathy," 83–84; Trall, *Hydropathic Encyclopedia*, 41.

47. Legan, "Hydropathy," 84–85.

48. Whorton, *Nature Cures*, 98–100.

49. Barbara Anne White, *The Beecher Sisters* (New Haven, CT: Yale University Press, 2003), 77–78.

50. Whorton, *Nature Cures*, 77; Catharine Beecher, *Letters to the People on*

Health and Happiness (New York: Harper, 1856), 117–18, 135–50; Catharine E. Beecher, "Hydropathy," *New York Observer and Chronicle*, October 24, 1846.

51. Phinney, *Water Cure*, 103–4.

52. Mary Gove Nichols, *A Woman's Work in Water Cure and Sanitary Education* (London: Nichols & Co., 1874), 20, 26.

53. Silver-Isenstadt, *Shameless*, 75.

54. Ibid., 76–80, 86–87; Edgar Allan Poe, "The Literati of New York City," *Godey's Magazine and Lady's Book*, July 1846, 16; Blake, "Mary Gove Nichols," 226.

55. Blake, "Mary Gove Nichols," 222.

56. Cayleff, *Wash and Be Healed*, 86–87, 90.

57. Marland and Adams, "Hydropathy at Home."

58. Mary Gove Nichols, *Experience in Water Cure* (New York: Fowler and Wells, 1849), 18.

59. Cayleff, *Wash and Be Healed*, 44–45; Marland and Adams, "Hydropathy at Home."

60. Cayleff, "Gender, Ideology, and the Water-Cure Movement," 87, 94.

61. Cayleff, *Wash and Be Healed*, 35.

62. Silver-Isenstadt, *Shameless*, 135–36, 154–55; Ronald G. Walters, *American Reformers, 1815–1860* (New York: Hill and Wang, 1978), 156–57.

63. "Dr. Elizabeth Blackwell," *Changing the Face of Medicine*, National Library of Medicine, http://www.nlm.nih.gov/changingthefaceofmedicine/physicians/biography_35.html.

64. Cayleff, "Gender, Ideology, and the Water-Cure Movement," 90.

65. Thomas Low Nichols, "American Hydropathic Institute," *Water-Cure Journal* 11, no. 4 (April 1851): 91.

66. Cayleff, *Wash and Be Healed*, 70.

67. Edward Johnson, *The Hydropathic Treatment of Diseases Peculiar to Women; and of Women in Childbed; with Some Observations on the Management of Infants* (London: Simpkin, Marshall, and Co., 1850), 125.

68. Cayleff, "Gender, Ideology, and the Water-Cure Movement," 85–87.

69. Ibid., 91.

70. Ibid., 2; Gleason quoted in ibid., 77.

71. J. R. LeMaster and James D. Vilson, *The Routledge Encyclopedia of Mark Twain* (New York: Routledge, 2012), 322.

72. Joan D. Hedrick, *Harriet Beecher Stowe: A Life* (London: Oxford University Press, 1995), 176–81.

73. Legan, "Hydropathy," 86.

74. Whorton, *Nature Cures*, 79–80.

75. Ibid., 80.

76. "Hyponatremia," *A.D.A.M. Medical Encyclopedia* (Bethesda, MD: US National Library of Medicine, 2011).

77. Jean-Jacques Rousseau, "Book Six," in *The Confessions* (London: Wordsworth, 1996), 220; Whorton, *Nature Cures*, 100–101.

78. "The Water Cure," *Boston Medical and Surgical Journal* 35, no. 18 (December 2, 1846).

79. Holmes, *Medical Essays*, 6.

80. James F. Light, *John William DeForest* (New York: Twayne, 1965), 29–31.

81. John Townsend Trowbridge, *My Own Story: With Recollections of Noted Persons* (New York: Houghton Mifflin, 1903), 197–99; Legan, "Hydropathy," 90–91.

82. Whorton, *Nature Cures*, 100.

83. Ibid., 99–100; Cayleff, *Wash and Be Healed*, 166–68.

84. Whorton, *Nature Cures*, 86–87.

85. Cayleff, "Gender, Ideology, and the Water-Cure Movement," 91.

86. Ibid., 94.

87. Legan, "Hydropathy," 91–92; Cayleff, "Gender, Ideology, and the Water-Cure Movement," 95.

88. Cayleff, *Wash and Be Healed*, 169.

89. J. H. Kellogg, "Hygeio-Therapy and Its Founder," in Ronald L. Numbers, *Prophetess of Health: A Study of Ellen G. White* (New York: Harper & Row, 1976), 66–67.

90. Cayleff, *Wash and Be Healed*, 99–100.

91. Ibid., 168–69.

92. Ibid., 171.

93. Ibid., 160–61.

94. Ibid., 162.

95. Blake, "Mary Gove Nichols," 230–33; "Feminism and Free Love," H-net, http://www.h-net.org/~women/papers/freelove.html.

96. Silver-Isenstadt, *Shameless*, 235–37.

97. Ibid., 241; Cayleff, *Wash and Be Healed*, 173–75.

98. Nina Rastogi, "Who Says You Need Eight Glasses a Day?," *Slate*, April 4, 2008, http://www.slate.com/articles/news_and_politics/explainer/2008/04/who_says_you_need_eight_glasses_a_day.html.

99. Whorton, *Nature Cures*, 191–92; Piers Edwards, "Sports and Recovery: End of the Ice Bath Age?," CNN.com, December 18, 2012, http://edition.cnn.com/2012/12/18/sport/feature-ice-baths.

100. Cayleff, *Wash and Be Healed*, 174.

CHAPTER FOUR: DILUTIONS OF HEALTH

1. Elizabeth Cady Stanton to Lucretia Mott (October 22, 1852) in *Women's Suffrage in America*, 2nd ed., ed. Elizabeth Frost-Knappman and Kathryn Cullen-DuPont (New York: Facts on File, 2005), 103.

2. Judith Wellman, *The Road to Seneca Falls: Elizabeth Cady Stanton and the First Woman's Rights Convention* (Urbana: University of Illinois Press, 2004), 158.

3. Kirschmann, *A Vital Force*, 29–30.

4. Whorton, *Nature Cures*, 49.

5. Hahnemann, *Organon*, 186–87.

6. Haller, *History of American Homeopathy*, 9–11; Kaufman, *Homeopathy in America*, 24.

7. Haller, *History of American Homeopathy*, 11–12; Kaufman, *Homeopathy in America*, 24.

8. Quoted in Peter Watson, *The German Genius: Europe's Third Renaissance, the Second Scientific* (New York: Harper Perennial Reprint, 2011), 176.

9. Quoted in Thomas Lindsley Bradford, "The Life of Hahnemann," *Homeopathic Recorder* 8 (August 1893): 346.

10. Whorton, *Nature Cures*, 51.

11. Ibid., 51.

12. Hahnemann, *Organon*, 45.

13. Haller, *History of American Homeopathy*, 12–14.

14. Hahnemann quoted in Lester S. King, *The Medical World of the Eighteenth Century* (Chicago: University of Chicago Press, 1958), 170–71.

15. Whorton, *Nature Cures*, 57; Robins, *Copeland's Cure*, 7–8.

16. Whorton, *Nature Cures*, 57.

17. Haller, *History of American Homeopathy*, 29–31.

18. Robins, *Copeland's Cure*, 7; Nadav Davidovitch, "Negotiating Dissent: Homeopathy and Anti-Vaccinationism at the Turn of the Twentieth Century," in Johnston, *Politics of Healing*, 13–15; Haller, *History of American Homeopathy*, 243–44.

19. Quoted in Porter, *Greatest Benefit to Mankind*, 391.

20. Whorton, *Nature Cures*, 52–54; Haller, *History of American Homeopathy*, 19–20.

21. Samuel Hahnemann to Dr. Stapf (September 11, 1813), in *British Journal of Homeopathy*, J. J. Drysdale and J. Rutherfurd Russell, eds. (London: H. Turner, 1845), 3:137–40.

22. Samuel Hahnemann, *Materia Medica Pura*, trans. Charles Hempel (New York: Radde, 1846), 1:vii.

23. Whorton, *Nature Cures*, 53–54.

24. Haller, *History of American Homeopathy*, 12–13; Robins, *Copeland's Cure*, 7.

25. Whorton, *Nature Cures*, 54–56; Kaufman, "Homeopathy in America," 100–101.

26. Hahnemann, *Materia Medica Pura*, 26–28, 29, 30, 39, 43; Whorton, *Nature Cures*, 56.

27. Whorton, *Nature Cures*, 72–73; Haller, *History of American Homeopathy*, 70–73.

28. Quoted in David W. Ramey et al., "Homeopathy and Science: A Closer Look," *Technology Journal of the Franklin Institute* 6, no. 1 (1999): 99.

29. Holmes, *Medical Essays*, 56.

30. Kaufman, *Homeopathy in America*, 31–32.

31. Whorton, *Nature Cures*, 57–58; Robins, *Copeland's Cure*, 10.

32. Hahnemann, *Organon*, 37, 38.

33. Kirschmann, *Vital Force*, 13.

34. Haller, *History of American Homeopathy*, 16.

35. Kirschmann, *Vital Force*, 18.

36. Hahnemann, *Organon*, 142.

37. Ibid., 143–45.

38. Samuel Hahnemann, "On the Effects of Coffee, from Original Observations," in *The Lesser Writings of Samuel Hahnemann*, ed. R. E. Dudgeon (New Delhi: B. Jain Publishers, 2004), 391–92.

39. Haller, *History of American Homeopathy*, 31–33; Samuel Hahnemann, *The Chronic Diseases: Their Specific Nature and Homeopathic Treatment* (New York: William Radde, 1845–46), 1:113–14.

40. Haller, *History of American Homeopathy*, 33–34.

41. Whorton, *Nature Cures*, 60; Haller, *History of American Homeopathy*, 28.

42. Haller, *History of American Homeopathy*, 98.

43. Ibid., 35–37.

44. William Harvey King, *History of Homeopathy and Its Institutions in America*, vol. 1 (New York: Lewis Publishing Company, 1905), 60–61; Kaufman, *Homeopathy in America*, 28.

45. Hering quoted in Arthur M. Eastman, "Life and Reminiscences of Dr. Constantine Hering," *Hahnemannian Monthly* 2 (June 25, 1917).

46. *Pennsylvania Biographical Dictionary* (St. Clair Shores, MI: Somerset Publishers, 1999), 554–55.

47. "Making Medicines from Poisonous Snakes," National Institutes of Health, Office of Science Education, http://science.education.nih.gov/animal research.nsf/Story1/Making+Medicines+from+Poisonous+Snakes; Whorton, *Nature Cures*, 61.

48. Haller, *History of American Homeopathy*, 124–27.

49. Anna Kobsar and Martin Eigenthaler, "NO Donors as Antiplatelet Agents," in Peng George Wang et al., eds., *Nitric Oxide Donors* (New York: John Wiley, 2005), 258–86; N. Marsh and A. Marsh, "A Short History of Nitroglycerine and Nitric Oxide in Pharmacology and Physiology," *Clinical Experimental Pharmacology and Physiology* 27 (April 2000): 314–15; Kaufman, "Homeopathy in America," 100–101.

50. Haller, *History of American Homeopathy*, 100–101.

51. Kaufman, *Homeopathy in America*, 29.

52. Quoted in William E. Kirtsos, "The Beginning of the American Institute of Homeopathy," AIH, http://homeopathyusa.org/home/about-aih/our-heritage-our-future.html.

53. Haller, *History of American Homeopathy*, 138–39, 176.

54. *Code of Ethics of the American Medical Association, adopted May, 1847* (Philadelphia: AMA, 1848), 18–19.

55. Michael Flannery, "Another House Divided: Union Medical Service and Sectarians During the Civil War," *Journal of the History of Medicine and Allied Sciences* 54 (1999): 490; Robins, Copeland's Cure, 18–19.

56. Kaufman, "Homeopathy in America," 102.

57. Whorton, *Nature Cures*, 68–69.

58. "Remarks of Dr. Dake," *Proceedings of the Fifteenth Annual Meeting of the American Institute of Homeopathy* 13 (1864): 131–32; Haller, *History of American Homeopathy*, 177–78.

59. Albert Bellows, A *Memorial to the Trustees of the Free City Hospital, With Statistics and Facts, Showing the Comparative Merits of Homeopathy and Allopathy, as Shown by Treatments in European Hospitals* (Boston: Clapp, 1863), 23–25; Whorton, *Nature Cures*, 64.

60. Hahnemann quoted in ibid., 56.

61. Hahnemann, *Organon*, 261.

62. Kirschmann, *Vital Force*, 33–35; Haller, *History of American Homeopathy*, 226.

63. Kirschmann, *Vital Force*, 34; Haller, *History of American Homeopathy*, 227–28, 247–49.

64. Haller, *History of American Homeopathy*, 228–32.

65. Ibid., 231–33.

66. Kirschmann, *Vital Force*, 31; Martin Bickman, "Transcendental Ideas: Definitions," *American Transcendentalism Web*, Virginia Commonwealth University, http://transcendentalism-legacy.tamu.edu/ideas/definitionbickman.html.

67. Kirschmann, *Vital Force*, 32; Dana Ullman, *The Homeopathic Revolu-

tion: Why Famous People and Cultural Heroes Chose Homeopathy (Berkeley, CA: North Atlantic Books, 2007), 67–68; N. Hirschorn and I. A. Greaves, "Louisa May Alcott: Her Mysterious Illness," *Perspectives in Biological Medicine* 50 (Spring 2007): 243–59.

68. Elizabeth Stuart Phelps, "What Shall They Do?," *Harper's New Monthly Magazine* (1877): 522.

69. Ibid., 523.

70. Frederick Wegener, "'Few Things More Womanly or More Noble': Elizabeth Stuart Phelps and the Advent of the Woman Doctor in America," *Legacy* 1, no. 22 (2005): 2–3.

71. Kirschmann, *Vital Force*, 40–41; George W. Swazey, "The Admission of Women," *Transactions of the American Institute of Homeopathy* (1869–70): 345.

72. Kirschmann, *Vital Force*, 74–75.

73. Duffy, *From Humors to Medical Science*, 290.

74. Anne C. Mastroianni, Ruth R. Faden, and Daniel D. Federman, *Women and Health Research: Ethical and Legal Issues of Including Women in Clinical Studies* (Washington, DC: National Academies Press, 1994), 46; Kirschmann, *Vital Force*, 77.

75. Kirsten Swinth, "Emily Sartain and Harriet Judd Sartain, MD: Creating a Community of Women Professionals," in *Philadelphia's Cultural Landscape*, Katherine Martinez and Page Talbott, eds. (Philadelphia: Temple University Press, 2000), 139–41.

76. Ibid., 143–45; Kirschmann, *Vital Force*, 62–63, 76–78.

77. Holmes, *Medical Essays*, 101.

78. Ibid., 203, ix-x.

79. Kaufman, *Homeopathy in America*, 32–33, 100–101.

80. Haller, *History of American Homeopathy*, 260.

81. Robins, *Copeland's Cure*, 27–28.

82. Ibid., 28; Kaufman, *Homeopathy in America*, 21–26.

83. Kaufman, "Homeopathy in America," 106.

84. William Holcombe, "What Is Homeopathy?," *North American Journal of Homeopathy* 13 (1865): 341–42; Haller, *History of American Homeopathy*, 266–69.

85. Rogers, "The Proper Place of Homeopathy."

86. Kirschmann, *Vital Force*, 24; Haller, *History of American Homeopathy*, 268–70.

87. Whorton, *Nature Cures*, 272; Mark Twain quoted in Harris L. Coulter, *Divided Legacy: The Conflict between Homeopathy and the American Medical Association*, vol. 3, *Science and Ethics in American Medicine, 1800–1914* (Berkeley, CA: North Atlantic Books, 1982), 288–89.

88. Kirschmann, *Vital Force*, 19; Alex Berman, "The Heroic Approach in 19th Century Therapeutics," *Bulletin of the American Society of Hospital Pharmacists* 11 (1954): 320–24.

89. Dan King, *Quackery Unmasked; or, a Consideration of the Most Prominent Empirical Schemes of the Present Time* (Boston: David Clapp, 1858), 132–33.

90. Holmes, *Medical Essays*, xiv.

91. Kirschmann, *Vital Force*, 113–20; Terri A. Winnick, "From Quackery to 'Complementary' Medicine: The American Medical Profession Confronts Alternative Therapies," *Social Problems* 52, no. 1 (February 2005): 40; Haller, *History of American Homeopathy*, 292–94.

92. Kirschmann, *Vital Force*, 114.

93. Anne Taylor Kirschmann, "Making Friends for 'Pure' Homeopathy," in Johnston, *Politics of Healing*, 31–33.

94. Julia M. Green, "Obituary," *Pacific Coast Homeopathic Bulletin* 12, no. 1 (January 1964).

95. "Homeopathy: An Introduction," National Center for Complementary and Alternative Medicine, http://nccam.nih.gov/health/homeopathy.

96. Hahnemann, *Organon*, 226.

CHAPTER FIVE: HYPNOTIZED

1. Rennie B. Schoepflin, "Christian Science Healing in America," in Gevitz, *Other Healers*, 193–94; Milmine, *Life of Mary Baker G. Eddy*.

2. Sidney Ochs, "A History of Nerve Functions: From Animal Spirits to Molecular Mechanisms," *Brain* 128, no. 1 (2005): 227–31; Finger, *Doctor Franklin's Medicine*, 220–22; Allen G. Debus, "Paracelsus and the Medical Revolution of the Renaissance," National Library of Medicine, http://www.nlm.nih.gov/exhibition/paracelsus/index.html; Jessica Riskin, "Franz Anton Mesmer (1734–1815)," *The Super-Enlightenment Authors*, digital collection, Stanford University Libraries, http://collections.stanford.edu/supere/page.action?forward=authors&section=authors.

3. Whorton, *Nature Cures*, 104–5; Haller, *American Medicine in Transition*, 101; Finger, *Doctor Franklin's Medicine*, 222.

4. Finger, *Doctor Franklin's Medicine*, 222; Whorton, *Nature Cures*, 104–5.

5. Whorton, *Nature Cures*, 105; Fuller, "Mesmerism," 207.

6. Fuller, "Mesmerism," 220.

7. Ibid., 207.

8. Franz Anton Mesmer, *Memoir of F. A. Mesmer on His Discoveries*, Jerome Eden, trans. (Mt. Vernon, NY: Eden, 1957), 55; Whorton, *Nature Cures*, 105.

9. Whorton, *Nature Cures*, 105; "Glass Armonica," *Benjamin Franklin: An*

Extraordinary Life, An Eclectic Mind, PBS, 2002, http://www.pbs.org/benfrank lin/l3_inquiring_glass.html.

10. Pattie, *Mesmer and Animal Magnetism*, 63–69; Turner, "Mesmeromania"; Jan Ehrenwald, *The History of Psychotherapy: From Healing Magic to Encounter* (New York: Jason Aronson, 1976), 221.

11. Mesmer quoted in Ehrenwald, *History of Psychotherapy*, 223.

12. Whorton, *Nature Cures*, 105–6.

13. Turner, "Mesmeromania."

14. Whorton, *Nature Cures*, 105–6; Turner, "Mesmeromania."

15. Finger, *Doctor Franklin's Medicine*, 234.

16. Whorton, *Nature Cures*, 106–7.

17. Alison Winter, *Mesmerized: Powers of Mind in Victorian Britain* (Chicago: University of Chicago Press, 1998), 171–72.

18. Lady Rosse quoted in Winter, *Mesmerized*, 257–58.

19. Harriet Martineau, *Letters on Mesmerism*, 2nd ed. (London: Edward Moxon, 1845), 7–8.

20. Fuller, *Mesmerism*, 6; Darnton, *Mesmerism*, 51.

21. Tim Fulford, "Conducting the Vital Fluid: The Politics and Poetics of Mesmerism in the 1790s," *Studies in Romanticism* 43, no. 1 (Spring 2004): 62–63.

22. Mesmer quoted in Alan Gauld, *A History of Hypnotism* (London: Cambridge University Press, 1995), 11–12.

23. John Gardner, *The Great Physician: The Connection of Diseases and Remedies with the Truths of Revelation* (London: J. Hatchard, 1843), 244.

24. Finger, *Doctor Franklin's Medicine*, 228.

25. Whorton, *Nature Cures*, 108.

26. Pattie, *Mesmer and Animal Magnetism*, 142–44.

27. Franklin et al., *Report of Dr. Benjamin Franklin*, 95.

28. Ibid., 87–88.

29. Ibid., 88–89, 102, 108–14.

30. Benjamin Franklin Bache quoted in Claude-Anne Lopez, "Franklin and Mesmer: An Encounter," *Yale Journal of Biology and Medicine* 66 (1993): 328.

31. Finger, *Doctor Franklin's Medicine*, 230–31.

32. Franklin et al., *Report of Dr. Benjamin Franklin*, 114, 117, 123.

33. Finger, *Doctor Franklin's Medicine*, 230–33; Fuller, *Mesmerism*, 7–10.

34. Wallace and Gach, *History of Psychiatry and Medical Psychology*, 558–59; Judith Pintar and Steven Jay Lynn, *Hypnosis: A Brief History* (Malden, MA: Wiley-Blackwell, 2008), 23–25.

35. Fuller, *Mesmerism*, 10–11; Darnton, *Mesmerism*, 58.

36. Fuller, *Mesmerism*, 10–11; Darnton, *Mesmerism*, 58.

37. Adam Crabtree, "The Transition to Secular Psychotherapy: Hypnosis and the Alternate-Consciousness Paradigm," in Wallace and Gach, *History of Psychiatry and Medical Psychology*, 557–59.

38. Fuller, *Mesmerism*, 11; Whorton, *Nature Cures*, 107–8.

39. Puységur quoted in Henri Ellenberger, *The Discovery of the Unconscious: The History and Evolution of Dynamic Psychiatry* (New York: Basic Books, 1970), 72.

40. Fuller, *Mesmerism*, 10–11.

41. Brian A. Harris and Melvin A. Gravitz, "An 1829 Eyewitness Account of Hypnotic Anesthesia in Major Surgery," *Bulletin of Anesthesia History* 26 (October 2008): 9.

42. Stephen E. Braude, *First Person Plural: Multiple Personality and the Philosophy of the Mind* (Lanham, MD: Rowman & Littlefield, 1995), 20–21; Martin Willis and Catherine Wynne, "Introduction," in *Victorian Literary Mesmerism*, Willis and Wynne, 1–3.

43. Whorton, *Nature Cures*, 108–9; James Braid and Arthur Edward Waite, *Braid on Hypnotism: The Beginnings of Modern Hypnosis* (New York: Julian Press, 1960); Adam Crabtree, *From Mesmer to Freud: Magnetic Sleep and the Roots of Psychological Healing* (New Haven, CT: Yale University Press, 1993), 155–62.

44. Fuller, *Mesmerism*, 16–17; Finger, *Doctor Franklin's Medicine*, 228.

45. Poyen, *Progress of Animal Magnetism*, 40–41.

46. William Stone, "Animal Magnetism," *Connecticut Current*, September 26, 1837.

47. Fuller, "Mesmerism and the Birth of Psychology," 209–10.

48. Ralph L. Rusk, ed. *The Letters of Ralph Waldo Emerson* (New York: Columbia University Press, 1939), 2:55.

49. Fuller, *Mesmerism*, 17–19; Whorton, *Nature Cures*, 110; Nadis, *Wonder Shows*, 88.

50. Fuller, *Mesmerism*, 19.

51. Poyen, *Progress of Animal Magnetism*, 55.

52. Fuller, *Mesmerism*, 20–21.

53. Whorton, *Nature Cures*, 110–11.

54. Fuller, *Mesmerism*, 78–85; Nadis, *Wonder Shows*, 88.

55. Fuller, *Mesmerism*, 33; Turner, "Mesmeromania."

56. Whorton, *Nature Cures*, 107; Turner, "Mesmeromania."

57. LaRoy Sunderland, *Confessions of a Magnetizer* (Boston: Redding, 1845).

58. Timothy Shay, *Agnes: or, The Possessed, A Revelation of Mesmerism* (Phil-

adelphia: T. B. Peterson, 1948), 3; Jerome M. Schneck, "Henry James, George Du Maurier, and Mesmerism," *International Journal of Clinical and Experimental Hypnosis* 26, no. 2 (1978): 76; Nadis, *Wonder Shows*, 89, 103.

59. Samuel Coale, "The Romance of Mesmerism: Hawthorne's Medium of Romance," *Studies in the American Renaissance* (1994): 273–74; Leland S. Person, *The Cambridge Introduction to Nathaniel Hawthorne* (New York: Cambridge University Press, 2007), 86.

60. Whorton, *Nature Cures*, 110–11; Joseph Philippe Francois Deleuze, *Practical Instruction in Animal Magnetism* (Fowler & Wells Co., 1886), 144.

61. Willis and Wynne, *Victorian Literary Mesmerism*, 129; "Mesmeric Mania and Clairvoyant Somnambulists in 19th Century America," *Annual Report to the Friends* (New York: Institute for the History of Psychiatry, 2007), 25–27; Poyen, *Progress of Animal Magnetism*, 144.

62. Madison Park, "HypnoBirthing: Relax While Giving Birth?," CNN.com, August 12, 2011, http://edition.cnn.com/2011/HEALTH/08/12/hypnobirth .pregnancy/index.html.

63. Elizabeth, "Remarks of a Female Mesmerist in Reply to the Scurrilous Insinuations of Dr. F. Hawkins, Dr. Mayo, and Mr. Wakley," *Zoist* 7 (London: Hippolyte Bailliere, 1850): 46, 47.

64. Fuller, *Mesmerism*, 30.

65. Whorton, *Nature Cures*, 112.

66. "Lectures on Mesmerism," *Boston Medical and Surgical Journal* 29, no. 3 (January 20, 1844): 466.

67. X. Y., "Animal Magnetism," *New-Hampshire Gazette*, July 5, 1841.

68. Whorton, *Nature Cures*, 111–13.

69. X. Y., "Animal Magnetism"; Sheila O'Brien Quinn, "Credibility, Respectability, Suggestibility, and Spirit Travel: Lurena Brackett and Animal Magnetism," *History of Psychology* (October 24, 2011): 2–3.

70. Fuller, *Mesmerism*, 56–59.

71. Phineas Taylor Barnum, *Struggles and Triumphs; or, Forty Years' Recollections of P. T. Barnum* (Buffalo, NY: Warren, Johnson & Co., 1872), 70–71.

72. Fuller, *Mesmerism*, 79–82, 118.

73. Whorton, *Nature Cures*, 116; Fuller, *Mesmerism*, 119.

74. Fuller, *Mesmerism*, 119–20.

75. Whorton, *Nature Cures*, 116–17; Fuller, *Mesmerism*, 120–21.

76. Robert E. Hales, *Textbook of Psychiatry*, 5th ed. (Arlington, VA: American Psychiatric Publishing, 2008), 622.

77. Dresser, *Quimby Manuscripts*, 30.

78. Ibid., 180.

79. Fuller, *Mesmerism*, 120–21; Whorton, *Nature Cures*, 117; Rosenberg, *Our Present Complaint*, 64.

80. Dresser, *Quimby Manuscripts*, 82.

81. Ibid., 78.

82. Whorton, *Nature Cures*, 117.

83. Dresser, *Quimby Manuscripts*, 83–85.

84. Whorton, *Nature Cures*, 118.

85. Dresser, *Quimby Manuscripts*, 52.

86. Quoted in Fuller, *Mesmerism*, 125.

87. Dresser, *Quimby Manuscripts*, 173.

88. Fuller, *Mesmerism*, 128–33; Whorton, *Nature Cures*, 118–19.

89. Fuller, *Mesmerism*, 131–32, 124.

90. Ibid., 137–38.

91. Georgine Milmine, "Mary Baker G. Eddy," *McClure's Magazine* 28 (1906–7): 509–13.

92. McDonald, "Mary Baker Eddy," 94–95; Whorton, *Nature Cures*, 121–22; Mary Baker Eddy, *Science and Health with a Key to the Scriptures* (Boston: Allison B. Stewart, 1912), 109, 187–89.

93. Whorton, *Nature Cures*, 123.

94. Ibid., 123–25; Eddy quoted in Georgine Milmine and Willa Cather, *The Life of Mary Baker G. Eddy and the History of Christian Science* (Lincoln: University of Nebraska Press, 1993), 118.

95. Christian Science Publishing Society, *A Century of Christian Science Healing* (Boston: Christian Science Publishing Society, 1966), 48–49, 58; Whorton, *Nature Cures*, 124.

96. Whorton, *Nature Cures*, 124; "Writing Science and Health," Longyear Museum, http://www.longyear.org/mary_baker_eddy/teacher/en_extra_writing.

97. Edmund Andrews, "Christian Science," *Journal of the American Medical Association* 32 (1899): 581.

98. "Phases of Christian Science," *Journal of the American Medical Association* 33 (1899): 297.

99. Ambrose Bierce, *Devil's Dictionary* (Cleveland: World Publishing, 1948), 139.

100. "Mrs. Mary Baker Eddy, Boston," *Cincinnati Daily Gazette*, June 8, 1882.

101. Gillian Gill, *Mary Baker Eddy* (New York: Perseus, 1998), 289.

102. Richard Cabot, "One Hundred Christian Science Cures," *McClure's Magazine* 31 (1908): 472–76; Whorton, *Nature Cures*, 124–26.

103. Whorton, *Nature Cures*, 125–27.

104. Rev. M. W. Gifford, *Christian Science against Itself* (Cincinnati: Jennings and Pye, 1902), 74, 258.

105. Rev. Gray, *The Antidote to Christian Science or How to Deal with It from the Bible and Christian Point of View* (New York: Fleming H. Revell, 1907), 52.

106. Edgar L. Wakeman, "Wakeman's Wanderings," *Concord Evening Monitor*, January 17, 1891; Ralph Wallace Reed, "A Study of the Case of Mary Baker G. Eddy," *Cincinnati Lancet-Clinic* 104 (October 15, 1910): 360; McDonald, "Mary Baker Eddy," 98–100.

107. McDonald, "Mary Baker Eddy," 105–6.

108. "Global Membership," *Christian Science*, http://christianscience.com/church-of-christ-scientist/about-the-church-of-christ-scientist/global-membership.

109. Rennie B. Schoepflin, "Christian Science Healing in America," in Gevitz, *Other Healers*, 197.

110. Fuller, *Mesmerism*, 175.

111. Ibid., 145–46, 153–56.

112. Ralph Waldo Trine, *In Tune With the Infinite* (New York: Crowell Co., 1897), 16, i.

113. Frank C. Haddock, *Mastery of Self for Wealth, Power, Success* (Meriden, CT: Pelton, 1928), *Project Gutenberg*, http://www.gutenberg.org/ebooks/4286.

114. Fuller, *Mesmerism*, 164–67.

115. Sara Y. Krakauer, *Treating Dissociative Identity Disorder: The Power of the Collective Heart* (Philadelphia: Brunner-Routledge, 2001), 5–10.

CHAPTER SIX: SELLING SNAKE OIL

1. James Frank Dobie, *Rattlesnakes* (Austin: University of Texas Press, 1982), 75–76; Dan Hurley, *Natural Causes: Death, Lies and Politics in America's Vitamin and Herbal Supplement Industry* (New York: Broadway Books, 2006), 1–2; Gene Fowler, *Mavericks: A Gallery of Texas Characters* (Austin: University of Texas Press, 2008), 97–100; Joe Schwarcz, "Why Are Snake-Oil Remedies So-Called?," *Gazette* (Montreal), February 23, 2008, http://www.canada.com/montrealgazette.

2. Nadis, *Wonder Shows*, 6.

3. Harold B. Gill, *The Apothecary in Colonial Virginia* (Williamsburg: Colonial Williamsburg, 1972), 44.

4. Sally Lansdell Osborn, "Delights of Daffy," Medicine at the Margins conference paper, University of Glamorgan (Wales), April 15, 2011, http://phdpanacea.wordpress.com/2011/08/20/the-delights-of-daffy/.

5. Young, *Medical Messiahs*, 14–15.

6. John Parascandola, "Patent Medicines and the Public's Health," *Public Health Reports* 114, no. 4 (July–August 1999): 320.

7. Young, "Patent Medicine," 96–99.

8. Anderson, *Snake Oil*, 35–36; Kellie Patrick Gates, "PennDOT Archaeologists Uncover Historic Dyottville Glass Works," PlanPhilly, January 20, 2012, http://planphilly.com/penndot-archaeologists-uncover-historic-dyottville-glass-works (accessed April 18, 2012).

9. Sivulka, *Soap, Sex, and Cigarettes*, 34.

10. Lydia Pinkham quoted in Stage, *Female Complaints*, 46.

11. Ibid., 17–23; "Lady with a Compound," *American Journal of Nursing* 59, no. 6 (June 1959): 854.

12. Stage, *Female Complaints*, 27–28.

13. Virginia G. Drachman, *Enterprising Women: 250 Years of American Business* (Chapel Hill: University of North Carolina Press, 2002), 42–44; ibid., 30–31.

14. Daniel Pinkham quoted in "News," *Lynn (MA) Daily Item*, January 23, 1893.

15. Drachman, *Enterprising Women*, 43; Haller, *American Medicine in Transition*, 269–70; Stage, *Female Complaints*, 31.

16. Young, "Patent Medicine," 99–103.

17. Stage, *Female Complaints*, 52, 89–90; John King, *The American Dispensatory*, 10th ed. (Cincinnati: Wistach, Baldwin, and Co., 1876), 79.

18. Jacob Bigelow, MD, "On Self Limited Diseases," paper presented to the Massachusetts Medical Society (May 27, 1835), repr. in *Medical America in the Nineteenth Century: Readings from the Literature*, ed. Gert H. Brieger (Baltimore: Johns Hopkins University Press, 1972), 99, 103–4.

19. Stage, *Female Complaints*, 55–56.

20. Richard Swiderski, *Calomel in America: Mercurial Panacea, War, Song, and Ghosts* (Boca Raton, FL: BrownWalker Press, 2012), 59–60; Cohen, "Medical Social Movements," 59–63.

21. "Editor's Table," *Cincinnati Lancet and Observer* 6 (June 1836), 376.

22. Stage, *Female Complaints*, 61–62.

23. Shaw, "History of the Comstock Patent Medicine Business," 24–25; Stage, *Female Complaints*, 62–63; Anderson, *Snake Oil*, 37.

24. Stage, *Female Complaints*, 32.

25. Jacob Appel, "Physicians Are Not Bootleggers: The Short, Particular Life of the Medicinal Alcohol Movement," *Bulletin of the History of Medicine* 8, no. 2 (July 10, 2008): 355–86; ibid., 32, 62.

26. Stage, *Female Complaints*, 90.

27. Young, "Patent Medicine," 103.

28. Stage, *Female Complaints*, 40–41; Young, "Patent Medicines," 102–3.

29. Stage, *Female Complaints*, 17, 40–41.

30. Sivulka, *Soap, Sex, and Cigarettes*, 34–35; Troesken, "Elasticity of Demand," 25–27.

31. *Boston Daily Times* quoted in Michael Schudson, *Discovering the News: A Social History of American Newspapers* (New York: Basic Books, 1978), 23; Parascandola, *Sex, Sin, and Science*, 320.

32. Stage, *Female Complaints*, 100; Parascandola, *Sex, Sin, and Science*, 320; Anderson, *Snake Oil*, 44.

33. American Medical Association, *Nostrums and Quackery: Articles on the Nostrum Evil, Quackery, Reprinted, with Additions and Modifications, from* The Journal of the American Medical Association, vol. 1 (Chicago: American Medical Association Press, 1912), 364.

34. Stage, *Female Complaints*, 102–3.

35. Drake Holcombe, "Private Die Proprietaries," *Weekly Philatelic Gossip* 113 (June 1842): 375.

36. Charles Austin Bates, *Good Advertising* (New York: Holmes Publishing, 1896), 439.

37. Erika Janik and Matthew B. Jensen, "Giving Them What They Want: The Reinhardts and Quack Medicine in Wisconsin," *Wisconsin Magazine of History* 94 (Summer 2011): 31–32.

38. Parascandola, *Sex, Sin, and Science*, 320–21; Brooks McNamara, "The Indian Medicine Show," *Educational Theatre Journal* 23, no. 4 (December 1971): 432.

39. "Medicated Almanacs," *New York Times*, January 16, 1860, ProQuest Historical Newspapers: *New York Times* (1851–2008), accessed April 11, 2012.

40. Shaw, "History of the Comstock Patent Medicine Business," 30–31.

41. Stage, *Female Complaints*, 93.

42. Master Specialist, *Home Private Medical Advisor*.

43. Sivulka, *Soap, Sex, and Cigarettes*, 35.

44. Nadis, *Wonder Shows*, 20–21.

45. "Popularizing Science," *Nation* 4, no. 80 (January 10, 1867): 32.

46. George Park Fisher, ed., *Life of Benjamin Silliman, M.D., L.L.D.*, vol. 2 (New York: Charles Scribner and Co., 1866), 1–2.

47. As quoted in John C. Greene, "Protestantism, Science and American Enterprise: Benjamin Silliman," in *Benjamin Silliman and His Circle*, ed. Leonard G. Wilson (New York: Science History Publishing, 1979), 22.

48. Nadis, *Wonder Shows*, 22–23.

49. Anderson, *Snake Oil*, 6.

50. Nadis, *Wonder Shows*, 10, 23–27, 35–45.

51. Ibid., 29–30, 35–36.

52. Ibid., 32–39.

53. Porter, *Quacks*, 84–85; Nadis, *Wonder Shows*, 30, 36; Starr, *Social Transformation of American Medicine*, 48.

54. Starr, *Social Transformation of American Medicine*, 128; "Facts for Sick Women," *Breckenridge News* (Cloverport, KY), October 20, 1909.

55. Stage, *Female Complaints*, 45–46; "Lady with a Compound," *American Journal of Nursing*, 855.

56. Steven Seidman, "The Power of Desire and the Danger of Pleasure: Victorian Sexuality Reconsidered," *Journal of Social History* 24 (Autumn 1990): 50–51; Ellen Bayuk Rosenman, "Body Doubles: The Spermatorrhea Panic," *Journal of the History of Sexuality* 12, no. 3 (July 2003): 366.

57. Master Specialist, *Home Private Medical Advisor*.

58. A. C. Umbreit, "The Reinhardts and Their Frauds," 12, in "Medical Institute Investigation 1907," *Wisconsin Governor, Investigations, 1851-1959*, series 81, box 18, folder 6, Wisconsin Historical Society; Consumer Price Index Calculator, Bureau of Labor Statistics, http://www.bls.gov/data/inflation_calculator.htm.

59. Starr, *Social Transformation of American Medicine*, 127–28; Umbreit, *Pending Medical Legislation*, 12; Umbreit, "The Reinhardts and Their Frauds," 12–13, 14.

60. "Code of Ethics, Adopted May, 1847," American Medical Association (Philadelphia: Turner Hamilton, 1871), 15.

61. Henry H. Tucker, "'The True Physician': An Address Delivered before the Graduating Class of the Medical College of Georgia, at Its Annual Commencement" (Augusta, GA: E. H. Pughe, 1867), 7.

62. Starr, *Social Transformation of American Medicine*, 128–29.

63. *New York Times*, May 7, 1875, ProQuest Historical Newspapers: *New York Times* (1851–2008), accessed April 11, 2012.

64. Haller, *American Medicine in Transition*, 269–70.

65. Rosenman, "Body Doubles," 389; William H. Helfand, *Quack, Quack, Quack: The Sellers of Nostrums in Prints, Posters, Ephemera, and Books* (Hamden, CT: Winterhouse Editions, 2002), 22.

66. Stage, *Female Complaints*, 103–4.

67. Norman Gevitz, "Three Perspectives on Unorthodox Medicine," in Gevitz, *Other Healers*, 9; Starr, *Social Transformation of American Medicine*, 129–30.

68. *American Lancet*, "Can the Advertisements in a Reputable Medical Jour-

nal Promote Quackery," *Journal of the American Medical Association* 22 (Chicago: American Medical Association, 1894), 957–58.

69. "Physicians' Advertisements," *Boston Medical and Surgical Journal* (1866): 303–4.

70. Dr. Hunter, "Dr. Hunter on Quacks and Quackeries," *New York Daily Times*, October 27, 1855, ProQuest Historical Newspapers: *New York Times* (1851–2008), accessed April 11, 2012.

71. Porter, *Quacks*, 16–18.

72. Troesken, "Elasticity of Demand," 5–6; Starr, *Social Transformation of American Medicine*, 18; Porter, *Quacks*, 31, 47.

73. Troesken, "Elasticity of Demand," 32; Starr, *Social Transformation of American Medicine*, 128.

74. Porter, *Quacks*, 11–12, 17–19, 23, 30–31.

75. Ibid., 30–31; Guenter B. Risse, "Introduction," in Risse, *Medicine without Doctors*, 1–4.

76. Troesken, "Elasticity of Demand," 17–19; Anne Cooper Funderburg, *Sundae Best: History of Soda Fountains* (Bowling Green, OH: Bowling Green State University Popular Press, 2002), 93–94, 72; Barbara Mikkelson, "Cocaine-Cola," Snopes.com, May 19, 2011, http://www.snopes.com/cokelore/cocaine.asp; "Advertising and Branding," Patent Medicine Exhibit, Hagley Museum and Library, Wilmington, DE, http://www.hagley.org/library/exhibits/patentmed/history/advertisingbranding.html; Joe Nickell, "'Pop' Culture: Patent Medicines Become Soda Drinks," *Skeptical Inquirer* 35 (January/February 2011), http://www.csicop.org/si/show/pop_culture_patent_medicines_become_soda_drinks/.

77. Nancy Tomes, "The Great American Medicine Show Revisited," *Bulletin of the History of Medicine* 79, no. 4 (2005): 635; Anderson, *Snake Oil*, 31; Young, *Medical Messiahs*, 20.

78. FDA, "A History of the FDA and Drug Regulation in the United States," http://www.fda.gov/AboutFDA/WhatWeDo/History/default.htm; Julie Donohue, "A History of Drug Advertising: The Evolving Roles of Consumers and Consumer Protection," *Milbank Quarterly* 84, no. 4 (2006): 663–64; Stage, *Female Complaints*, 170–71.

79. Umbreit, *Pending Medical Legislation*, 12.

80. Umbreit, "The Reinhardts and Their Frauds," 16–17; "The Reinhardt Case Concluded: The End of a Long Fight for the Protection of the Public Against Imposition," *Journal of the American Medical Association* 51 (October 3, 1908): 1144–49.

81. "The Reinhardt Case Concluded."

82. "Williams' Electric Batteries," image on *Quackery: A Brief History of*

Quack Medicines and Peddlers, http://www.authentichistory.com/1898–1913/ 2-progressivism/8-quackery/index.html (December 23, 2012).

83. Peter Conrad and Valerie Leiter, "From Lydia Pinkham to Queen Levitra: Direct-to-Consumer Advertising and Medicalization," in Simon J. Williams et al., eds., *Pharmaceuticals and Society: Critical Discourses and Debates* (Malden, MA: Blackwell, 2009), 18–23; Dominick L. Frosch et al., "A Decade of Controversy: Balancing Policy with Evidence in the Regulation of Prescription Drug Advertising," *American Journal of Public Health* 100, no. 1 (January 2010): 24–25, 31.

CHAPTER SEVEN: MANUAL MEDICINE

1. B. J. Palmer, *The Science of Chiropractic: Its Principles and Philosophies,* 4th ed. (Davenport, IA: Palmer School of Chiropractic, 1920), 59–61; D. D. Palmer, *Text-Book of the Science, Art, and Philosophy of Chiropractic, for Students and Practitioners* (Portland, ME: Portland Printing House, 1910), 10, 18; Wardwell, "Chiropractors," in Gevitz, *Other Healers,* 157–58.

2. Moore, *Chiropractic in America,* 4.

3. Ibid., 15.

4. Hippocrates, "On the Articulations," trans. Francis Adams, online at Internet Classics Archive, http://classics.mit.edu/Hippocrates/artic.html.

5. Moore, *Chiropractic in America,* 15–17; Pettman, "History of Manipulative Therapy."

6. Moore, *Chiropractic in America,* 15–16; Richard Dean Smith, "Avicenna and the *Canon of Medicine*: A Millennial Tribute," *Western Journal of Medicine* 133 (October 1980): 368.

7. James Caulfield, "Mrs. Mapp, The Female Bone-setter," in *Portraits, Memoirs, and Characters, of Remarkable Persons, from the Revolution in 1688 to the End of the Reign of George II: Collected from the Authentic Accounts Extant,* vol. 4 (London: T. H. Whiteley, 1820), 70–77; Moore, *Chiropractic in America,* 16–17.

8. Paul Slack, "Mirrors of Health and Treasures of Poor Men: The Uses of the Vernacular Medical Literature of Tudor England," in *Health, Medicine, and Mortality in the Sixteenth Century,* ed. Charles Webster (Cambridge, UK: Cambridge University Press, 1979), 237.

9. Moore, *Chiropractic in America,* 16–17.

10. J. Paget, "Cases That Bonesetters Cure," *British Medical Journal* 1 (1867): 1–4.

11. Moore, *Chiropractic in America,* 17.

12. Leonard F. Peltier, MD, *Fractures: A History and Iconography of Their Treatment* (San Francisco: Norman Publishing, 1990), 4–5; Whorton, *Nature Cures,* 144.

13. Whorton, *Nature Cures*, 143.

14. Ibid., 142–43.

15. Gevitz, "Osteopathic Medicine," in Gevitz, *Other Healers*, 125.

16. Still, "Osteopathy."

17. Walter, *Women and Osteopathic Medicine*, 6–7.

18. Pettman, "History of Manipulative Therapy."

19. Whorton, *Nature Cures*, 144; Walter, *Women and Osteopathic Medicine*, 8–9.

20. Cohen, "Medical Social Movements," 76; Whorton, *Nature Cures*, 144.

21. Still, "Osteopathy," 2.

22. Whorton, *Nature Cures*, 145.

23. Cohen, "Medical Social Movements," 76.

24. Still, *Autobiography*, 287.

25. Still, "Osteopathy," 3.

26. Still, *Autobiography*, 371.

27. Ibid., 219, 310.

28. Pettman, "History of Manipulative Therapy."

29. Still, "Osteopathy," 4.

30. Whorton, *Nature Cures*, 148–50.

31. Still, *Osteopathy: Research and Practice*, 338.

32. Still, *Autobiography*, 32.

33. Whorton, *Nature Cures*, 149.

34. Ibid., 150.

35. A. T. Still, "Differences Between Osteopathy and Massage," in George Webster, *Concerning Osteopathy* (Norwood, MA: Plimpton Press, 1917), 93.

36. Emmons Rutledge Booth, *History of Osteopathy, and Twentieth Century Medical Practice* (Cincinnati: Press of Jennings and Graham, 1905), 33.

37. Gevitz, "Osteopathic Medicine," in Gevitz, *Other Healers*, 129–30.

38. Arthur Hildreth, *The Lengthening Shadow of Dr. Andrew Taylor Still* (Kirksville, MO: Journal Printing, 1942), 31.

39. Cohen, "Medical Social Movements," 78–79, 81–83; Baer, "Divergence and Convergence," 184.

40. Quoted in Walter, *Women and Osteopathic Medicine*, 12.

41. Lara Vapnek, *Breadwinners: Working Women and Economic Independence, 1865–1920* (Carbondale: University of Illinois Press, 2009), 11–13.

42. Whorton, *Nature Cures*, 151; Walter, *Women and Osteopathic Medicine*, 13; Still, *Autobiography*, 156.

43. Still, *Autobiography*, 155.

44. Walter, *Women and Osteopathic Medicine*, 12.

45. Wardwell, *Chiropractic*, 52–53.

46. Moore, *Chiropractic in America*, 6–12.

47. Gielow, *Old Dad Chiro*, 47–48.

48. Wardwell, *Chiropractic*, 53.

49. Whorton, *Nature Cures*, 167.

50. Gielow, *Old Dad Chiro*, 44, 47.

51. Moore, *Chiropractic in America*, 14.

52. Whorton, *Nature Cures*, 167.

53. Gielow, *Old Dad Chiro*, 79; ibid., 168.

54. Wardwell, *Chiropractic*, 56.

55. Moore, *Chiropractic in America*, 19.

56. Ibid., 21.

57. Wardwell, "Chiropractic," in Gevitz, *Other Healers*, 189; Whorton, *Nature Cures*, 169–71; Moore. *Chiropractic in America*, 21–22.

58. Whorton, *Nature Cures*, 170–71.

59. Palmer, *The Chiropractic Adjustor*, 21–22, 380.

60. Ibid., 558; Whorton, *Nature Cures*, 173.

61. Whorton, *Nature Cures*, 173.

62. Martin, "The Only Truly Scientific Method of Healing," 213.

63. Still, *Autobiography*, 208.

64. Whorton, *Nature Cures*, 146.

65. Andrew T. Still, "Body and Soul of Man," 2 (1903), Andrew Taylor Still Papers, Missouri Digital Heritage, http://cdm.sos.mo.gov/u?/atsu,736.

66. Whorton, *Nature Cures*, 146.

67. Ibid., 171–72.

68. Palmer, *The Chiropractic Adjustor*, 835–39.

69. Whorton, *Nature Cures*, 172.

70. Moore, *Chiropractic in America*, 105–6.

71. Whorton, *Nature Cures*, 174; Wardwell, *Chiropractic*, 59; Susan Smith-Cunnien, "Without Drugs or Knives: The Early Years of Chiropractic," *Minnesota History* 59, no. 5 (Spring 2005): 202.

72. Palmer quoted in Moore, *Chiropractic in America*, 108.

73. Oakley Smith, *Naprapathy Genetics: Being a Study of the Origin and Development of Naprapathy* (Chicago: printed by the author, 1932), 5–6.

74. Matthew Brennan, "Perspectives on Chiropractic Education in Medical Literature, 1910–1933," *Chiropractic History* 3 (1983): 285–88.

75. Whorton, *Nature Cures*, 185–87.

76. "Chiropractic Candor," *Journal of the American Medical Association* 75 (November 19, 1920): 1276.

77. Whorton, *Nature Cures*, 186–87; Wardwell, "Chiropractors," in Gevitz, *Other Healers*, 158–59; Moore, 46–49; Thomas Lamar, "From Broadcasting to Podcasting: Chiropractic Is on the Air!," part I, Spinal Column Radio, http://spinalcolumnradio.com/2010/02/05/from-broadcasting-to-podcasting-chiropractic-is-on-the-air-part-1/; "Chiropractic Candor," *Journal of the American Medical Association*, 1276.

78. Whorton, *Nature Cures*, 152.

79. Still, *Autobiography*, 321–22.

80. Whorton, *Nature Cures*, 152–53; Cohen, "Medical Social Movements," 93–94.

81. Laughlin quoted Baer, *Biomedicine and Alternative Healing Systems*, 54, 53.

82. Ibid., 53–55.

83. Ibid., 72–73; Moore, *Chiropractic in America*, 94–98.

84. Cohen, "Medical Social Movements," 93–99.

85. Russell Gibbons, *Chiropractic History: Lost, Strayed or Stolen* (Davenport, IA: Palmer College Student Council, 1976), 13-14.

86. Gevitz, "Osteopathic Medicine," in Gevitz, *Other Healers*, 132–34.

87. Ibid., 134–35.

88. Still, *Autobiography*, 395–96.

89. Cohen, "Medical Social Movements," 106.

90. Wardwell, *Chiropractic*, 58–63.

91. Cohen, "Medical Social Movements," 106; Whorton, *Nature Cures*, 182–84.

92. Wardwell, *Chiropractic*, 68–69.

93. Whorton, *Nature Cures*, 182–83; Wardwell, *Chiropractic*, 67.

94. Palmer, *The Chiropractic Adjustor*, 146, 256, 695.

95. John Wesley, *Primitive Physick*, 14th ed. (Philadelphia, 1770), 57, 61–62.

96. Harvey Green and Mary Elizabeth Perry, *The Light of the Home: An Intimate View of the Lives of Women in Victorian America* (New York: Pantheon, 1983), 138–39.

97. Leica Claydon et al., "Dose-specific Effects of Transcutaneous Electrical Nerve Stimulation (TENS) on Experimental Pain: A Systematic Review," *Clinical Journal of Pain* 27 (September 2011): 635–47; Richard M. Dubinsky and Janis Miyasaki, "Assessment: Efficacy of Transcutaneous Electrical Nerve Stimulation in the Treatment of Pain in Neurologic Disorders," *Neurology* 74 (January 12, 2010): 173–76.

98. "Mr. Frank X. Trudell," *Anaconda (MT) Standard*, March 31, 1907, 12; Moore, *Chiropractic in America*, 23–25, 31–41.

99. Moore, *Chiropractic in America*, 22–23; Starr, *Social Transformation of American Medicine*, 54–58.

100. Cohen, "Medical Social Movements," 100; Whorton, *Nature Cures*, 159–60.

101. B. J. Palmer, *The Philosophy of Chiropractic* (Davenport, IA: Palmer School of Chiropractic, 1909), 5:6.

102. I. D. Coulter, "Chiropractic and Medical Education: A Contrast in Models of Health and Illness," *Journal of the Canadian Chiropractic Association* 27, no. 4 (December 1983): 153.

103. James B. Campbell et al., "Chiropractic and Vaccination: A Historical Perspective," *Pediatrics* 105, no. 4 (April 1, 2000), http://pediatrics.aappublica tions.org/content/105/4/e43.full; Martin, "Chiropractic and the Social Context of Medical Technology," 814.

104. Moore, *Chiropractic in America*, 142–49.

105. Cohen, "Medical Social Movements," 82–83.

106. Twain quoted in Ober, *Mark Twain and Medicine*, 160–63.

107. "Topics of the Times," *New York Times*, May 31, 1905, ProQuest Historical Newspapers: *New York Times* (1851–2008), accessed March 9, 2012.

108. Richard Newton, "Is There Any Good in Osteopathy?," *American Medicine* 6 (1903): 616–17; Whorton, *Nature Cures*, 152–53.

109. John R. Musick, "Healing Without Medicine," *Godey's Magazine*, October 1895, 380.

110. "Mark Twain, Osteopath: Appears at Public Hearing Before Assembly Committee," *New York Times*, February 28, 1901.

111. Baer, *Biomedicine and Alternative Healing Systems*, 61.

112. Charles Warner, *Quacks* (Jackson, MS: printed by the author, 1930), 97.

113. "The Menace of Chiropractic: Practically No Educational Qualifications Necessary for Matriculation in Chiropractic Colleges," *Journal of the American Medical Association* 80 (March 10, 1923): 715–16.

114. Morris Fishbein, *The Medical Follies: An Analysis of the Foibles of Some Healing Cults* (New York: Boni and Liveright, 1925), 61.

115. J. F. Hart, "Did D. D. Palmer Visit A. T. Still in Kirksville?," *Chiropractic History* 17, no. 2 (1997): 49–55.

116. George Creel, "Making Doctors While You Wait," *Harper's Weekly* (April 3, 1915): 321.

117. "Don't Drug Yourself to Death," advertisement, *St. Paul (MN) Dispatch*, August 27, 1904.

118. Still, *Osteopathy: Research and Practice*, 433; Centers for Disease Control, "Diphtheria," *Pinkbook*, http://www.cdc.gov/vaccines/pubs/pinkbook/down loads/dip.pdf; Whorton, *Nature Cures*, 153; Moore, *Chiropractic in America*, 80–81.

119. "Dr. D. D. Palmer Goes to Jail," *Davenport (IA) Democrat & Leader*, March 27, 1906; Gielow, *Old Dad Chiro*, 67, 99–104.

120. Moore, *Chiropractic in America*, 76.

121. Baer, "Divergence and Convergence," 185–86.

122. "Mark Twain, Osteopath," *New York Times*, February 28, 1901.

123. Whorton, *Nature Cures*, 154–55, 158–60; Cohen, "Medical Social Movements," 102–4.

124. Whorton, *Nature Cures*, 159–60; Andrew Taylor Still, "An Appeal to the Thinking Osteopaths of the Profession," *Journal of the American Osteopathic Association* 15 (1915–16): 52.

125. Whorton, *Nature Cures*, 182; H. L. Mencken, *Prejudices: Sixth Series* (New York: Octagon, 1977), 224.

126. Whorton, *Nature Cures*, 163; Cohen, "Medical Social Movements," 110–12.

127. Gevitz, "Osteopathic Medicine," in *Other Healers*, 153–55; Cohen, "Medical Social Movements," 115–16.

128. Raymond J. Roberge and Marc. R. Roberge, "Overcoming Barriers to the Use of Osteopathic Manipulation Techniques in the Emergency Department," *Western Journal of Emergency Medicine* 10, no. 3 (August 2009), http://www.ncbi.nlm.nih.gov/pmc/articles/PMC2729220/; S. M. Johnson, M. E. Kurtz, and J. C. Kurtz, "Variables Influencing the Use of Osteopathic Manipulative Treatment in Family Practice," *Journal of the American Osteopathic Association* 97, no. 2 (February 1997): 86; Whorton, *Nature Cures*, 179; Cohen, "Medical Social Movements," 120–22, 144–45; Rosenberg, *Our Present Complaint*, 123.

129. Baer, "Divergence and Convergence," 180–81; Cohen, "Medical Social Movements," 145–46; Shawn A. Silver, "'Thanks, but no thanks': How Denial of Osteopathic Service in World War I and World War II Shaped the Profession," *Journal of the American Osteopathic Association* 112 (February 1, 2012): 93–97.

130. Baer, *Biomedicine and Alternative Healing Systems*, 52, 56–57; Eileen L. DiGiovanna et al., *An Osteopathic Approach to Diagnosis and Treatment*, 3rd ed. (New York: Lippincott, Williams & Wilkins, 2005), 8.

131. Cohen, "Medical Social Movements," 145; Baer, *Biomedicine and Alternative Healing Systems*, 50–52.

132. Baer, *Biomedicine and Alternative Healing Systems*, 74.

133. Gevitz, "Osteopathic Medicine," in *Other Healers*, 186–89.

134. J. Licciardone, R. Gamber, and K. Cardarelli, "Patient Satisfaction and Clinical Outcomes Associated with Osteopathic Manipulative Treatment," *Journal of the American Osteopathic Association* 102 (January 2002): 13; M. Pomykala, B. McElhinney, B. L. Beck, and J. E. Carrerio, "Patient Perception of

Osteopathic Manipulative Treatment in Hospitalized Setting: A Survey-Based Study," *Journal of the American Osteopathic Association* 108 (November 2008): 665–66.

135. Deanna M. Rothwell, Susan J. Bondy, and J. Ivan Williams, "Chiropractic Manipulation and Stroke: A Population-Based Case-Control Study," *Stroke* 32 (2001): 1055, 1059–60; J. David Cassidy et al., "Risk of Vertebrobasilar Stroke and Chiropractic Care," *Journal of Manipulative and Physiological Therapeutics* 32 (February 2009): S208.

136. Baer, *Biomedicine and Alternative Healing Systems*, 82–84.

137. B. J. Palmer quoted in Wardwell, *Chiropractic*, 74.

CHAPTER EIGHT: THE FALL AND RISE OF ALTERNATIVE MEDICINE

1. Thomas Lindsley Bradford, *History of the Homeopathic Medical College of Pennsylvania* (Lancaster, PA: T. B. & H. B. Cochran, 1898), 279–80; Naomi Rogers, *An Alternative Path: The Making and Remaking of Hahnemann Medical College* (New Brunswick, NJ: Rutgers University Press, 1998), 80; Naomi Rogers, "The Proper Place of Homeopathy: Hahnemann Medical College and Hospital in the Age of Scientific Medicine," *Pennsylvania Magazine of History and Biography* 108, no. 2 (April 1984): 179; Philadelphia College of Pharmacy Alumni Association, "Senior Class News," *Alumni Report* 30, issues 1–9 (1894): 36–38.

2. Cayleff, *Wash and Be Healed*, 169–70; Duffy, *From Humors to Medical Science*, 167–69.

3. Rosenberg, *Our Present Complaint*, 118–20.

4. Duffy, *From Humors to Medical Science*, 216–17; ibid., 119.

5. Whorton, "From Cultism to CAM," 292–94; Cayleff, *Wash and Be Healed*, 168–70.

6. Abraham Flexner, *Medical Education in the United States and Canada: A Report to the Carnegie Foundation for the Advancement of Teaching* (New York: Carnegie Foundation for the Advancement of Teaching, 1910), 157; Whorton, *Nature Cures*, 226–27; Claire Johnson and Bart Green, "100 Years after the Flexner Report," *Journal of Chiropractic Education* 24, no. 2 (Fall 2010): 145–50.

7. Mike Mitka, "The Flexner Report at the Century Mark: A Wake-Up Call for Reforming Medical Education," *Journal of the American Medical Association* 15 (April 23, 2010): 1465–66.

8. Duffy, *From Humors to Medical Science*, 209–13.

9. Whorton, *Nature Cures*, 226–27.

10. Duffy, *From Humors to Medical Science*, 212–13.

11. Flexner, *Medical Education in the United States*, xiv.

12. Martin, "Chiropractic and the Social Context of Medical Technology," 815; Meryl S. Justin, "The Entry of Women into Medicine in America: Education and Obstacles, 1847–1910," Hobart and William Smith Colleges, http://www.hws.edu/about/blackwell/articles/womenmedicine.aspx; Flexner quoted in Morantz-Sanchez, *Sympathy and Science*, 343; Starr, *Social Transformation of American Medicine*, 124.

13. Morantz-Sanchez, *Sympathy and Science*, 65–66, 88–89, 244–49.

14. Oliver Wendell Holmes, "Notes," *Maryland Medical Journal* 10 (1883): 424.

15. Morantz, "Women in the Medical Profession," 163–64.

16. Kirschmann, *Vital Force*, 119–21; Morantz, "Women in the Medical Profession," 167; Dodson quoted in Morantz-Sanchez, *Sympathy and Science*, 253; Starr, *Social Transformation of American Medicine*, 124.

17. Morantz-Sanchez, *Sympathy and Science*, 70; Kirschmann, *Vital Force*, 119–21; Morantz, "Women in the Medical Profession," 167.

18. Edward Clarke, *Sex in Education; or, a Fair Chance for Girls* (Boston: James R. Osgood and Company, 1875), 17–18, 31–36.

19. Stille quoted in Kimmel, "Men's Response to Feminism," 268.

20. Ibid., 270.

21. Ibid., 269–71.

22. Morantz, "Women in the Medical Profession," 165–67.

23. Whorton, "From Cultism to CAM," 299–300; Robins, *Copeland's Cure*, 223–24.

24. Robins, *Copeland's Cure*, 223–24, 238, 241.

25. Twain quoted in Ober, *Mark Twain and Medicine*, 241.

26. Rosenberg, *Our Present Complaint*, 123.

27. Ibid., 122–23.

28. Bara Fintel, Athena T. Samaras, and Edson Carias, "The Thalidomide Tragedy: Lessons for Drug Safety and Regulation," *Science in Society* (July 28, 2009), http://scienceinsociety.northwestern.edu/content/articles/2009/research-digest/thalidomide/title-tba; Duffy, *From Humors to Medical Science*, 241–43.

29. Whorton, "From Cultism to CAM," 300–301.

30. Ibid., 300–2.

31. Johnston, "Introduction," *Politics of Healing*, 3.

32. Cassedy, *Medicine in America*, 191; Reed, *Healing Cults*, 67–71.

33. Robins, *Copeland's Cure*, 242.

34. Whorton, "From Cultism to CAM," 302.

35. Rustum Roy, "Science and Whole Person Medicine: Enormous Potential

in a New Relationship," *Bulletin of Science, Technology, and Society* 22, no. 5 (October 2002): 377; Rosenberg, *Our Present Complaint*, 118.

36. American Holistic Medical Association statement in Whorton, "From Cultism to CAM," 287.

37. Ibid., 287–88, 302–4.

38. "Holistic Health Hard to Define," *Milwaukee Journal* (May 21, 1979), parts 2 and 3.

39. Whorton, "From Cultism to CAM," 301–3.

40. Astin, "Why Patients Use Alternative Medicine"; Rosenberg, *Our Present Complaint*, 113–14; Goldstein, *Alternative Health Care*, 8.

41. Martin, "Chiropractic and the Social Context of Medical Technology," 814.

42. Alex Berman, "The Heroic Approach in 19th-Century Therapeutics," in Leavitt and Numbers, *Sickness and Health in America*, 81–82.

43. Centers for Disease Control and Prevention, "Chronic Diseases and Health Promotion," http://www.cdc.gov/chronicdisease/overview/index.htm.

44. Martin, "'The Only Truly Scientific Method of Healing,'" 209.

45. More, Fee, and Parry, *Women Physicians and the Cultures of Medicine*, 10–11.

46. Cohen, "Medical Social Movements," 62–64; Duffy, *From Humors to Medical Science*, 169–70.

47. Goldstein, *Alternative Health Care*, 6.

48. Patricia M. Barnes, Barbara Bloom, Richard L. Nahin, *Complementary and Alternative Medicine Use Among Adults and Children: United States, 2007, National Health Statistics Report* 12 (Washington, DC: Centers for Disease Control: December 10, 2008), http://nccam.nih.gov/sites/nccam.nih.gov/files/news/nhsr12.pdf..

49. James Whorton, "The Homeopathy Debate," *The Alternative Fix, Frontline*, posted November 4, 2003, http://www.pbs.org/wgbh/pages/frontline/shows/altmed/themes/homeopathy.html.

50. Astin, "Why Patients Use Alternative Medicine."

51. Charles Vincent and Adrian Furnham, *Complementary Medicine: A Research Perspective* (Chichester, UK: Wiley & Sons, 1997), 119–21.

52. Montaigne quoted in Hunter, "A Question of Faith," 125–28.

53. Holmes, *Medical Essays*, 1.

54. Maj-Britt Niemi, "Placebo Effect: A Cure in the Mind," *Scientific American*, February 25, 2009, http://www.scientificamerican.com/article.cfm?id=placebo-effect-a-cure-in-the-mind.

55. Hunter, "A Question of Faith," 126–27.

56. "Just the Placebo Effect?," *Science in School* 21, http://www.sciencein school.org/2011/issue21/placebo.

57. Hunter, "A Question of Faith," 125–28.

58. "Think Yourself Better," *Economist*, May 19, 2011, http://www.economist .com/node/18710090; Ted Kaptchuk, "The Placebo Effect in Alternative Medicine: Can the Performance of a Healing Ritual Have Clinical Significance?," *Annals of Internal Medicine* 136, no. 11 (June 4, 2002): 817; Aijing Shang et al., "Are the Clinical Effects of Homeopathy Placebo Effects? Comparative Study of Placebo-Controlled Trials of Homeopathy and Allopathy," *Lancet* 366, no. 9487 (August 2005): 726–32.

59. J. Bruce Moseley et al., "A Controlled Trial of Arthroscopic Surgery for Osteoarthritis of the Knee," *New England Journal of Medicine* 347 (July 11, 2002): 81–88.

60. Steve Silberman, "Placebos Are Getting More Effective. Drugmakers Are Desperate to Know Why," *Wired*, September 2009, http://www.wired .com/medtech/drugs/magazine/17–09/ff_placebo_effect?currentPage=all.

61. Goldstein, *Alternative Health Care*, 10–11; Johnston, "Introduction," *Politics of Healing*, 4.

62. Owsei Temkin, *Double Face of Janus and Other Essays in the History of Medicine* (Baltimore: Johns Hopkins University Press, 1977), 16.

63. Walter Johnson, *Homeopathy: Popular Exposition and Defence of Its Principles and Practices* (Simpkin, Marshall, and Co., 1852), 8.

64. Forbes quoted in "Miscellany," *Medical Times* 15 (London: J. Angerstein Carfrae, 1846), 115.

BIBLIOGRAPHY

Anderson, Ann. *Snake Oil, Hustlers and Hambones: The American Medicine Show*. Jefferson, NC: McFarland, 2000.

Astin, John A. "Why Patients Use Alternative Medicine: Results of a National Study." *Journal of the American Medical Association* 279, no. 19 (1998): 1548–53. http://www.ncbi.nlm.nih.gov/pubmed/9605899.

Baer, Hans A. *Biomedicine and Alternative Healing Systems in America: Issues of Class, Race, Ethnicity, and Gender*. Madison: University of Wisconsin Press, 2001.

———. "Divergence and Convergence in Two Systems of Manual Medicine: Osteopathy and Chiropractic in the United States." *Medical Anthropology Quarterly* 1, no. 2 (June 1987): 176–93.

Blake, John B. "Mary Gove Nichols, Prophetess of Health." *Proceedings of the American Philosophical Society* 106 (June 29, 1962): 219–34.

Cassedy, James H. *Medicine in America: A Short History*. Baltimore: Johns Hopkins University Press, 1991.

Cayleff, Susan E. "Gender, Ideology, and the Water-Cure Movement." In *Other Healers*, edited by Norman Gevitz.

———. *Wash and Be Healed: The Water-Cure Movement and Women's Health*. Philadelphia: Temple University Press, 1987.

Cohen, Marcine J. "Medical Social Movements in the United States, 1820–1982: The Case of Osteopathy." PhD diss., University of Wisconsin-Madison, 1983.

Colbert, Charles. *A Measure of Perfection: Phrenology and the Fine Arts in America*. Chapel Hill: University of North Carolina Press, 1998.

Darnton, Robert. *Mesmerism and the End of the Enlightenment in France.* Cambridge, MA: Harvard University Press, 1968.

Dresser, Horatio, ed. *The Quimby Manuscripts.* New York: Thomas Crowell, 1921.

Duffy, John. *From Humors to Medical Science: A History of American Medicine.* 2nd ed. Urbana: University of Illinois Press, 1993.

Fenster, Julie M. *Mavericks, Miracles and Medicine: The Pioneers Who Risked Their Lives to Bring Medicine into the Modern Age.* New York: Carroll & Graf, 2003.

Finger, Stanley. *Doctor Franklin's Medicine.* Philadelphia: University of Pennsylvania Press, 2006.

———. *Minds behind the Brain: A History of the Pioneers and Their Discoveries.* New York: Oxford University Press, 2000.

———. *Origins of Neuroscience: A History of Explorations in Brain Function.* New York: Oxford University Press, 1994.

Flannery, Michael. "The Early Botanical Medical Movement as a Reflection of Life, Liberty, and Literacy in Jacksonian America." *Journal of the Medical Library Association* 90, no. 4 (October 2002): 442–54.

Franklin, Benjamin, et al. *Report of Dr. Benjamin Franklin, and Other Commissioners.* London: Johnston, 1785. Reprinted in *Foundations of Hypnosis.* Edited by Maurice M. Tinterowd. Springfield, IL: Charles C. Thomas, 1970.

Fuller, Robert C. *Mesmerism and the American Cure of Souls.* Philadelphia: University of Pennsylvania Press, 1982.

———. "Mesmerism and the Birth of Psychology." In *Pseudoscience and Society,* edited by Arthur Wrobel.

Gevitz, Norman. "Osteopathic Medicine: From Deviance to Difference." In *Other Healers,* edited by Norman Gevitz.

———, ed. *Other Healers: Unorthodox Medicine in America.* Baltimore: Johns Hopkins University Press, 1988.

Gielow, Vern. *Old Dad Chiro: Biography of D. D. Palmer, Founder of Chiropractic.* Davenport, IA: Bawden Brothers, 1981.

Goldstein, Michael S. *Alternative Health Care: Medicine, Miracle, or Mirage?* Philadelphia: Temple University Press, 1999.

Greenblatt, Samuel H. "Phrenology in the Science and Culture of the 19th Century." *Neurosurgery* 37, no. 4 (October 1995): 790–804.

Hahnemann, Samuel. *Organon of the Rational Art of Healing.* Translated by C. E. Wheeler. New York: E. P. Dutton, 1913.

Haller, John S., Jr. *American Medicine in Transition, 1840–1910.* Urbana: University of Illinois Press, 1981.

————. *The History of American Homeopathy: The Academic Years, 1820–1935.* New York: Pharmaceutical Press, 2005.

————. *Medical Protestants: The Eclectics in American Medicine, 1825–1939.* Carbondale: Southern Illinois University Press, 1994.

————. *The People's Doctor: Samuel Thomson and the American Botanical Movement, 1790–1860.* Carbondale: Southern Illinois University, 2000.

Holmes, Oliver Wendell. *Medical Essays, 1842–1882.* New York: Houghton Mifflin, 1892.

Hooker, Worthington. *Physician and Patient; or, a Practical View of the Mutual Duties, Relations and Interests of the Medical Profession and the Community.* New York: Baker and Scribner, 1849.

Hunter, Philip. "A Question of Faith: Exploiting the Placebo Effect Depends on Both the Susceptibility of the Patient to Suggestion and the Ability of the Doctor to Instill Trust." *EMBO (European Molecular Biology Organization) Reports* 8, no. 2 (February 2007): 125–28.

Johnston, Robert D., ed. *The Politics of Healing: Histories of Alternative Medicine in Twentieth-Century North America.* New York: Routledge, 2004.

Kaufman, Martin. "Homeopathy in America: The Rise and Fall and Persistence of a Medical Heresy." In *Other Healers*, edited by Norman Gevitz.

————. *Homeopathy in America: The Rise and Fall of a Medical Heresy.* Baltimore: Johns Hopkins University Press, 1971.

Kimmel, Michael S. "Men's Response to Feminism at the Turn of the Century." *Gender & Society* 1, no. 3 (September 1987): 261–83.

Kirschmann, Anne Taylor. *A Vital Force: Women in American Homeopathy.* New Brunswick, NJ: Rutgers University Press, 2004.

Leavitt, Judith Walzer, and Ronald L. Numbers, eds. *Sickness and Health in America: Readings in the History of Medicine and Public Health.* Madison: University of Wisconsin Press, 1978.

Lebergott, Stanley. "Wage Trends, 1800–1900." In *Trends in the American Economy in the Nineteenth Century*, by the Conference on Research in Income and Wealth. Vol. 24. Washington, DC: National Bureau of Economic Research, 1960.

Legan, Marshall Scott. "Hydropathy, or Water Cure." In *Pseudoscience and Society*, edited by Arthur Wrobel.

Marland, Hilary, and Jane Adams. "Hydropathy at Home: The Water Cure and Domestic Healing in Mid-Nineteenth-Century Britain." *Bulletin of the History of Medicine* (Fall 2009): 499–529.

Martin, Steve C. "Chiropractic and the Social Context of Medical Technology, 1895–1925." *Technology and Culture* 34, no. 4 (October 1993): 808–34.

———. "The Only Truly Scientific Method of Healing: Chiropractic and American Science, 1895–1990." *Isis* 85, no. 2 (June 1994): 207–27.

The Master Specialist [pseud.]. *The Home Private Medical Advisor.* Miner Library Rare Books and Archives, University of Rochester. Milwaukee: Wisconsin Medical Institute, c. 1903.

McDonald, Jean A. "Mary Baker Eddy and the Nineteenth-Century 'Public' Woman: A Feminist Reappraisal." *Journal of Feminist Studies in Religion* 2, no. 1 (Spring 1986): 89–111.

Milmine, Georgine. *The Life of Mary Baker Eddy and the History of Christian Science.* New York: Doubleday, 1909. http://www.archive.org/details/lifeof marybakergoomilmuoft.

Moore, Stuart. *Chiropractic in America: The History of a Medical Alternative.* Baltimore: Johns Hopkins University Press, 1992.

Morantz, Regina Markell. "Women in the Medical Profession: Why Were There So Few?" *Reviews in American History* 6, no. 2 (June 1978): 163–70.

Morantz-Sanchez, Regina. *Sympathy and Science: Women Physicians in American Medicine.* New York: Oxford University Press, 1985.

More, Ellen S., Elizabeth Fee, and Manon Parry, eds. *Women Physicians and the Cultures of Medicine.* Baltimore: Johns Hopkins University Press, 2009.

Nadis, Fred. *Wonder Shows: Performing Science, Magic, and Religion in America.* New Brunswick, NJ: Rutgers University Press, 2005.

Numbers, Ronald L. "Do-It-Yourself the Sectarian Way." In *Medicine without Doctors,* edited by Guenter B. Risse.

Ober, K. Patrick. *Mark Twain and Medicine: "Any Mummery Will Cure."* Columbia: University of Missouri Press, 2003.

Palmer, B. J. *The Chiropractic Adjustor: A Compilation of the Writings of D. D. Palmer,* 1st ed. Davenport, IA: Palmer School of Chiropractic, 1921.

Parascandola, John. *Sex, Sin, and Science: A History of Syphilis in America.* New York: Praeger, 2008.

Pattie, F. A. *Mesmer and Animal Magnetism.* Hamilton, NY: Edmonston, 1994.

Paul, Annie Murphy. *The Cult of Personality Testing: How Personality Tests Are Leading Us to Miseducate Our Children, Mismanage Our Companies, and Misunderstand Ourselves.* New York: Simon and Schuster, 2005.

Pettman, Erland. "A History of Manipulative Therapy." *Journal of Manual and Manipulative Therapy* 15, no. 3 (2007): 165–74.

Phinney, H. F., ed. *The Water Cure in America: Over Three Hundred Cases of Various Diseases Treated with Water.* New York: Fowler and Wells, 1852.

Porter, Roy. *The Greatest Benefit to Mankind: A Medical History of Humanity.* New York: W. W. Norton, 1999.

————. *Quacks: Fakers and Charlatans in Medicine*. Stroud, UK: Tempus, 2003.

Poyen, Charles. *Progress of Animal Magnetism in New England*. Boston: Weeks, Jordan, 1837.

Reed, Louis S. *The Healing Cults: A Study of Sectarian Medical Practice*. Chicago: University of Chicago Press, 1932.

Risse, Guenter B., ed. *Medicine without Doctors: Home Health Care in American History*. New York: Science History Publications, 1977.

Robins, Natalie S. *Copeland's Cure: Homeopathy and the War between Conventional and Alternative Medicine*. New York: Knopf, 2005.

Rogers, Naomi. "The Proper Place of Homeopathy: Hahnemann Medical College and Hospital in an Age of Scientific Medicine." *Pennsylvania Magazine of History and Biography* 108, no. 2 (April 1984): 179–201.

Rosenberg, Charles E. *Our Present Complaint: American Medicine, Then and Now*. Baltimore: Johns Hopkins University Press, 2007.

Rothstein, William G. "The Botanical Movements and Orthodox Medicine." In *Other Healers*, edited by Norman Gevitz, 29–51.

Shaw, Robert B. *History of the Comstock Patent Medicine Business and Dr. Morse's Indian Root Pills*. Smithsonian Studies in History and Technology 22. Washington, DC: Smithsonian Institution Press, 1972.

Silver-Isenstadt, Jean L. *Shameless: The Visionary Life of Mary Gove Nichols*. Baltimore: Johns Hopkins University Press, 2002.

Simpson, Donald. "Phrenology and the Neurosciences: Contributions of F. J. Gall and J. G. Spurzheim." *ANZ Journal of Surgery* 75 (2005): 475–82.

Sivulka, Juliann. *Soap, Sex, and Cigarettes: A Cultural History of American Advertising*. Belmont, CA: Wadsworth, 1997.

Stage, Sarah. *Female Complaints: Lydia Pinkham and the Business of Women's Medicine*. New York: W. W. Norton, 1979.

Starr, Paul. "Medicine, Economy and Society in Nineteenth-Century America." *Journal of Social History* 10 (1977): 588–606.

————. *The Social Transformation of American Medicine: The Rise of a Sovereign Profession and the Making of a Vast Industry*. New York: Basic Books, 1984.

Stern, Madeline B. *Heads and Headlines: The Phrenological Fowlers*. Norman: University of Oklahoma Press, 1972.

Still, Andrew T. *Autobiography of Andrew T. Still*. Kirksville, MO: printed by the author, 1897.

————. *Osteopathy: Research and Practice*. Kirksville, MO: printed by the author, 1910.

————. "Osteopathy: Some of the Circumstances and Personal Experiments Which Led to Treating Bodily Ills without Drugs." *Ladies Home Journal* article and correspondence, c. 1907. Andrew Taylor Still Papers, Missouri Digital Heritage. http://cdm.sos.mo.gov/u?/atsu,1003.

Thomson, Cyrus, ed. *Learned Quackery Exposed; or, Theory According to Art, as Exemplified in the Practice of the Honorable Doctors of the Present Day.* Syracuse, NY: Lathrop and Dean, Printers, 1843.

Thomson, Samuel. *A Narrative of the Life and Medical Discoveries of Samuel Thomson: Containing an Account of His System of Practice, and the Manner of Curing Disease with Vegetable Medicine. . . .* 8th ed. Columbus, OH: Pike, Platt, 1832.

———. *A New Guide to Health, or Botanic Family Physician.* London: Simpkin, Marshall, 1849.

Thurs, Daniel Patrick. *Science Talk: Changing Notions of Science in American Culture.* Piscataway, NJ: Rutgers University Press, 2008.

Tomlinson, Stephen. "Phrenology, Education, and the Politics of Human Nature: The Thought and Influence of George Combe." *History of Education* 26, no. 1 (March 1997): 1–22.

Trall, Russell Thacher. *The Hydropathic Encyclopedia: A System of Hydropathy and Hygiene.* Vol. 2. New York: Fowlers and Wells, 1854.

Troesken, Werner. "The Elasticity of Demand with Respect to Product Failures; or Why the Market for Quack Medicines Flourished for More Than 150 Years." National Bureau of Economic Research Working Paper no. 15699 (January 2010), http://www.nber.org/papers/w15699.

Turner, Christopher. "Mesmeromania, or, the Tale of the Tub." *Cabinet* 21 (Spring 2006). http://www.cabinetmagazine.org/issues/21/turner.php.

Umbreit, A. C. *Pending Medical Legislation: Brief on Certain Bills Pending before the Legislature of 1907: Senate Bills Numbers 314 S, 315 S, 449 S, 416.* Madison, WI: State Board of Medical Examiners, 1907.

Vogel, Morris J., and Charles E. Rosenberg, eds. *The Therapeutic Revolution: Essays in the Social History of American Medicine.* Philadelphia: University of Pennsylvania Press, 1979.

Wallace, Edwin R., IV, and John Gach, eds. *History of Psychiatry and Medical Psychology: With an Epilogue on Psychiatry and the Mind-Body Relation.* New York: Springer, 2008.

Walter, Georgia Warner. *Women and Osteopathic Medicine: Historical Perspectives.* Kirksville, MO: A. T. Still Memorial Library, 1994.

Wardwell, Walter. Chiropractic: *History and Evolution of a New Profession.* St. Louis: Mosby, 1992.

Wardwell, Walter I. "Chiropractors: Evolution to Acceptance." In *Other Healers,* edited by Norman Gevitz.

Wesley, John. *Primitive Physick: Or, an Easy and Natural Method of Curing Most Diseases*. 14th ed. (Philadelphia, 1770).

Whorton, James C. "From Cultism to CAM." In *Politics of Healing*, edited by Robert D. Johnston.

———. *Nature Cures: The History of Alternative Medicine in America*. New York: Oxford University Press, 2002.

Willis, Martin, and Catherine Wynne, eds. *Victorian Literary Mesmerism*. New York: Editions Rodopi, 2006.

Wrobel, Arthur, ed. *Pseudoscience and Society in Nineteenth-Century America*. Lexington: University Press of Kentucky, 1987.

Young, Dwight L. "Orson Squire Fowler: To Form a More Perfect Human." *Wilson Quarterly* (Spring 1990): 120–27.

Young, James Harvey. *The Medical Messiahs: A Social History of Health Quackery in Twentieth-Century America*. Princeton, NJ: Princeton University Press, 1967.

———. "Patent Medicine and the Self-Help Syndrome." In *Medicine without Doctors*, edited by Guenter B. Risse.

Note: Page numbers in *italics* indicate illustrations.

610 JAN
Janik, Erika.
Marketplace of the marvelou